Physical Activity and Aging

ROY J. SHEPHARD

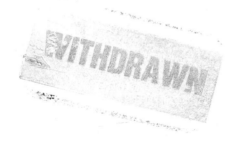

CROOM HELM LONDON

© 1978 Roy J. Shephard
Croom Helm Limited, 2-10 St John's Road, London SW11

British Library Cataloguing in Publication Data

Shephard, Roy J.
   Physical activity and aging.
   1. Aged — Health and hygiene
   I. Title
   613.7'044   RA777.6

   ISBN 0-85664-541-9

Printed in Great Britain by offset lithography by
Billing & Sons Ltd, Guildford, London and Worcester

CONTENTS

PREFACE

Aging might seem a depressing theme for a book. Stephen Leacock, the Canadian humourist, suggested: 'About the only good thing you can say about it is, it's better than being dead.' Nevertheless, it is a topic we can hardly avoid. A combination of a rapidly falling birth rate and the conquest of acute disease is confronting many governments with the practical problems of a rapidly expanding geriatric population. Individually, we must also face old age and make our personal adaptation to it. I was startled recently to hear one of my daughters acknowledge that she was getting old. At the ripe age of seventeen, her judgement was based on the fact that she now knew the former pop stars discussed in the evening paper under the heading 'Whatever became of . . .'. Most of us first begin to appreciate aging in its social context — the weddings of our friends give place to christenings, marriages of the younger generation, and then a geometrically increasing progression of funerals! As we approach the half century, the limitations of our own bodies become painfully apparent. Books are suddenly printed in abominably small type, friends mumble in a ridiculously unintelligible fashion, and even the weekly bag of groceries becomes a burden. For the first time in our lives, we appreciate the significance of research that promises to halt or even reverse the inexorable loss of body function.

The problems of a geriatric society are felt most acutely by the older social democracies of Western Europe, and it may seem presumptuous even to discuss questions of senescence from the comfort of a young nation such as Canada. Our one claim to geriatric fame is Pierre Joubert. Joubert was a French Canadian bootmaker, born in Charlesbourg, Quebec on 15 July 1701. Despite recent legends from the Caucasus, Joubert retains the distinction of attaining the greatest authenticated age in the world. He died in Quebec City on 16 November 1814, having lived for 113 years, 124 days. Dr Tache, official statistician to the Canadian government of 1870, made a careful examination of his credentials, and concluded that the proofs were irrefutable. His story underscores the challenge of geriatric investigation. Fewer people are dying in early old age. But despite two centuries of earnest research, we remain unable to check the underlying process of senescence; still, there is a ceiling of 112-114 years that apparently cannot be surpassed.

The present book makes no attempt to solve this ultimate mystery. Rather, it explores how far we can improve our adaptation to the early part of old age through an increase of personal fitness. Research is presented that suggests such an approach holds a great potential, not only for the extension of personal happiness, but also for the avoidance of national bankruptcy. The substantial but scattered information on physical activity and aging is drawn together into a single volume that should appeal not only to the gerontologist but also to many other scientists interested in human performance — the physiologist, the physical educator, the ergonomist and the physiotherapist. In preparing the book, I have drawn frequently upon the wisdom and experience of a number of close colleagues and co-investigators; it is a great pleasure to acknowledge my debts to Dr Terence Kavanagh, Medical Director of the Toronto Rehabilitation Centre, Dr Cope Schwenger, Professor of Health Administration at the University of Toronto, and two exceptional graduate students, Dr Kenneth Sidney and Mr Veli Niinimaa.

The general plan of the book is evident from the page of contents. After discussing definitions and techniques, the aging of cells and of organs is reviewed in the specific context of physical activity. The normal activity patterns of the old person are examined, together with their attitudes to physical exercise, and the implications for nutrition are discussed. A training plan for the elderly is considered, and the likely response of the body to increased activity is indicated. The elderly athlete is presented as an extreme case of sustained training. Final chapters review the interactions of physical activity with some of the common diseases of old age, and the economic implications of an aged and increasingly dependent population.

No easy solutions are found to the overall decline in biological function. However, the point is made that quite moderate training can set back the deterioration of physiological work capacity by an average of eight to nine years; assuming a much smaller change in death rates, this would reduce by two thirds the proportion of the population who must accept a final period of physical incapacitation. If the present book does no more than encourage senior citizens and their advisers to exploit this important possibility, the labour of its writing will be well repaid.

Toronto, 1977   Roy J. Shephard

1 INTRODUCTION

Scope of Text

From early antiquity, medical science has been fascinated by the gradual loss of function that occurs with aging. One compelling reason for this interest has been the universality of the aging process, its threat extending to both the eager investigators and their anxious patrons. The philosopher's stone was sought not only to translate base metals into gold, but also to yield an elixir that would allow the alchemist leisure to contemplate his new found wealth (Comfort, 1963).

Taoists believed that the secret lay in preserving the essence of life (the semen), and sages such as Wei Po-Yang (second century AD) claimed substantial extension of their life span through a combination of detachment from worldly cares and a complicated ritual of general and sexual gymnastics. If in fact the Chinese philosophers attained longevity, this reflected their privileged place in society, and the year 1978 still finds us far from success in our search for a general elixir of life. We can induce small extensions of life-span in experimental animals by changes in diet or environmental temperature, and by treatment with antioxidant chemicals. Nevertheless, the strategy of geriatric medicine remains the piecemeal treatment of senile disability rather than any more general attempt to slow the rhythm of a seemingly limited duration biological clock (Comfort, 1973).

Partly because many fundamental questions of aging have yet to be resolved, the main focus of the present book is upon the practical problems of human aging rather than theories describing the decline and fall of the common fruit-fly (Drosophila). While it is superficially attractive to be able to study senescence in many generations of insects over a short time interval, observations such as deterioration in the cuticle of an arthropod have less than immediate relevance to the urgent problems of a growing geriatric population. The emphasis of this volume is further upon aging in an active man, rather than the senescence that can be detected through studies of basal function, and the behaviour of the whole body is discussed in preference to observations at the cellular and sub-cellular levels, for the issue of prime concern to society is whether a senior citizen can meet the physical demands of independence during everyday life.

In this introductory chapter, we will attempt a definition of aging, propose a classification of the elderly, and deal with such practical issues of experimental design as the selection of 'normal' subjects, the choice between cross-sectional and longitudinal studies, and the statistical distribution of geriatric data.

Subsequent chapters will examine cellular aspects of aging, changes of gross function, normal activity patterns of the elderly, techniques for increasing the activity of the senior citizen, specific characteristics of the elderly athlete, the general impact of physical activity upon the pathology of aging and goals for a geriatric society.

The Definition of Aging

While it is possible to describe certain manifestations of aging at the cellular and the sub-cellular levels of organisation the overall process is best defined in terms of man as a whole. Two related concepts are a diminished capacity to regulate the internal environment (impaired homeostasis), and a reduced probability of survival.

Homeostasis

Rowlatt & Franks (1973) explained senescence as 'a progressive loss in the individual of physiological adaptability to the environment culminating in death'. Their view can be illustrated in terms of the reaction to a severe haemorrhage; the chance of death following a given blood loss increases logarithmically with age (Simms, 1942). Presumably, the feedback mechanisms stabilising the blood volume of a younger person are no longer fully operative in the elderly. Similar impairment of control mechanisms develops in many other homeostatic systems, including the regulation of blood sugar (Silverstone *et al.*, 1957) and of body temperature (Pickering, 1936; Burch *et al.*, 1942). The old person thus becomes progressively more vulnerable to environmental threats, and mortality is increased by extremes of heat and cold. In the United Kingdom, for example, many senior citizens still develop hypothermia, sometimes with fatal consequences. One problem is that through a deterioration of sensory receptors and loss of central information processing an old person may develop an inappropriate thermal preference, not realising that he is becoming chilled (Watts *et al.*, 1972; Fox *et al.*, 1973). Such hazards are compounded by a limited ability to increase metabolism and to minimise heat loss (Wagner *et al.*, 1974).

While a severe cold challenge can develop because of a limited income or failure to detect a falling house temperature, in the modern

North American world of air-conditioned buses and subway cars, enclosed shopping malls and centrally-heated homes, such difficulties are not very prevalent. Indeed, the main threat to homeostasis can come from within the body. Physical activity increases the demands on many body systems by a factor of at least ten, and a complicated series of feedback loops must be activated to conserve the constancy of the internal environment. In reviewing the biology of aging, it thus seems particularly appropriate to consider data in the context of the performance of external work.

Survival

Other factors being equal, the overall survival prospects of an individual depend on his capacity for homeostasis. However, if there were no senescence, homeostasis would be equally well-developed at all ages. Deaths due to accidents, disease and other forms of stress would then occur in random fashion, with a constant percentage of the residual population dying over each successive time interval (Figure 1.1). This type of curve is found in some animal species that are exposed to a hazardous environment, since very few individuals survive to the age of senescence. The alternative possibility is to live in a well-protected environment, where most of the deaths are due to senescence. The survival curve then has a relatively rectangular form, with a sudden drop in the percentage of survivors once a critical age has been passed. In practice, most survival curves have a form that is intermediate between these two extremes.

Mathematicians have found much amusement in trying to fit equations to such data. The first attempt was by Gompertz (1825). He suggested that the mortality rate R_m at time t was given by an exponential function related to the number of survivors n and a hypothetical mortality rate R_0 typical of zero time:

$$R_m = -\frac{1}{n} \times \frac{dn}{dt} = R_0 e^{\alpha t} .$$

A linear function should thus be obtained by plotting the logarithm of the death rate against age (Figure 1.2), the rate of aging being indicated by the slope constant α.

Other authors have attempted to improve on his formula by adding a second component of mortality A that is independent of age:

$$R_m = R_0 e^{\alpha t} + A .$$

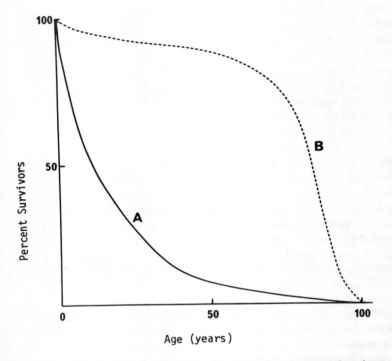

Figure 1.1   Survival Curves. Population A is showing a constant and random mortality due to natural causes. Population B is showing a sudden increase of mortality with the onset of senescence.

A third suggestion has been to allow an initial interval of early adulthood b before senescence begins to take effect:

$$R_m = R_0 e^{\alpha(t - b)} \ .$$

However, it seems unlikely that any simple formula will do more than approximate the complex interactions between environment and senescence. For example, such factors as the development of immunity to common diseases and the learning of caution in the operation of a motor vehicle will distort the semi-logarithmic plot, leading to an underestimation of aging from Gompertz-type curves.

Improvements in environmental conditions reduce the frequency and extent of challenges to homeostasis, thus displacing the Gompertz

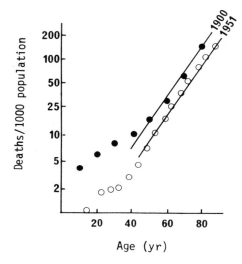

Figure 1.2   Gompertz plots relating deaths/1,000 population (logarithmic scale) and age of population. Data for USA, 1900 and 1951 (after Shock, 1967).

curve to the right (Figure 1.2) without much change in the slope of the relationship (Shock, 1967). While some authors have interpreted this as a reduction of physiological age, there is little question that the real explanation lies in the decreased environmental challenge. If the population of 1951 had been confronted with the environment of 1900, they would not have survived any better than their forbears!

One final complication may be noted. In most countries, the environment has changed perceptibly while subjects have been aging. The slope of the Gompertz relationship thus reflects the combined influence of senescence and alterations in the environment.

Classification of the Aged

Group Classifications

Dividing points in any system of age classification show a direct relationship to the age of the speaker or the writer. Many of my undergraduate students would propose quite seriously that a thirty-year-old person could be included in a study of elderly subjects! Even published reports on the exercise tolerance of the elderly are too commonly based on people in the age range 40-60 years. This makes the research easier and safer to conduct. But from my particular vantage point, the individuals that have been studied no longer seem old!

Function provides a more objective basis of categorisation. Shakespeare suggested this many years ago when he traced the 'seven ages of man' (*As You Like It*, Act 2, Scene 5). There was the inevitable progression from childhood — the mewling infant and the whining schoolboy — to the young adult — the sighing lover and the vigorous soldier. Then came the archetype of middle age — the paunchy justice, effective and affluent but with the first warning signs of functional deterioration. Old age was represented by the lean and slipper'd pantaloon, with spectacles on nose and shrunk shank. Finally, there was second childishness — extreme senescence, sans teeth, sans eyes, sans taste, sans everything. In a somewhat analagous manner, we may distinguish the following classes:

Middle age: the second half of a person's working career (e.g. age 40-65 years)

Old age: the immediate post-retirement period, when there is usually no gross impairment of function or homeostasis (e.g. age 65-75 years, sometimes described as young old age)

Very old age: a stage when there is usually some functional impairment, but the individual can still live a relatively independent life (e.g. 75-85 years, sometimes described as middle old age)

Extreme old age: a stage where institutional and/or nursing care is usually needed (e.g. age 85 years and over, sometimes described as old old age).

The age boundaries separating the several functional categories are naturally flexible, and show some cultural differences. Thus the average age of retirement varies substantially from one country to another (Table 1.1). Within a given country, there are also differences in expected behaviour from one era to another and from one socioeconomic group to another. For example, the traditional Eskimo remains extremely fit and active until his son has become a skilled hunter; thereafter, he has the privilege of choosing the best items from the game won by his son, and his own physical condition shows a rapid deterioration.

We will have some occasion to refer to problems encountered by the middle-aged towards the end of their working careers. However, our main focus will be on the 'young' old person, retired but without gross

Table 1.1   Retirement age in selected countries. Figure in brackets
shows female retirement age when this differs from that of men
(Schwenger, 1976)

Country	Retirement age (normal, 1974)		Country	Retirement age (normal, 1974)	
Australia	65	(60)	Israel	65	(60)
Austria	65	(60)	Italy	60	(55)
Belgium	65	(60)	Japan	60	(55)
Bulgaria	65	(60)	Luxembourg	65	(60)
Canada	65		Netherlands	65	
Czechoslovakia	60	(53-57)	New Zealand	60 or 65	
Denmark	67	(62)	Norway	67	
Finland	65		Poland	65	(60)
France	60		Portugal	65	(62)
Germany (DR)	65	(60)	Romania	60	(55)
Germany (FR)	65	(60)	Spain	65	
Great Britain	65	(60)	Sweden	67	
Greece	62	(57)	Switzerland	65	(62)
Hungary	60	(55)	USA	65	
Iceland	67		USSR	60	(55)
Ireland	65		Yugoslavia	60	(55)

functional impairment. This target group has both the time and the
capacity to undertake vigorous exercise, and through a suitably graded
programme of increased physical activity it may well taste the elixir
of youth, holding back the final years of declining function and
institutional care.

Individual Classifications

It is a matter of experience that not all individuals age at the same rate.
Some 70-year-old subjects are completely bed-ridden, while some
90-year-olds are extremely lively members of their respective communities. It is thus useful to superimpose upon the group classification
some statement regarding the biological age of the individual.

    Techniques of measuring biological age in the elderly are still far
from standardised (Comfort, 1969; Bourlière, 1973; Linn, 1975).
The need is for a test battery of sufficient diversity to describe the
aging of the organism as a whole. Individual measurements must be
simple yet reliable, with a regular and sufficient change to detect over
a span of five or ten years. Finally, appropriate statistical techniques

must be used to combine all of this information into a single expression of biological age. Among the measurements suggested by Comfort are anthropometric data (standing, sitting and trunk height, biacromial diameter, weight and hair-greying score), physiological tests (vital capacity, tidal volume, maximum voluntary ventilation, blood pressure, heart size and grip strength), observations on bone and connective tissue (osteoporotic index, skin elasticity and nail calcium), sensory tests (visual acuity, dark adaptation, vibrometry and audiometry), biochemical data (serum cholesterol, albumin, copper, elastase, RNA[ase]), cellular characteristics (lymphocyte RNA/DNA, serum growth promotion, clonal viability, auto-antibody titres), intelligence tests (Wechsler test, digit span, digit symbol, vocabulary) and psycho-motor tests (reaction time, light extinction test). Linn (1975) proposed that ratings should be based on a cumulative illness score. Each of thirteen body systems was rated on a five-point clinical scale. The cumulative burden of pathology reduced the individual's adaptability, and Linn found that the overall score gave a good prediction of subsequent mortality.

Problems of Experimental Technique

Use of Human Subjects

The use of human subjects greatly increases the relevance of aging studies, but at the same time it creates several technical problems for the investigator (Andres, 1974). Pure bred species are unknown, seriously hampering the possibilities of genetic research. Diet and other environmental conditions cannot be controlled as in an animal cage. There are severe limitations on the tissues that can be biopsied. Sampling problems are created through the need for informed consent. Disease-free colonies of humans are unknown, and it is thus necessary to distinguish aging from the effects of disease. Man is the longest-lived of the mammals, and a longitudinal experiment requires thirty or forty times as long to complete in man as in a rat. Finally, because of sampling problems, data may not conform to normal distribution curves. We will now explore several of these issues in more detail.

Problems Arising from 'Informed Consent'

Completion of a full battery of aging tests can require many hours of careful observations on a single individual. Results are thus commonly reported for a small sample of 'normal' subjects who are presumed representative of the general population under study.

The experimental ideal would be a randomly selected sample, stratified by age, sex, occupation and so on. However, ethical considerations dictate that those examined be volunteers (Shephard, 1972) who have given their informed consent to all required procedures without any form of coercion. Assuming such standards to be observed, the goal of near 100 per cent response (Cochrane, 1954) becomes unrealistic. In a small community where there is a good rapport between laboratory and villagers, response rates of up to 90 per cent can be realised, but in large cities much poorer figures are usual. Bailey *et al.* (1974) had a nurse select names from the Saskatoon telephone directory, inviting the individuals contacted to attend the laboratory for a simple stepping test of fitness with electrocardiogram; about a third of the group refused the offer, and of the remainder almost half made some excuse why they could not attend during the period of the survey. A study of physical and mental health among the old people of Edinburgh commenced with an approach to the subject through his family physician (Milne *et al.*, 1971b). This technique could possibly apply unwarranted pressure on some individuals. Nevertheless, the response rate was only 65 per cent, with 28.5 per cent refusals; 6 per cent of those selected died before examination, and 0.5 per cent had moved out of the survey area.

Unfortunately, even a small percentage of refusals can distort the composition of a supposed normal sample. Certain types of experiment attract the neurotic individual (Shephard & Kemp, unpublished report, Porton Down). If there is the promise of a medical examination or an exercise electrocardiogram, recruits may include an undue proportion of subjects who are anxious about their health. On the other hand, tests of functional competence and of fitness appeal to those with above average health. The problem can be illustrated by a recent survey of Eskimos living in the Canadian arctic (Shephard, 1977b, 1978). A team of exercise physiologists saw 224 of the 335 villagers (Table 1.2). Ignoring individuals crippled by congenital disease of the hip, poliomyelitis or a recent coronary attack, there yet remained a much higher proportion of villagers with pulmonary disease among those not seen (56/111) than among those volunteering for functional assessment (48/224). This difference was due largely to subjects with minor manifestations of tuberculous disease (primary tuberculosis or hilar calcification); apparently villagers with abnormalities in their chest radiograph were cautious about participating in this type of study. A medical team subsequently visited the same village, offering a comprehensive physical examination. They thus had occasion to

Table 1.2   A comparison between the health of Eskimos volunteering for functional testing and nursing station records for those who chose not to volunteer (Shephard, 1977b, 1978)

	Volunteers		Non-volunteers	
Total sample	224	(100%)	111	(100%)
Normal health	176	(78.6%)	49	(44.1%)
Primary tuberculosis or hilar calcification	20	(8.9%)	34	(30.6%)
Secondary tuberculosis fibrosis or emphysema	28	(12.5%)	22	(19.8%)
Crippled	—		5	(4.5%)
Recent coronary attack	—		1	(0.9%)

Table 1.3   Lung function data as determined on Eskimo villagers. Results obtained by observers with physiological and medical orientation (Shephard, 1977b, 1978)

Variable	Subjects observed only by physiologists	Subjects observed by both groups		Subjects observed only by physicians
		physiologists' data	physicians' data	
Vital capacity				
adult males	4.92 l. (N = 28)	4.87 l. (N = 41)	4.94 l. (N = 41)	4.41 l. (N = 41)
females	3.59 l. (N = 44)	2.82 l. (N = 5)	2.80 l. (N = 5)	2.66 l. (N = 24)
One sec. forced expiratory volume				
adult males	3.86 l. (N = 28)	3.69 l. (N = 41)	3.64 l. (N = 41)	3.14 l. (N = 41)
females	2.83 l. (N = 44)	1.99 l. (N = 5)	1.98 l. (N = 5)	1.88 l. (N = 24)

repeat the tests of pulmonary function previously carried out by the physiology team (Table 1.3). Where subjects were common to the two surveys, results were closely comparable. However, the physicians attracted a sample of men with poorer function than the common group, while the physiologists saw a sample of women with better function than that of those attending both examinations.

Such problems are more serious in the elderly than in young subjects, since the proportion of volunteers diminishes as the sample becomes older (Cochrane, 1954). In the Eskimo survey (Shephard, 1977b, 1978), the physiologists saw 77 per cent of the boys, 65 per cent of the girls, 67 per cent of men aged 20-39, 56 per cent of women aged 20-39, 41 per cent of the older men and 48 per cent of the older women.

Because of difficulties in obtaining a random sample, some authors have preferred to use 'captive' populations, such as the residents of old folks' homes or hospitals. In such situations, it is extremely difficult to maintain free and informed consent, and obvious biases are introduced relative to the general population of elderly individuals.

Effects of Disease

Descriptions of aging usually refer to changes of function anticipated in healthy subjects. However, there are several important limitations to this approach. One difficulty is the very fine line that separates normal aging from disease (Bourlière, 1973). For example, almost all older subjects show some degree of atherosclerosis, but in only a proportion has this advanced to the point where anginal pain or frank myocardial infarction has resulted. Korenchevsky (1961) suggested that pathological changes could be distinguished on the basis of their potential for treatment; this is probably a valid distinction, with the proviso that effective treatment has yet to be discovered for many of the pathologies that affect the elderly.

A second problem is that a high proportion of elderly samples are afflicted by clinically diagnosable disease. The residue of healthy individuals may thus be over-weighted by that sub-sample of the general population who enjoy an unusual longevity. Brown & Shephard (1967) examined 62 middle-aged and elderly female departmental store employees. Only 33 were given a clean bill of health, and 17 were affected by conditions influencing cardio-respiratory performance; diagnoses included hypertension, rheumatic carditis, anaemia, thyroidectomy, bronchitis, healed tuberculosis and retropulsion of a cervical intervertebral disc. In the 40-49 age group, the maximal oxygen intake of the diseased women was only 90.1 per cent of that for the healthy subjects, and in the 50-59 group the average for the diseased subjects had dropped to 86.5 per cent of that for the healthy individuals. The effect on lung function test results is even larger. Anderson *et al.* (1968)

established multiple regression equations relating vital capacity to height and age. The prediction formulae for normal men and for those with a history of respiratory disease were as follows:

$$VC_{normal} = -4.21 + 0.0563 \ (H, cm) - 0.0174 \ (A, yr)$$
$$VC_{disease} = -3.47 + 0.0563 \ (H, cm) - 0.0483 \ (A, yr)$$

Thus at the age of 65, the predicted vital capacity for a man of 170 cm height would be 4.23 l. BTPS if he were healthy, but only 2.96 l. if he had a history of chest disease (70.0 per cent of the normal prediction). Corresponding formulae for women were:

$$VC_{normal} = -5.12 + 0.0545 \ (H, cm) - 0.0105 \ (A, yr)$$
$$VC_{disease} = -4.25 + 0.0545 \ (H, cm) - 0.0362 \ (A, yr)$$

At the age of 65, a healthy woman with a height of 155 cm would have a predicted vital capacity of 2.65 l. BTPS, compared with 1.85 l. in a subject reporting previous chest disease (69.8 per cent of the normal prediction). Reported function scores for the elderly can thus differ markedly, depending on the care which has been taken to exclude diseased subjects from the sample tested.

A related issue is exposure to tobacco and various environmental insults. Experimental volunteers are often a health conscious group who do not smoke. They are also likely to be drawn mainly from middle and upper socio-economic groups, with less than average exposure to air contaminants both at home and at work. The course of aging in that proportion of the population who use tobacco and/or are exposed to high concentrations of air pollutants is thus likely to be less favourable than indicated by many experimental samples.

Cross-Sectional Versus Longitudinal Data

It is an almost impossible task to follow a group of subjects from birth to death. Most observers have thus compared results in subjects of differing ages (the cross-sectional approach), or have followed cohorts of varying initial age for periods of five to ten years (the semi-longitudinal approach).

Andres (1974) has pointed out that when determining the rate of aging of a variable, the standard error of the slope varies inversely as D (the duration of the study), and inversely as the square root of the number of observations. On theoretical grounds, it is thus as effective to space six examinations over ten years as to crowd twenty

examinations into five years. However, for many physiological variables
15 or even 20 years of testing may be needed to define the rate of aging
of individual subjects with acceptable accuracy.

A cross-sectional survey has the advantages of cheapness and ease of
administration. Some of the disadvantages can be illustrated by
considering data for standing height. It is well recognised that aging is
associated with some shortening of stature, due to compression of
intervertebral discs and increasing kyphosis of the spine. In one sample
of Toronto men (Shephard & Brown, 1968), the average height
decreased from 175.3 cm at age 18 to 170.2 cm at age 54, while in a
group of Eskimos (Rode & Shephard, 1971) the change was from 166.7
cm at age 25 to 163.4 cm at 45 and 164.3 cm in a small sample surviving to 55. However, factors other than aging contributed to these
differences. Successive generations of adults have become progressively
taller (Tanner, 1962; Skrobak-Kaczynski & Lewin, 1976), due to better
living conditions and improvements in diet; this 'secular trend' has
amounted to 1 cm per decade in Britain, and has been even faster
among groups such as the Lapps (Skrobak-Kaczynski & Lewin, 1976)
and the Eskimos (Rode & Shephard, 1976). On the other hand, tall
and thin subjects tend to live longer than those who are short and fat
(Spain *et al.*, 1963; Damon *et al.*, 1969), so that death has a selective
effect increasing the average height of older groups of subjects. Other
causes of change are a selective migration of taller or shorter people
(Miall *et al.*, 1967) and an alteration in the genetic composition of a
population through intermarriage with other groups (Jamison, 1970).

How large are these effects relative to the true change of stature in
the individual? Büchi (1950) followed six cohorts of men for nine
years each. Height increased by 0.5 cm between the ages of 20 and 29,
remained unchanged from the ages of 30 to 45, and thereafter declined
rapidly. Miall *et al.* (1967) had somewhat similar findings in a semi-
longitudinal study of families from the Rhondda Fach (a Welsh mining
community) and the nearby Vale of Glamorgan (an agricultural and
dormitory community). Height remained relatively constant to age 40,
but thereafter there was an accelerating decline, so that by the age
of 70 losses relative to age 25 amounted to 1.7 cm for Vale men, 3.6
cm for Rhondda men, 3.5 cm for Vale women, and 4.3 cm for
Rhondda women. Cross-sectional data (Figure 1.3) would have
indicated losses of 6-7 cm over the same period. The discrepancy
(average 3.3 cm) reflects mainly the secular trend, with some migration
of tall men from the mining villages (Illsley *et al.*, 1963).

In terms of height measurements, there can be little argument that

a semi-longitudinal survey is necessary. Nevertheless, the longitudinal
approach also has its problems. The interest of subjects must be secured
and maintained over a long period, and this predisposes to recruitment
of a health conscious minority of the total population. Some of the
sample will develop inter-current disease, and must then be eliminated.
Ideally, observers and techniques should remain constant throughout
the study. The apparent magnitude of something as simple as a skinfold thickness can change by up to 25 per cent if it is measured by a
different technician or even a different design of fat caliper. If the
constancy of methodology is assured, there remains the hazard that
laboratory procedures considered acceptable at the outset of an
investigation will have become seriously dated before all of the required
information has been collected. Finally, the enthusiasm of the principal
investigator must be preserved and the impatience of the granting
agency must be withstood over the long period while figures are
accumulating.

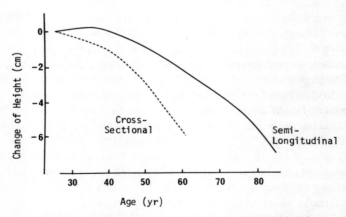

Figure 1.3   Differences in the rate of change of standing height with age as seen
in semi-longitudinal and cross-sectional data. Observations of Miall *et al.* (1967)
on men living in the Rhondda Fach.

Unfortunately, longitudinal surveys are not as immune from secular
trends as some observers have assumed. In our present context, let us
examine habitual activity and aging. As a subject gets older, his level of

daily activity falls (Figure 1.4). Part of this trend reflects the decline
of activity that has accompanied aging in every century, but there is a
substantial additional element that reflects a general change in
community habits secondary to automation, widespread use of the
automobile and the introduction of power appliances. Longitudinal
study of activity related variables such as the maximum oxygen intake
may thus show an unrealistically rapid loss of function (Hollmann,
1966; Dehn & Bruce, 1972).

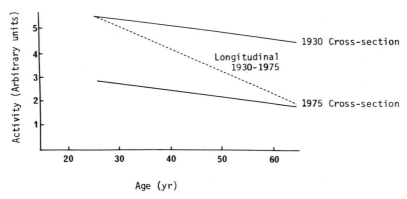

Figure 1.4   Diagram to illustrate the influence of a secular trend to reduced
habitual activity. In a longitudinal study, the usual decline of physical activity
with age is exaggerated.

Normality of Data

Most physiologists tacitly assume that their numerical data conform
to normal (Gaussian) distribution curves, allowing a description of
results as means and standard deviations. In fact, examples of departures from a normal distribution are found at all ages. Body weight,
for instance, has a marked rightward skewing even in childhood
(Jéquier *et al.*, 1977). However, atypical distributions become more
prevalent as a population ages. It is thus desirable to apply formal tests
for the normality of data, and where necessary to apply normalising
techniques such as a logarithmic transformation prior to undertaking
a detailed statistical analysis of results.

Bearing in mind these various items of philosophy and technique,
we may now proceed to the more detailed examination of exercise
and aging.

2 CELLULAR CONSIDERATIONS

Although the main emphasis of this book is upon the aging of gross function, a brief consideration of cellular changes may contribute to our understanding of aging phenomena in the whole man. Topics to be reviewed in this chapter include the genetics of aging, theories concerning its molecular basis, the metabolism of the aging cell, tissue energy reserves and micro-structural changes.

The Genetics of Aging

Aging as an Inherited Characteristic

Most authors now accept aging as a universal characteristic of normal cells (Hayflick, 1974). Early reports of 'immortal' tissue cultures (Carrel, 1912) can probably be attributed to an infiltration by abnormal, cancer-like cells. Human fibroblasts, for example, are capable of about fifty divisions before they die out. Cells taken from older animals show a capacity for fewer divisions than cultures taken from younger individuals. Exhaustion of the potential for cell division could thus be a facet of aging in some tissues, although it is obviously irrelevant to muscle and nerve (where cell division has already ceased).

Despite improvements in the life-expectancy of the average man, the maximum human life-span has apparently remained unchanged at about 112-114 years throughout the last three centuries (Pitskelauri, 1966; Timiras, 1972; Rockstein, 1974). The form of the mortality curve has thus moved progressively from an exponential towards a rectangular shape (Figure 1.1). Nevertheless, there continue to be substantial individual variations of longevity, and there is reason to believe that at least a part of such interindividual differences reflects genetic factors rather than an unequal exposure to environmental stress.

One pointer towards inheritance is a very consistent sex difference of longevity (Table 8.1, p. 269), shown not only by humans but also by many animal species (Rockstein, 1974). A second strand of evidence comes from life insurance statistics. Dublin *et al.* (1949) pointed out a strong association between survival of the parents and the mortality of immediate male offspring (Table 2.1). Unfortunately, the association could reflect not only the transmission of specific genetic information but also the acquisition of a certain life-style from the parents. As an example of the latter, we may instance the prospective study of the Framingham community in the US; this found an above anticipated proportion of cigarette smokers not only among 'coronary' victims, but also in their children (Margolis *et al.*, 1974).

Table 2.1 Mortality among men purchasing life insurance policies, classified according to survival of parents (based on data of Dublin *et al.*, 1949)

Age of insurance purchaser	Subsequent mortality (1899/1905 — 1939) (per cent of expected value)		
(years)	Both parents dead	One parent dead	Both parents alive
20-29	121.2	106.9	94.0
30-39	115.6	101.9	88.8
40-49	111.8	91.9	78.5
50-64	104.1	84.6	73.3

More convincing documentation of genetic influences is provided by comparisons of identical (monozygotic) and non-identical (hetero-zygotic) twins. Kallman & Sander (1948) found that if identical twins died between the ages of 60 and 75 years, the average intra-pair difference in the age at death was 47.6 months for the males and 24.0 months for the females. For the non-identical twins, corresponding intra-pair differences were much larger, 107.9 months for the males and 88.7 months for the females. However, it could be argued that the identical twins experienced unusually comparable environmental conditions over much of their life-span, and that they also suffered more grief than the heterozygotes on bereavement. While it is thus reasonable to conclude that genetic factors have some influence on longevity, it is virtually impossible to estimate the extent of this influence.

Evolutionary Pressures and the Programmed Theory of Aging

Given that there is an inherited component to longevity, some authors have argued that evolutionary pressures would lead to the programmed aging of a species. Their reasoning has been that prolonged survival of an individual after procreation of a sufficient number of offspring would place an excessive burden on the finite resources of a given habitat. Variants showing unusual longevity would thus tend to be eliminated by the forces of natural selection.

If life-span is increased, the total number of a species that can be supported must fall. This reduces the number of potential gene combinations, and thus the possibility of adapting to environmental change. On the other hand, if the life-span is shortened excessively, few members of the species survive to reproduce. From the evolutionary point of view, each type of creature thus has an optimum life-span, determined by the time to reproductive maturity, the number of offspring, and the likelihood of their survival to reproductive maturity (Wilson, 1974).

Rubner (1908) drew attention to an inverse relationship between life-span and energy expenditure per gram of body tissue. Such a relationship might suggest that an excessive rate of metabolism leads to a build-up of errors or an exhaustion of biochemical mechanisms. However, more detailed examination of the Rubner relationship has shown the importance of brain size; man, for instance, lives about four times as long as would be predicted from his weight (Frolkis, 1968). Presumably, a well developed brain gives him a better chance to cope with deleterious changes occurring elsewhere in the body.

Evolution may influence the development of senescence in other ways. If a deleterious gene cannot be eliminated through natural selection, it is possible that its effects may be postponed until after reproduction is complete (Medawar, 1957). Some genes may also exert several effects on an individual. If reproductive or early adaptive capacity is enhanced, such genes may be selected even though they carry serious disadvantages for later life. Thus the human brain is undoubtedly a striking product of evolution. The fact that the neurons do not divide allows the development of a sophisticated memory, with major advantages when adapting to a multiplicity of environments. However, the post-mitotic state carries one big handicap; if a fault develops in a brain cell, it cannot be replaced. Thus, aging leads to a progressive deterioration of cerebral function.

Some authors have objected that no one has yet demonstrated a gene that will accelerate aging. In fact, the concept of a 'programmed' life-span carries no *a priori* views on how this has been accomplished. Many of the molecular mechanisms discussed below could serve as a biological clock, causing a loss of function in one or more key groups of cells; the resulting loss of adaptability to environmental change could then give rise to the exponential increase of mortality associated with aging.

The Molecular Basis of Aging

General Considerations

Comfort (1973) has suggested that aging is fundamentally a question of information loss. This may express itself as an alteration in the characteristics of an inert material such as collagen, in the injury or death of cells that can no longer multiply (for example, the brain neurons), and in a loss of vigour, injury or death of cells that are still capable of multiplying.

One possible explanation of such changes would be an accumulation of 'noise' in the system, with consequent errors in homeostasis and in the copying of key molecules. The problem could be a chemical alteration in the master-template of protein synthesis (deoxyribonucleic acid, DNA), induced by radiation, chemical damage or failure of normal mechanisms for template repair. The error could also arise elsewhere in the chain of protein transcription (other constituents of the chromosome, ribonucleic acid-RNA, or protein synthetases).

Alternatively, there could be an exhaustion of functional potential with maturation, perhaps as a consequence of 'over-differentiation' of the cell. A situation could develop where the rate of production of enzymes and/or large structural molecules became less than their rate of failure, with disastrous consequences for cell function.

Lastly, function might be disturbed by the accumulation of undesirable substances within the cell. Large molecules might be altered sufficiently to escape normal turnover and replacement mechanisms. Elimination might also be circumvented because complexes had been formed with vital constituents of the cell. Some materials might even accumulate as simple precipitates.

Such diverse mechanisms open the field to equally diverse treatments of aging. Noise accumulation could perhaps be reduced by shielding a person physically or chemically from environmental stresses likely to modify mechanisms of protein synthesis. Exhaustion of vital constituents might be avoided by having the person live at a slower pace. Finally, compounds might be devised to help the elimination of debris from within the cell.

Protein Synthesis and Mutation

A brief description of protein synthesis is necessary to an understanding of mutations. Each of the chromosomes in the body carries a multiplicity of 'genes' in the form of specific DNA molecules. An individual DNA molecule consists of two complementary chains of nucleotides, held together by hydrogen bonds. When nuclear protein is to be formed, the two chains separate and a new complementary nucleotide chain is built alongside each of the two original components. Cellular proteins are built up from amino acids carried by soluble RNA; sites of synthesis are the ribosomes of the cytoplasmic reticulum, and the template is provided by messenger RNA which has first been matched to the reference template of the nuclear DNA.

A somatic cell may carry as many as 15,000 genes, and of these only some 3,000 are essential to its normal functioning, at least at maturity (Szilard, 1959). The course of life seems marked by a progressive build-up of abnormal DNA molecules. As the affected cells multiply, such errors accumulate in an exponential fashion. Factors contributing to the phenomenon include spontaneous hydrolysis of the DNA molecule, irradiation, exposure to chemical agents and the development of cross-linkages between molecules. Many of the simpler faults due to hydrolysis and cross-linkage can be corrected by standard repair mechanisms (endonucleases, repair polymerases and ligases). From the viewpoint of aging, only permanent damage is important, and even this must develop rapidly enough to produce significant effects in relation to the normal life-span. The type of event under consideration occurs in random (stochastic) fashion, allowing mathematicians the fun of building models to calculate likely totals of 'faults' and 'hits' (Szilard, 1959; Failla, 1960). A 'fault' was originally conceived as a mutation of one of the 3,000 genes essential to normal cell function. A 'hit' rendered inactive all of the genes on a single chromosome. According to this hypothesis, a mutation was recessive, and a cell only became inoperative if the error was brought to light by inactivation of both of a given pair of genes, for example if the homologous chromosome had already received a 'hit' or was carrying a 'fault' at some point.

There are many technical objections to such a simple explanation. Heterozygotes and hybrids generally live longer than homozygotes and inbred varieties of animal, whereas the hypothesis would lead us to expect more masking of mutations and less difficulty in copying protein in the homozygote. The mathematicians also complain of difficulty in fitting the concept of point mutations to an explanation of such statistics as male/female differences in the rate of aging (Maynard Smith, 1959), and the concept of more extensive damage is supported by observations using chemical mutagens (Alexander, 1967). Sinex (1974) has argued that most mutations are in fact dominant rather than recessive, and that they occur in control genes rather than in the genes which themselves hold the code for enzyme structure. Nevertheless, the simple visual image of 'faults' and 'hits' provides a convenient model for envisaging changes induced by irradiation and cross linkage. There has also been some recent experimental proof of the error concept, at least in lower species. Harrison & Holliday (1967) created artificial errors by feeding fruit flies an amino-acid analogue similar to but not identical with that normally incorporated into protein. The flies given the analogue died prematurely. Again, amoebae normally exist in mortal and immortal forms. However, if the protoplasm of an immortal amoeba is contaminated with a small quantity of protoplasm from a mortal amoeba, the characteristics of aging soon begin to appear (Muggleton & Danielli, 1968).

Effects of Irradiation

Kunze (1933) was the first to attribute aging to an accumulation of radiation-induced mutations; he blamed exposure to cosmic radiation. It was soon appreciated that the observed frequency of mutations was rather larger than would have been predicted from the average radiation exposure, but the discrepancy was explained on the basis of irradiation during pre-natal life, when the sensitivity to radiation was much greater (Failla, 1960).

The harmful effects of radiation seem due to the formation of free radicals, in which electron pairs have been separated temporarily into two independently moving electrons (Pryor, 1973). Thus, when water is irradiated, the reaction is

$$H_2O \longrightarrow {}^{\bullet}H + {}^{\bullet}OH + e^-_{aq}$$

(where e^-_{aq} is a hydrated electron).

Since the free radicals are no longer complimentary, they have a large increase of free energy, and this allows them to attack adjacent molecules. In the body, the first steps (Sinex, 1974) are probably the formation of an excited form of oxygen ('singlet oxygen') and superoxide (O_2^-):

$$e^-_{aq} + O_2 \longrightarrow {}^{\bullet}O_2^-$$

$$O_2^- + H^+ \longrightarrow {}^{\bullet}HO_2$$

Even in the absence of radiation, some free radicals are formed from oxygen during normal mitochondrial metabolism (Commoner *et al.*, 1957); other sources are the interaction of metallic ions with cellular components, and ozone exposure. The atypical and hyperactive forms of oxygen go on to react with the body tissues (auto-oxidation), disrupting normal gene structure (Brooks *et al.*, 1973). Comfort (1964) has set the average irradiation for a chromosome break at 19 rad, and the mean lethal dose for an interphase human cell at 86 rad. The free radicals cause additional havoc by reacting with the unsaturated fatty acids of organelle membranes (mitochondria, microsomes, ribosomes) and cell surfaces. The damaged fat is cleared away by special scavenger enzymes, and lysozomes, leaving the cell filled with an unwanted and insoluble residue, the age pigment lipofuscin (Gordon, 1974). Chemists are now developing drugs that can clear the pigment, at least from nerve cells (Nandy, 1968). However, there is little evidence that accumulation of the pigment in itself leads to any impairment of cellular function (Spiegel, 1972).

In terms of the whole animal, irradiation could have at least four possible effects upon survival (Comfort, 1964). It could present simply an additional environmental hazard, decreasing the percentage of individuals surviving for a given time interval irrespective of their age. It could cause aging to develop prematurely, displacing the Gompertz plot (Figure 1.2) towards the left, without changing its slope. It could also modify the subsequent rate of aging, so that the Gompertz relationship showed a steeper slope. Lastly, it could produce an all or none type of damage, certain members of a population incurring defects that caused their immediate or premature death while the remainder of the sample enjoyed an unchanged rate of aging.

The results of some animal studies conform to the second model, radiation inducing precocious aging (Neary *et al.*, 1957). If the exposure is chronic in character, there appears to be a partial saturation of the vulnerable cell components, since early doses have the largest effects; nevertheless, such experiments show not only precocious aging but also some steepening of the subsequent mortality slope (Sacher *et al.*, 1958). There have been few observations in man. One early paper suggested that the lives of radiologists were curtailed by as much as 5.2 years relative to the general population (Warren, 1956). However, the method of data handling used in this report was soon vigorously attacked by statisticians (Court-Brown & Doll, 1958). The latter authors found no evidence of premature death in radiologists; nor did they consider the causes of death as unusual, except for a small excess of skin tumours dating from the early days of radiology, when protection of the workers had been minimal. A large number of the Japanese people were exposed to a heavy dose of ionising radiation during the two atomic explosions at the end of World War II; however, not much can be learnt from the subsequent mortality experience of the exposed populations, since the communities concerned have undergone rapid social change in the post-war period.

We may conclude that the damage induced by irradiation and by chemical mutagens bears a superficial resemblance to aging, both at the molecular level and in terms of overall mortality experience. With the exception of radiation sickness and certain neoplastic diseases, the causes of death are as in natural aging, but the time of death is moved forward. Closer examination of individual lesions reveals certain points of distinction. For example, the cataracts found after irradiation are very different from the normal senile cataract (Alexander & Connell, 1963). A more serious argument against invoking irradiation as a total explanation of aging is the limited value of anti-oxidant treatment. If molecular senescence were due to the ravages of free radicals, one would anticipate that aging could be delayed substantially by the use of anti-oxidants such as Vitamins C and E and the commercial preservatives added to many food products. Animal experiments do show some positive effects from anti-oxidant therapy, but the required doses are heroic, and the typical benefit (a 15-20 per cent retardation of aging) is much less than could have been obtained simply by a curtailment of food intake. Since body weight is generally reduced by the massive use of anti-oxidants, it is by no means clear that these compounds are acting against free radicals. Other, indirect mechanisms such as a reduction of appetite or a change in the toxicity of laboratory food may be involved. A final difficulty is presented by the immortality of the germ cells (the ova and the spermatozoa). If radiation causes cumulative errors that reduce viability, how are we to explain the fact that the germ cells escape this hazard and survive in healthy form from one generation to the next?

Cross-Linkage

The concept of a progressive, age-related deterioration in macromolecules has quite a long history. The loss of elasticity with aging first focused attention on the connective tissue, and it was postulated that the body colloids underwent a slow dehydration as a person became older (Růzička, 1924). More recently, enquiry has centred around the development of cross-linkages between macro-molecules. The usual agents responsible for such bonding are free radicals, liberated by radiation and chemical mutagens; in its current form, the cross-

linkage hypothesis thus has much in common with concepts of senescence based upon mutation and irradiation. However, it should be
noted that cross-linkages can develop not only in DNA, but also in
many of the other large molecules of the body.

Bjorksten (1974) has illustrated the likely sequence of events in a
DNA filament. Initially, the cross-linkage is attached to only one
strand of the nucleoside (Figure 2.1). Defence mechanisms cannot
detach the cross-link, but they are able to excise the affected segment
of the nucleoside chain, using its partner as a template for accurate
resynthesis of the damaged zone. With the link swinging freely, it can
soon become attached to the second nucleoside strand. If repair is not
rapid enough to avert this danger, the cell may still excise the mal-
formed segment, but now the damage has become irreversible, since
there is no longer a residual template to allow accurate replacement
of the missing amino acids. In some instances, the cross-linkage may
remain in place. At the next cell division, separation of the nucleoside
chains is incomplete, and a Y-shaped monstrosity is formed. Usually,
this is lethal for the cell in question, although on occasion it may be
able to mutate successfully.

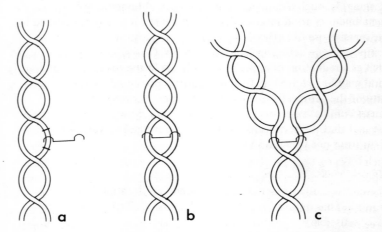

Figure 2.1   Three possible consequences of cross-linkage: (a) single DNA
filament repaired by excision of affected segment; (b) both DNA filaments
affected, linkage irreversible, so that when cell division is attempted a Y-shaped
non-viable monstrosity (c) is formed (after Bjorksten, 1974).

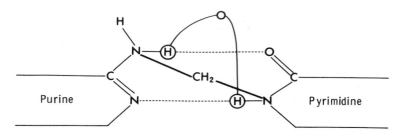

Figure 2.2   Example of cross-linkage. Two nucleosides are linked by weak hydrogen bonds (dotted lines) connecting purine and pyrimidine molecules. Formaldehyde reacts with the two hydrogen atoms to form water and a strong methylene bridge between the purine and the pyrimidine (after Watson & Crick, 1953).

The chemical basis of cross-linkage is shown in Figure 2.2. In this example, the aggressor is a molecule of formaldehyde (CH_2O), but it could equally well be a free radical. The two nucleoside chains of the DNA molecule are normally held together by weak hydrogen bonds, linking for instance the purine and pyrimidine radicals. However, in the presence of a migrant formaldehyde molecule, the bonding hydrogen atoms combine with the oxygen of the formaldehyde to yield water, and a strong methylene (CH_2) bridge is established between the purine and the pyrimidine radicals.

Cross-linkage may not only unite the two nucleoside chains of the DNA, but may also bind the DNA more closely to its associated protein within the chromosome. This has the effect of repressing its capacity to induce enzyme formation (Speigel, 1972).

Other large intra- and extra-cellular molecules may undergo cross-linkage, with the formation of complex and dense structures that cannot be cleared away by the normal enzyme systems of the body. Such linkages provide a likely basis for the proteinaceous amorphous deposits such as hyalin and amyloid that accumulate with aging. The chemical processes seem analogous to those described for DNA. Changes in collagen have received extensive study. Young collagen consists of three helical chains, twisted about one another to form a super helix, and held together rather loosely by hydrogen bonds between the carbonyl, imino and amino groups of adjacent chains. Cross-linkage leads to the formation of dimers (rigid bonding of two chains) and trimers (rigid bonding of three chains). Aging certainly leads to an increase in the dimer and trimer content of collagen (Hall, 1973), but there is little evidence that this change influences the overall well-being of the individual (Spiegel, 1972).

Other evidence for the cross-linkage concept follows the lines discussed in previous sections. One big weakness of the hypothesis is the limited effect of anti-oxidants and other agents that should modify the rate of cross-linkage.

Auto-Immunity

The immune system of the body is remarkable in that it initiates a brisk reaction against any foreign protein, but at the same time it recognises and spares the protein of its owner. At one time it was suggested that 'hits' from radiation or some other source modified the nature of body constituents to the point where they became 'other than self', provoking an immune response (Comfort, 1964) with death of the affected cells (Walford, 1969). The main objection to this viewpoint was that insufficient protein was altered to cause any substantial immunological reaction.

A second possibility is that the antigenic characteristics of certain cells are modified by viral infection rather than by a 'hit' from a free radical (Liburd *et al.*, 1973). In this regard, it is known that if female mice are infected at birth with Coxsackie virus, their median life-span is shortened by some five months. However, infected males live some thirteen months longer than anticipated, mainly because the virus inhibits the normal tendency of the young mice to kill each other (Hotcin & Sikova, 1970).

A third and more credible hypothesis is that aging leads to a partial failure of the normal mechanisms of immunity, with a breakdown of the usual systems that distinguish vital from foreign protein molecules (Burnet, 1959; Bjorksten, 1974). On this last concept, one mutation and subsequent rapid multiplication of the abnormal anti-body-producing cell could cause widespread damage.

There is some evidence of a decline in normal immunological function as a person becomes older (Heidrick & Makinodan, 1972), although this begins rather later than the normal onset of aging (Adler, 1974). In a more direct test of the auto-immune hypothesis, Walford (1964) succeeded in extending the life-span of mice by use of an immuno-suppressant (Imuran), but the increase of longevity was less than could have been accomplished by simple dietary restriction. The prevalence of auto-immune conditions such as generalised rheumatoid arthritis also increases with age, although it remains puzzling why the condition is twice as common in women as in men.

Is the site of mutation on the sex-related X chromosome, and do women have twice as many antibody-producing cells as men? If so, we would anticipate that they would not only encounter problems from auto-immune disease, but that they would also have a greater resistance to infection than men (Burch, 1963). Of more significance in the present context, they should also age twice as fast as men. This is so obviously at variance with common experience that it seems difficult to accept auto-immunity as the principal cause of aging.

'Wear and Tear' and Exhaustion

The longevity of most man-made pieces of equipment varies inversely with use. Early gerontologists thus found it logical to postulate 'wear and tear' (*Abnutzungstheorie*) as a basis for aging.

It still seems reasonable to anticipate mechanical deterioration of some structures such as bones, joints and blood vessels. The original concept was of a mechano-chemical deterioration in cell colloids. This is rather at variance with the present-day view of the living cell as a dynamic system where there is a continuous modification and rebuilding of individual elements. The rate of 'turnover' of liver and serum proteins, for example, is such that a given molecule has a half-life averaging no more than ten days (Bender, 1953). Nevertheless, radioactive tracer studies have shown that some constituents of muscle and brain are very stable, and rarely if ever turn over (Nordgren *et al.*, 1969). There is also evidence that a given enzyme has only a finite life-span (Theorell *et al.*, 1951). After it has processed a given number of reactions, it is exhausted. Thus, as an animal becomes older, the proportion of actively functioning molecules falls (Gershon & Gershon, 1970). In body cells that are still capable of division, enzymes can be replaced at mitosis. In post-mitotic cells such as nerve and muscle, it is harder to see how enzymes can be regenerated. Since human nerve cells live for seventy to one hundred years, we must suppose either that neural enzymes are very resistant to spoilage, or that the neurons have developed some non-mitotic mechanism for the replacement of such molecules.

Animal experiments lend some credibility to the concept of enzyme exhaustion, since longevity can be reduced by devices that increase metabolic activity, such as exposure to a high environmental temperature (Loeb & Northrup, 1917) or severe cold (Johnson *et al.*, 1961). Equally, survival is increased by a drop of metabolism with hibernation or dietary restriction (Ross, 1961). However, the relevance of such observations to human longevity is questionable. In the dietary experiments, for example, the animals are caged, and those whose food supply is limited do not grow as large as those on an unrestricted diet. Further, the extension of life-span occurs mainly before the animals have reached maturity (Barrows & Beauchene, 1970).

In man, Pearl (1928) found a higher mortality in outdoor workers of social class V (the heavy manual labourers) than in the other four categories of employee. However, it is difficult to separate the high probable energy expenditure of the class V men from their more general socio-economic disadvantages. Studies of athletes (Chapter 6) have suggested little relationship between a high level of physical activity and longevity. Even assuming that there is some association between the average rate of metabolism and life-span, this does not provide unique proof that enzyme exhaustion has arisen through an increase of biochemical turnover. Other potential aging processes such as cross-linkage and copying errors may also have been accelerated by an increase of cellular activity.

The cessation of ovulation at the menopause is associated with substantial changes of endocrine balance, and perhaps for this reason many authors have sought a relationship between aging and exhaustion of the endocrine system. While morphological changes can be seen in certain of the endocrine glands as a person becomes older, it is difficult to decide whether such changes are cause or effect. Certainly, there is no evidence that the majority of endocrine-secreting cells become post-mitotic, nor can the picture of senescence be established in an experimental animal by removal of any of its endocrine glands. Administration of androgens and oestrogens can reverse some of the secondary stigmata of aging; in women, for example, beard growth can be halted, atrophy of the vaginal epithelium corrected, and a youthful elasticity restored to the skin. There may also be more general anabolic effects, including an increased synthesis of protein with a net retention of nitrogen. However, the typical course of aging in eunuchs is a strong argument that the sex hormones have no fundamental role in the prevention of senescence. The most probable endocrine source of general disability would be an impairment of function in the pituitary gland, since this is linked by feedback loops with many other endocrine organs. Some authors have seen their caloric restriction experiments as a form of dietary hypophysectomy. Any action of procaine on aging has also been attributed to a mild activation of the pituitary-adrenal system (Green, 1959). However, there seems little evidence of a direct relationship between aging and pituitary function.

Accumulation of Debris

There is much literature to document a progressive intracellular accumulation of both calcium and pigment with aging (Lansing, 1951). Such changes are probably consequences rather than the prime cause of aging. The lipofuscin, for example, is probably an end-product of the peroxidation of lipids by free radicals (Toth, 1968). Nevertheless, the life-span of one group of ciliated water creatures, the rotifers, can be extended if they are kept in a calcium poor medium. Advocates of procaine therapy (Aslan, 1974) have also seized upon the concept of calcium accumulation (Officer, 1974). In man, calcium accumulates irreversibly in the cell membrane as this undergoes an age-related decrease in its phospholipid content. Apparently, procaine hydrochloride can compete for and release the irreversibly bound calcium (Seeman, 1972), thus restoring a normal pattern of cell function.

Conclusion

The very multiplicity of hypotheses concerning the cellular basis of aging emphasises the point that no current view offers a complete and unique explanation of the known facts of gerontology. Nor does it seem likely that future research will reveal a unitarian concept. The death of an individual cell is a cumulative response to life's insults — exposure to free radicals, viruses and auto-antibodies, accumulation of debris and deterioration in the constancy of the external environment. Likewise, death of the whole organism is the end-result of a progressive deterioration of function; death or malfunction of key cells gives an ever poorer homeostatic response, until a minor infection, a sudden exertion or a change in the external environment become sufficient to terminate life. The corollary of this viewpoint is that research will not suddenly discover some treatment that confers immortality. Rather, longevity will be extended by a series of small steps, as means are found to mitigate one or other of the various factors that currently contribute to malfunction and death of individual cells.

Metabolism of the Aging Cell

Overall Metabolism

In view of the exhaustion of enzyme systems and the deterioration in mechanisms for their repair, one would anticipate an overall decline in metabolic activity with age. Dubois (1927) found such a trend, although there was considerable individual variation in his data, 'probably depending on the degree of senility'. Calloway (1964) went further, describing senescence as a 'decline in the production of free energy in a living system'. More recent research has cast some doubt on this traditional view. Interpretation of results is complicated by age-related changes in body composition, since metabolism is usually expressed per kg of body weight or per m^2 of body surface area. Durnin (1973) estimated that after allowance for the increase of adipose tissue, the resting metabolism in the seventh and eighth decades of life would be 10 per cent lower than in the third decade. Shock (1955) related his oxygen consumption figures to body water, and on this basis he found no age-related trend.

Cellular Metabolism

A decrease of enzyme activity could reflect not only a lack of the active protein, but also a failure of homeostasis, the local environment (pH, ionic concentration, concentration of activators and inhibitors or temperature) being unfavourable to the enzyme in question. Most measurements of enzyme activity have been made under 'static' conditions, rather than in the actual environment that exists at a given age; although the latter type of observation is more difficult to undertake, it may have more significance for the understanding of senescence (Finch *et al.*, 1969; Adelman, 1970).

Studies of the digestive secretions show a steady decline in the ptyalin content of saliva, the pepsin content of gastric juice and the proteolytic power of the pancreatic juice as a person becomes older. However, pancreatic amylase and lipase decrease but little with age (Timiras, 1972).

Kritchevsky *et al.* (1970) made serial cultures of human fibroblasts obtained from Dr Hayflick. The overall oxygen consumption of the tissue showed no change from the middle of its life-span (26th-27th generation) to towards its end (44th generation). Equally, the glucose utilisation remained unimpaired. Towards the end of the culture's life-span, the glycogen content of the cells increased, perhaps because the synthesis of carbohydrate stores was proceeding normally, while the rate of cell division had slowed. The protein content of the cells also rose. Lactic acid dehydrogenase and alkaline phosphatase activity continued unaltered, but the acid phosphatase activity was markedly augmented. This last enzyme is one of the lysozome scavengers that attempts to clear up intracellular debris.

Other authors have made detailed metabolic studies of the liver (Timiras, 1972) and the red cell (Bertolini, 1966). Some 50 per cent of the liver enzymes that have been measured show no change with age; of the remainder, 25 per cent show an increase and 25 per cent a decrease of activity. Changes reflect mainly an alteration in the cellular composition of the tissue classed as liver. For example, macrophage infiltration accounts for an increase of cathepsins (Timiras, 1972).

In the post-mitotic cells of the central nervous system, there are age-related decreases in both choline acetylase and choline esterase activity, more obvious in the spinal cord than in the cerebrum or the cerebellum. However, at least a part of this change can again be attributed to a modification of cell population, since there is an increase in the relative amount of white matter in the spinal cord with aging.

Some workers have reported age-related decreases in the oxygen consumption of tissue slices (Barrows *et al.*, 1960). However, the cause is far from clear. Although the total number of mitochondria per cell may be less than in a younger tissue, the remaining mitochondria all seem fully functional. Again, the explanation may well be a change in the relative proportions of different cells within the tissue, since the decrease is most evident in tissues that suffer a loss of mass or a decrease of cell number.

Specific Changes in Locomotor Enzymes

Rockstein (1972) studied flight mechanisms in the male house-fly (Musca domestica). Aging was associated with a progressive loss in the ability to fly. There were related decreases in the activity of at least three key enzymes: (i) Intramitochondrial magnesium-activated ATP[ase]. This enzyme is concerned with the transfer of energy from adenosine triphosphate, ATP, to the proteins actin and myosin as they join to form actomyosin during a muscular contraction. (ii) Cytochrome c oxidase. This enzyme is a vital link in the chain reaction of oxidative metabolism. (iii) Extramitochondrial NAD dependent alpha-glycero-phosphate dehydrogenase. This enzyme is needed for the resynthesis of ATP through a reaction dependent on the co-enzyme NAD (Nicotinamide adenine dinucleotide).

It is uncertain how far these observations apply to the function of mammalian muscles. However, there have been reports of a decrease in ATP[ase] activity in elderly rats (Rockstein & Brandt, 1961; Edington & Edgerton, 1976), and Schmukler & Barrows (1966) have also noted an age-related loss of lactic dehydrogenase activity. In general, one might anticipate greater vulnerability to aging in post-mitotic muscle than in the liver, since the latter tissue can replace cells that are defective

(Barrows, 1966).

Tissue Energy Reserves

Nature of Energy Reserves

The ability of muscle to develop and sustain a contraction is dependent on the intracellular liberation of energy which can be applied to the bonding of its constituent proteins actin and myosin:

$$\text{Actin} + \text{Myosin} + \text{Energy} \longrightarrow \text{Actomyosin} + \text{Muscle Shortening}$$

The immediate source of energy is found in the high energy phosphate compound adenosine triphosphate, ATP. Breakdown of a single gram-mole of ATP to adenosine diphosphate, ADP, yields some 10-12 kCal of energy:

$$\text{ATP} \longrightarrow \text{ADP} + \text{Phosphate} + 10\text{-}12 \text{ kCal} \ .$$

Unfortunately, intramuscular stores of ATP are extremely limited (in man, about 5 mmol/kg), and they are thus rapidly exhausted. The first available additional resource is another high energy phosphate compound, creatine phosphate, CP. This interacts with the ADP, allowing a resynthesis of ATP:

$$\text{CP} + \text{ADP} \longrightarrow \text{ATP} + \text{C} \ .$$

Intracellular reserves of creatine phosphate are also quite small (about 15 mmol/kg), and once these have been depleted further energy must be liberated by the breakdown of stored foods. The muscle cell contains substantial quantities of its two principal fuels, glycogen and fat. In the absence of oxygen, the glycogen is broken down to pyruvate, and this tends to accumulate as lactic acid. However, the falling intracellular pH inhibits several of the enzymes concerned with glycolysis (particularly phosphorylase and phosphofructokinase), so that after a brief period the reaction is halted unless oxygen is available for breakdown of the accumulating lactic acid to carbon dioxide and water.

Margaria and his associates (Di Prampero, 1971) have thus distinguished three phases of physical activity (Table 2.2):

(i)   The alactate debt: this comprises reactions that have occurred prior to lactate accumulation. It reflects largely the splitting of ATP and CP, with some contribution from oxygen stored in the red pigment of muscle (myoglobin).

(ii) The lactate debt: the breakdown of glycogen to pyruvate, with accumulation of lactic acid.

(iii) The oxygen conductance: the subsequent steady delivery of oxygen to the active tissues.

To permit comparison of the three terms, it is convenient if they are each expressed as a power (equivalent oxygen conductance) and as a capacity (equivalent volume of oxygen).

Table 2.2   Energy resources, expressed in terms of the equivalent oxygen conductance and oxygen capacity (based on Di Prampero, 1971)

Energy resource	Maximum power ml/kg min		Maximum capacity ml/kg		Time to exhaustion sec	
	age 25	age 65	age 25	age 65	age 25	age 65
Alactate system	165	90	22	? 15	8	? 10
Lactate system	68	? 54	45	40	40	? 45
Oxygen conductance	45	30	Infinity		Almost infinity	

Effects of Aging

Modern techniques of muscle biopsy allow direct determinations of ATP, CP and glycogen stores in human muscle. Unfortunately, there seem to have been few observations on elderly people. Apart from the obvious difficulties of obtaining volunteers for biopsy, there is the practical problem that intracellular energy reserves can be depleted quite markedly by habitual inactivity. Thus, if old people were studied and low values were found, it would still be unclear whether this reflected aging *per se* or whether it was due to a low level of daily physical activity.

There are less direct methods of estimating the extent of energy stores. Margaria (1966b) suggested that anaerobic power (the rate of the alactate mechanism) could be evaluated by timing a person as he worked against gravity in sprinting up a flight of stairs. Scores for his test decrease from an oxygen equivalent of 165 ml/kg min in a young adult to about 90 ml/kg min in a person aged 65 years. However, it seems fair comment that a young person is more easily persuaded to engage in such vigorous activity. Many old people have a fear of stumbling, due to poor vision and instability of the knee joints. Even if problems of motivation can be overcome, stiffness of the joints and lack of recent familiarity with the required exercise may lead to a poor performance. The loss of intracellular function is thus likely to be less than indicated by the Margaria test.

The phosphagen molecules, CP and ATP, are resynthesised by a breakdown of glycogen to pyruvate and lactate. Elderly people show a marked creatinuria, and D.A. Hall (1973) has thus deduced that there may be difficulty in the rebuilding of creatine phosphate stores. The capacity of the lactate mechanism is most commonly studied by collecting a specimen of arterial blood 1½-2 minutes following maximum exertion. In a young adult, terminal lactate concentrations of 11-13 mmol/l (100-120 mg/100 ml) are usually attained. In a 65 year old, limiting values are often much smaller. Some authors have set the ceiling of the elderly subject as low as 7 mmol/l (60 mg/100 ml). Our experience (Sidney & Shephard, 1977) suggests that the lesser accumulation of lactate in the old people is partly a question of motivation. With sufficient persuasion, figures of 8-10 mmol/l (90-110 mg/100 ml) are possible. The residual difference from the young adult does not necessarily reflect a deficiency of anaerobic capacity at the cellular level, since the experimental determinations of lactate have been made on blood rather than muscle specimens. In an old person, the ratio of muscle mass to blood volume is usually smaller than in a young adult, and the lactate also escapes less readily into the blood stream, thus blunting peak intra-arterial concentrations.

The steady oxygen conductance is usually measured by having a person walk or run uphill on a treadmill at a progressively increasing slope until exhaustion is attained. Again, old people may not be as well motivated as those who are younger, but in this test the plateauing of oxygen consumption with a further increase of treadmill slope provides a check on the validity of the data. Most reports suggest that the old person has only about two thirds the oxygen transporting power of the average 25-year-old (Chapter 3).

The approximate times required for exhaustion of the alactate and lactate mechanisms have been established in young adults (Table 2.2). In view of the decrease in ATP^{ase} activity, some slowing of the reactions might be anticipated with age, but, unfortunately, no accurate figures are yet available for the extent of such changes.

Stores of Glycogen and Fat

Anaerobic activity can continue only while the muscle cell has an internal supply of carbohydrate. An average young person has a muscle glycogen content of about 1.4g/100g of wet tissue, and this is exhausted over some 100 minutes of strenuous activity (Hultman, 1971). The liver contains a further 100g of glycogen, and in vigorous effort this can be mobilised at a rate of 1-2g/min (Rowell, 1971).

There do not seem to have been any *in vivo* measurements of muscle and liver glycogen concentrations in elderly people. Some post-mortem studies have found relatively high glycogen levels; this has been thought a reflection of the liability of the elderly to diabetes mellitus, with associated high blood sugar readings. Liver and kidney glycogen can accumulate to the point of forming visible vacuoles, apparently without effect on cellular function (Timiras, 1972).

Intramuscular stores of triglyceride are not particularly extensive. Figures for the young adult (Saltin, 1974) range from 5-30 mmol/kg of wet muscle (1.3-7.7 g/kg), the highest concentrations being found in the mitochondria-rich slow twitch muscle fibres. As much as a quarter of the energy requirements of exhausting endurance activity are met from fat metabolism and it is thus likely that intracellular reserves will be depleted at least as fast as the glycogen stores. Thereafter, exercise depends largely on the mobilisation and transport of fat from adipose tissue, and there is evidence that this can have a rate-limiting effect on physical activity even in a young person (Lloyd, 1966).

Observations on intracellular fat in the elderly have been limited mainly to the examination of pathological and post-mortem specimens. Tissues such as the heart, liver and kidney may show an unusual accumulation of fat (fatty degeneration or fatty metamorphosis). Although potentially a reversible phenomenon, it is often followed by cell death. Among suggested explanations, we may note an increased transport of fat from the periphery, an increased capture of circulating chylomicrons, an increased synthesis of fat by the liver, and a decreased utilisation of fat associated with respiratory impairment and impending death of the tissue. A further possible factor is an alteration in the form of stored fat; in a healthy young person, much of the available lipid is in a dispersed 'micellar' form, not detected by light microscopy or standard fat stains. However, if phospholipid production is impaired, it can become transformed into visible fat globules.

We have noted above the accumulation of pigments such as

lipofuscin in the aging cell. Lipofuscin has a high fat content, and is thought to be formed by the peroxidation of lipid/protein mixtures. Heart muscle contains almost no lipofuscin up to the age of ten years, but thereafter there is a steady increase of some 0.3 per cent per decade, so that if a person lives to the age of 90 years, his heart has 6-7 per cent of its intracellular volume occupied by the pigment (Strehler *et al.*, 1959). One early study of skeletal muscle noted that the age pigment accumulated preferentially in the muscles concerned with locomotion (Kny, 1937). This is a little surprising, since the muscles in question have a high proportion of fast twitch fibres; under normal circumstances, the fast twitch fibres contain less mitochondria and less stored triglyceride than the slow twitch fibres concerned with slow movements and maintenance of body posture. There is at present no evidence that the lipofuscin impairs function; indeed heart muscle that is well impregnated with the pigment retains a normal capacity for hypertrophy (Timiras, 1972). However, in view of the current emphasis on the adoption of a diet rich in unsaturated fat, it is worth noting that a large intake of vegetable oil leads to the formation of ceroid, a form of lipofuscin, and this can accumulate in atherosclerotic plaques.

One indication that aging gives a lesser reserve of fuel for sustained activity is provided by Epshtein (1968). He subjected young (eight to ten month) and old (thirty to thirty-two month) white rats to twelve hours of repeated electrical stimulation or swimming to exhaustion. In the young animals metabolism was sufficiently well maintained that there were no changes in the intramuscular concentrations of adenosine triphosphate (ATP) and creatine phosphate (CP) over the exercise bouts. However, in the old rats there was a substantial depletion of the high energy phosphate compounds. After muscle stimulation, ATP concentrations dropped from 33.6 mg/100 ml to 27.1 mg/100 ml, while CP decreased from 12.2 to 9.2 mg/100 ml. After swimming to exhaustion, even larger changes were seen, from 28.5 to 14.6 mg/100 ml (ATP) and from 8.5 to 4.0 mg/100 ml (CP).

Micro-Structural Alterations

Some of the micro-structural alterations that accompany aging have already been discussed — an increase of glycogen storage, fatty infiltration or degeneration, and the accumulation of age pigments. Topics to be discussed here include changes in the water content of the tissues, in the formed elements of connective tissue, in cell structure and in cell turnover rate.

Water Content

As a cell ages, it becomes less efficient at retaining its potassium and excluding extracellular sodium. It is still debated how far this reflects a change of membrane permeability, and how far it is due to a decline in cellular respiration with an associated weakening of the 'sodium pump' (Timiras, 1972). Intracellular water accumulates particularly in the mitochondria and in the endoplasmic reticulum. It leads to a slight oedema, or 'cloudy swelling'. The phenomenon is seen most frequently in the renal tubular cells, hepatic cells and cardiac muscle fibres. As with fatty change and glycogen accumulation, it is difficult to draw a clear line between aging and pathology. Certainly, water accumulation is slight until a cell is near to death. It is also necessary to exclude more general causes of oedema such as congestive heart failure, hypoproteinaemia, renal disease and hormonal malfunctions before blaming the cloudy swelling on the aging process.

Some authors have drawn attention to the paradox of shrivelled skin in the elderly. How can this be reconciled with hyperhydration? Estimates of total body water (Friis-Hansen, 1965) show a small decrease, from perhaps 55 per cent of body weight at age 25 to 47 per cent at age 85 years, but this change reflects largely an increase in the percentage of body fat over the same period. Other considerations are a change in cell population (specific cells being replaced by fibroblasts) and a redistribution of water between intra- and extracellular compartments of the body. Andrew (1968) noted a positive correlation between a decrease of protoplasmic units such as muscle fibres and an increase in the proportion of extracellular to total body water.

Connective Tissue

(i)   General considerations   The elements of connective tissue comprise cells (principally fibroblasts), collagen, elastin, a polysaccharide ground substance and (in the elderly) pseudoelastin (Hall, 1968) and cellulose (Hall & Saxl, 1961). Age alters both the relative proportions and also the properties of the various constituents. This is due partly to functional changes in the fibroblasts secreting the tissue, and partly to subsequent alterations in molecules that have a slow turnover rate.

(ii)   Collagen   Aging leads to an increase in the density and the stability of collagen. We have noted above that cross-linkage is one important reason for such changes. Long before the formal demonstration of such linkages, their existence had been inferred through the

experiments of Verzar (1964) and his associates. It had been demonstrated that as collagen aged, progressively more drastic methods were
needed for its extraction (Jackson, 1959); furthermore, if a tendon
was denatured by heat or by chemical reagents, the force required to
prevent its subsequent shortening increased with age. More recent
information is based on X-ray diffraction and electron microscopic
studies, mainly of the small fraction of collagen that is easily
dissolved; much less is known about the structure of the highly polymerised and relatively insoluble residue (Milch, 1966). An increase of
cross-linkages has been demonstrated for mouse skin (Heikkinen &
Kulonen, 1964), but Bakerman (1964) has queried whether aging
produces an equal increase of highly polymerised collagens in man.

    One alternative method of investigation is to look at collagen turn-
over rates. The formation of cross-linked polymers should protect
collagen molecules against breakdown by collagenases. The synthesis
of single collagen molecules continues while viable fibroblasts remain
in a tissue, but the turnover rate is usually very slow. Neuberger *et al.*
(1951) set the half life of a typical molecule as roughly equal to the
half life of the animal. Collagen breakdown is indicated by the urinary
excretion of hydroxyproline, but unfortunately the quantities
involved are so small that detection is difficult. For example, Hall
(1973) has set the mean loss of skin collagen in males at 15 $\mu g/mm^2$
per decade! Adolescents excrete about seven times as much hydroxyproline as adults, and this is presumptive evidence that the adult fibres
are gaining some protection from cross-linkage. Reed & Hall (cited by
Hall, 1973) have reported that skin, bone and intervertebral disc
collagen all show a diminished susceptibility to collagenase with aging.
However, a further imponderable is a possible age-related change in
collagenase activity. It is well recognised that this enzyme can become
active when needed for the remodelling of scar tissue or the involution
of the uterus following pregnancy, and it is conceivable that failure of
repressor mechanisms could lead to activation of the enzyme in the
elderly. Such a situation could explain a biphasic change in tissue
elasticity — early stiffening with cross-linkage, and later weakening by
increased collagenase activity. An alternative basis for a biphasic aging
response might be a loss of activity in tissue enzymes producing
aldehydes, thus causing a secondary decrease in the rate of cross-linkage
formation.

    The functional consequences of changes in the collagen molecule
have been studied by plotting stress/strain diagrams for various tissues
(Figure 2.3), and noting the elastic modulus (the slope of such

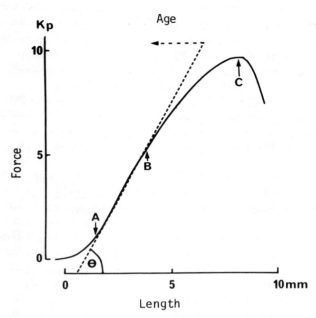

Figure 2.3 The influence of applied force on the length of a rabbit tendon (after Viidik, 1967). Up to point A, the fibres of the tendon are being straightened. Between points A and B, the tendon obeys Hooke's law, the modulus of elasticity being indicated by tan θ. Beyond point B, there is a progressive breakage of individual fibres, and at point C frank rupture of the tendon occurs. Aging increases the steepness of the force/length relationship.

relationships). Unfortunately, collagen obeys Hooke's law over only a very limited range of lengths, and perhaps for this reason the results reported have been conflicting. Fry *et al.* (1964) defined the extensibility of skin as its rate of stretching under constant load, and they noted that this index diminished as the collagen content of the tissue increased. Jansen & Rottier (1958) found little change in the stiffness of human abdominal skin with aging, while Ridge & Wright (1966) reported a biphasic change, stiffness increasing to 45 years of age, and diminishing thereafter. Elden (1966) developed a non-linear equation for elasticity, and concluded that the resultant 'elastic modulus' was not greatly modified by aging. In contrast, Viidik (1967) split the force/length relationship for rabbit tendon into its constituent parts, and found that the linear slope became steeper with age.

(iii)   Elastin   Elastin is some fifteen times as extensible as collagen, but the latter is twenty-five times stronger. The two types of fibre thus play a complementary functional role. Collagen provides strength and rigidity, protecting against over-extension of a part, while elastin confers the property of elasticity. Electron microscopy and X-ray diffraction studies do not usually reveal any characteristic structure for elastic tissue, and it is thus assumed that elastin fibres have a random orientation. Cross-linkages are formed through three amino acids — desmosine, isodesmosine and lysinonor-leucine (Franzblau *et al.*, 1966). Such binding produces even larger changes in the mechanical properties of the fibres than those seen in collagen when this undergoes cross-linkage.

With aging, elastic tissue frays, and the fibres undergo fragmentation, leaving little to be seen except a dispersed granular material. Fluorescence increases, and the colour becomes yellower. Chemical analysis shows a decreased water content, an increase of the three cross-linking amino acids, and sometimes deposition of calcium. While there are large changes in elasticity, it is difficult to be certain that this is due entirely to changes in the structure of the elastin; an increase in the viscosity of the ground substance may also play some role.

Some authors have found an increase in the overall elastin content of tissues with aging. However, this seems a reflection of methodological difficulties, particularly a confounding of elastin and pseudo-elastin. If modern techniques are used, a diminution of elastin content can be demonstrated (Hall, 1973).

(iv)   Pseudo-elastin   Elastin preparations from aged tissue contain a third protein, pseudo-elastin. In terms of amino acid composition, this is intermediate in structure between collagen and elastin. It is thought to be either a degradation product of collagen, or an incorrectly synthesised form of that protein. One could envisage a collagen molecule being broken down to the point of losing some of its characteristic amino and imino acids, yet retaining sufficient of its original form to allow reabsorption onto a standard template, where something closely akin to collagen would be laid down. The degree of departure from the normal collagen molecule apparently varies with the tissue and the site. Changes are particularly marked in the exposed dermis of the neck; here, the normal 64 nm cross-striations of the collagen molecule are completely obliterated by an adherent amorphous coating. The presence of this material seems responsible for reports that elderly people have an increased elastin content in many of their tissues.

(v) *Cellulose* Old and pathological connective tissue contains anisotropic fibres which have a central protein core surrounded by a pair of opposed helices of polysaccharide; the polysaccharide is indistinguishable from cellulose (Hall, 1973), while the protein core is similar to pseudo-elastin. The combination is immune to attacks from both collagenase and elastase.

(vi) *Polysaccharide* Protein/polysaccharide complexes play an important role in several tissues, including cartilage, skin and synovial fluid. Interstices in the network of linked chains of collagen are filled with polysaccharides, smaller fibres being glued to the larger by a cement continuous with the ground substance. The main polysaccharides of connective tissue are hyaluronic acid and chondroitin sulphate. The first is a highly viscous lubricant which allows elastic tissue, collagen fibres and muscle fibres to slide over each other with minimal friction. The chondroitin sulphate, on the other hand, functions as the cement. With aging, the collagen content of the tissues increases, but there is a decrease in both the content and the degree of polymerisation of the ground substance. This presumably reflects both a diminished formation of polysaccharide by the connective tissue cells, and a faster turnover of the ground substance. It can lead to a substantial reduction in the stability of material such as cartilage (Sylven & Malmgren, 1952). A loss of the plasticising function of the ground substance may also contribute to the increase of elastic modulus and make the tissue less permeable to nutrients.

However, it has been argued that in some tissues the loss of polysaccharide is more apparent than real, increased inter-chain binding making the material less accessible to normal methods of detection. After peroxidate oxidation, for example, certain of the polysaccharides can serve as cross-linking agents for both collagen and elastin fibres (Milch, 1966).

(vii) *Functional sequelae* It is obvious that the connective tissues make a major contribution to the dynamic properties of the body, and that an alteration in the relative proportions of the several constituents or in the mechanical properties of an individual constituent could create major problems for an elderly person who wished to exercise. Back and joint problems, tendon rupture and altered pressure/volume relationships for the lungs, heart and great vessels can all be traced at least in part to disturbances of connective tissue.

A typical aging sequence can be traced in the blood vessels. Frayed elastic fibres and degenerated smooth muscle are progressively replaced by collagen. Initially, the collagen fibres are arranged in parallel with the elastin, but after repeated cycles of elongation and contraction, they do not resist extension until a substantial force is applied. Again, whereas elastic tissue returns immediately to its original length after a distending force has been released, the collagen that replaces it shows much more hysteresis, retaining as much as two thirds of its elongation for a substantial period. There is a considerable increase in the capacity of the blood vessels as a person becomes older, making it more difficult to sustain a large central blood volume and a high cardiac output during vigorous exercise.

Cell Structure

Various modifications of cellular organelles accompany the aging process, although often the functional significance of such changes is unclear (Bakerman, 1969). The nucleus becomes larger and may show invagination of its membrane with various inclusions. The nucleoli are increased both in size and in number. The chromatin may show clumping, shrinking, fragmentation or dissolution, and there is an increased likelihood of finding chromosomal abnormalities. The cytoplasm shows an accumulation of pigments and sometimes of fat. There may be a depletion or sometimes an accumulation of glycogen. Other features include vacuole formation, the appearance of hyaline droplets, and alterations in the size, shape, cristal pattern and matrix density of the mitochondria.

Cell Turnover

We have noted already that muscle and nerve cells have lost the capacity to undergo cell division. Other cells retain this property until death, but nevertheless the time intervals between successive cell divisions may become progressively extended (Lesher & Sacher, 1968).

In tissue culture, one can distinguish three phases of cell turnover — early, rapid multiplication, a period of decreasing proliferation and eventual death. In the later generations of a culture, an ever-increasing proportion of the cells show nuclear abnormalities and chromosome aberrations. However, there is no clear relationship between the age of a donor and the age of the resultant culture. Furthermore, the length of life *in vitro* depends to some extent upon the type of culture medium that is used. One factor that can prolong life is the presence of some other variety of cells, raising the possibility of a need for 'feeder' cells that contribute essential nutrients the main tissue is incapable of synthesising (Rothfels *et al.*, 1963).

One form of cell growth that has been studied quite extensively in man is the production of red cells. Here, there is no clear evidence of aging, and if an old person is exposed to a hypoxic stress, he retains the ability to respond by an increased outpouring of red cells from his bone marrow (Das, 1969).

In the post-mitotic tissue of the brain, there is a progressive decrease of cell count with age. Gardiner (1950) also reported a 30 per cent reduction in the myelinated fibre population of the spinal cord by the age of 60-70 years, although Birren & Wall (1956) were unable to find parallel changes in the sciatic nerves of elderly rats. Brody (1955) made cell counts in various regions of the brain, and noted the greatest loss to occur in the superior temporal gyrus. While some cells die from cumulative metabolic errors, a second factor is anoxic death secondary to atherosclerosis of the cerebral blood vessels. McFarland (1963) has drawn attention to the parallel between the effects of oxygen lack in a young person and the mental changes of senescence; in his view, much of cerebral aging is an expression of progressive anoxia.

3 GROSS CHANGES OF FORM AND FUNCTION

As we turn from cellular and sub-cellular events to changes in gross form and function, it becomes much more difficult to distinguish true aging from the superimposed effects of environment and disease. The available data base refers largely to the sedentary and overfed population of North America, and in many instances it becomes necessary to report the actual capacity and power of physiological systems without forming a judgement as to whether the observed deterioration of performance is a necessary and inevitable accompaniment of aging.

Stature and General Body Form

Shortness of stature is a rather obvious external characteristic of an old person. We have already noted (Chapter 1) that this reflects both a secular trend towards an increase of standing height in subsequent generations and age-related changes in the spine: compression of the intervertebral discs, collapse of the vertebrae and increased bowing (kyphosis) of the vertebral column (Damon *et al.*, 1972). Secular trends can be distinguished from aging when the results of cross-sectional and longitudinal studies are compared (Figure 1.3). The decrease of stature due to senescence commences around 40 years of age, and accelerates to a loss of as much as 2 cm per decade between 60 and 80 years. Some authors have maintained that changes are greatest in those whose occupation has required them to carry heavy loads for many years; it may thus be significant that Miall *et al.* (1967) found a much more rapid loss of stature among men living in a mining community (Rhondda Valley) than in a farming and commuter region (Vale of Glamorgan).

Compression of the intervertebral discs is but one expression of more general changes in connective tissues with senescence (Chapter 2). In a young person, the intervertebral discs each comprise a rigid outer shell of fibrous tissue and fibro-cartilage (the annulus fibrosus) and a soft yellow core of pulpy elastic tissue (the nucleus pulposus). With aging, the latter becomes desiccated, and the disc collapses. This diminishes overall stature and allows an exaggeration of normal kyphosis. Other factors contributing to bowing of the spine include a weakening of the back muscles, physiological or pathological degeneration of the vertebrae ('senile osteoporosis'), and osteo-arthritis of the vertebral joints. Any increase of kyphosis augments postural work, particularly while maintaining an upright posture; in advanced cases, even the effort of supporting the head can become extremely fatiguing. Severe changes may also lead to distressing low back pain and respiratory problems.

Other well-recognised changes of body form include a decrease of sitting height, shoulder width and chest depth (although if the subject is emphysematous the normal appearance of the chest may be round – the so-called 'barrel' deformity, Mithoefer & Karetzky, 1968; Leeming, 1973 – since the subject has difficulty in expelling air from his lungs).

Changes of body circumferences due to loss of muscle and an increase of subcutaneous fat will be considered in the following section.

Body Composition

Cellular and sub-cellular changes of body composition have already been discussed (Chapter 2). In this section we shall examine gross changes, particularly increases of overall body weight and body fat and losses of muscle and bone.

Body Weight

An individual's weight usually climbs from 25 to 45 or 50 years of age, and thereafter begins a progressive decline (Bourlière & Parot, 1962; Kemsley *et al.*, 1962; Khosla & Lowe, 1967; Wyndham *et al.*, 1970; Bjelka, 1971; Timiras, 1972). The increase is generally due to an accumulation of fat and body weight is thus widely used as a simple index of obesity. In the usual cross-sectional type of survey, individual weights can be related to values that are 'ideal' from an actuarial point of view (Shephard, 1974b). Personal values may be distorted by a light body frame or heavy musculature, but the average excess usually gives a fair index of how fat a population is. When applying this simple approach to the problem of aging (Table 3.1), there are a number of pitfalls to avoid:

(i)   Many large series of body weight measurements have been collected for insurance purposes. The samples concerned are thus biased towards a favoured socio-economic group.

(ii)   Accumulation of body fat may be masked by a concomitant lightening of the bones and atrophy of the skeletal musculature (Pett & Ogilvie, 1956; Shock, 1961; Forbes & Hursh, 1963; Forbes & Reina,

Table 3.1   Influence of age on excess body weight (relative to the actuarial ideal, Shephard, 1974b) and thickness of subcutaneous fat (average of eight skinfold readings). Author's data for Canadians living in the Toronto area (cross-sectional material, Shephard, 1977d)

Age (yrs)	Men		Women	
	Excess weight (kg)	Skinfold (mm)	Excess weight (kg)	Skinfold (mm)
20-29	1.7 ± 8.7 (N = 78)	11.2 ± 5.9 (N = 78)	8.3 ± 5.3 (N = 6)	15.2 ± 3.8 (N = 6)
30-39	6.4 ± 8.5 (N = 66)	16.1 ± 10.6 (N = 65)	1.4 ± 5.3 (N = 18)	13.5 ± 5.2 (N = 18)
40-49	9.3 ± 9.5 (N = 75)	14.0 ± 5.8 (N = 76)	6.8 ± 8.4 (N = 37)	17.3 ± 5.4 (N = 38)
50-59	8.8 ± 7.7 (N = 60)	15.2 ± 6.7 (N = 63)	4.9 ± 7.2 (N = 22)	18.2 ± 5.1 (N = 23)
60-69	5.1 ± 7.3 (N = 9)	15.4 ± 2.7 (N = 10)	4.5 ± 9.5 (N = 14)	22.5 ± 7.9 (N = 11)

1970). Thus, in the example of Table 3.1, excess weight diminishes in the sixth and seventh decades, but the thickness of the subcutaneous fat layer remains unaltered or even increases; the weight loss is due to atrophy of lean tissue rather than loss of fat.

(iii)   Obese individuals have a higher mortality than those of 'ideal' body weight, either in their own right or because of an association between obesity and cardiovascular risk factors such as a high blood pressure or a high serum cholesterol (Friis Hansen, 1965; Norris *et al.*, 1963; Wessel *et al.*, 1963; Keys *et al.*, 1972; Ashley & Kannel, 1974). This can lead to a preponderance of lighter individuals in the older age categories.

(iv)   Ethical considerations require the examination of volunteers. In many types of experiment, the health conscious are more likely to volunteer than those who are unfit and obese; thus, the sample is likely to underestimate the average increase of body weight in an aging population.

(v)   Weight for height tables work well in the assessment of young individuals; however, the permissible weight may be underestimated if there has been a substantial reduction of stature with aging.

A second method of assessing an individual's weight is to ask him how much he has gained since the age of 25 years; the main source of any weight increase over this period is likely to be fat, but because of factor (ii), the extent of fat accumulation will be underestimated by the response to such a question.

Skinfold Measurements

Skinfold measurements provide a simple means of determining whether departures from 'ideal' body weight are due to adipose tissue or muscle. The data is often presented as the sum or the average of a series of skinfold readings. Alternatively, prediction formulae such as those of Durnin (Durnin & Rahaman, 1967; Durnin & Womersley, 1974) can be used to estimate the percentage of body fat from the skinfold thicknesses, or a combination of folds and circumferences. The advantage of calculating body fat is that one may then proceed to estimate lean body mass. However, it is by no means certain that formulae developed in one part of the world such as Glasgow work well when applied to the plumper citizens of North America.

Irrespective of the method of data treatment, it is important that the observer be well-trained in the technique of skinfold measurement; unless great care is taken, inter-observer errors of 25 per cent are liable to occur, particularly when measuring very fat subjects. A standard design of calipers must also be used, either the Harpenden or the Lange instrument. Both of these devices exert a standard pressure of $10g/mm^2$ over face plates of $35 \ mm^2$ area. Finally, in elderly subjects there is some tendency for the skin to move independently of the underlying fat, and it is thus vital to ensure that both skin and subcutaneous tissue are introduced between the jaws of the calipers.

At most of the common measurement sites (Table 3.2) sex differences in the thickness and distribution of subcutaneous fat persist into old age (Edwards, 1951; Ljunggren, 1963; Pářizková, 1963, 1964; Young, 1965). Some authors have suggested that men accumulate fat at a faster rate than women, so that sex differences diminish progressively with age (Skerlj *et al.*, 1953; Young, 1965). This is true if attention is directed to the lower part of the abdomen (Table 3.2). However, if data for 7-10 folds are averaged, the men show a 25 per cent gain, and the women a 51 per cent gain between the ages of 25 and 65 years. The women show a particularly large deposition of fat on the shin, chest, waist, hips and thighs (Skerlj *et al.*, 1953; Shephard *et al.*, 1969); certain of these differences can be brought out by factor analysis of the skinfold readings (Shephard *et al.*, 1969).

There have been suggestions that after 65 years of age, the amount of subcutaneous fat declines (for example, Bourlière & Parot, 1962). It remains uncertain how far such trends reflect alterations in the

Table 3.2   Skinfold thicknesses at selected body sites. Values for elderly subjects compared with readings for a young adult approximating the actuarial 'ideal' body weight (Shephard, 1972)

Body site	Male skinfold thickness							
	1	2	3	4 (mm)	5	6	7	10 %
Chin	5.8	8.5	8.5	7.0	7.6	7.3	9.3	+ 39
Subscapular	11.9	11.8	18.0	15.0	17.2	14.8	16.8	+ 31
Triceps	7.8	9.9	14.0	7.0	7.1	5.9	8.3	+ 12
Suprailiac	12.7	10.5	17.0	14.0	16.7	10.1	14.2	+ 8
Waist	14.3	18.6	21.0	30.0	26.6	25.1	17.5	+ 62
Suprapubic	11.0	—	21.5	—	—	—	24.9	+ 111
Chest	12.0	—	16.5	14.0	15.1	19.8	24.2	+ 49
Thigh	—	13.3	—	6.0	6.9	7.9	15.4	—
Calf	—	7.0	—	7.0	7.2	3.4	7.2	—
Knee	8.6	—	9.5	—	—	—	14.0	+ 37
Average and number of folds	10.4 (8)	11.3 (7)	15.8 (8)	11.5 (10)	12.4 (10)	10.6 (10)	16.2 (8)	+ 25

	Female skinfold thickness					
	1	4	8	9 (mm)	7	10 %
Chin	7.1	11.0	10.8	13.4	12.1	+ 67
Subscapular	11.3	18.0	22.6	21.4	18.0	+ 77
Triceps	15.6	15.0	28.0	15.3	20.6	+ 26
Suprailiac	14.6	21.0	22.8	31.1	18.1	+ 59
Waist	15.3	32.0	35.8	32.1	23.0	+ 101
Suprapubic	20.5	—	37.9	33.8	31.7	+ 68
Chest	8.6	16.0	14.5	22.3	18.1	+ 106
Thigh	—	13.0	32.7	—	29.1	—
Calf	—	16.0	—	—	20.0	—
Knee	11.8	—	11.5	25.9	30.0	+ 90
Average and number of folds	13.9 (8)	16.2 (10)	22.1 (12)	24.4 (8)	21.1 (8)	+ 51

References

1. Young adult (Shephard, 1972)
2. Lee & Lasker (1959)
3. Shephard *et al.* (1969)
4. Pářizková (1963, 1964)
5. Pářizková & Eiselt (1966)
6. Pářizková & Eiselt (1968) — trained subjects
7. Sidney *et al.* (1977)
8. Young *et al.* (1963); Young (1965)
9. Brown & Shephard (1967)
10. Average score for elderly subjects, expressed as a percentage increment over values for young normals of same sex.

relative proportions of deep and superficial fat (Durnin & Womersley, 1974) or are simply an artefact of population sampling. If there is a true fat loss, this could be due to the nutritional problems of extreme age (loss of interest in cooking, lack of teeth or dentures and poor gastro-intestinal absorption of food).

Body Fat Determinations

There are a number of more direct procedures for the determination of total body fat, but none are completely satisfactory in elderly subjects.

Underwater weighing is widely considered to be the reference procedure. However, there are considerable technical difficulties in applying this method to the aged. In a young person, it is possible to make a rapid weighing while submerged, and to estimate the buoyancy of residual lung gas as a fixed percentage of the individual's vital capacity measured under more comfortable conditions. The residual gas volume is much more variable in the elderly, and it thus becomes necessary to make direct measurements by the helium dilution method while submerged. Equilibration of helium with the lung gas may take many minutes. During this time the head must be kept underwater and a waterproof seal must be maintained about a rubber mouthpiece. The test thus becomes severely taxing for an edentulous subject. Having determined body density, it is still necessary to predict the corresponding body composition. In essence, the formulae that are used consider the body as having adipose and lean tissue compartments, each with a fixed density estimated from the dissection of cadavers. With senescence, changes of bone density and alterations in the cell population and structure of other lean tissues inevitably cause departures from the standard density figures, with corresponding errors in the estimates of body fat.

A second method used in a number of studies of senior citizens has been to determine the naturally occurring isotope ^{40}potassium, using a whole body counter (McNeill & Green, 1959). Since most of the body potassium is inside the muscle cells, the counts recorded give an indication of muscle mass and (less directly) of total lean body mass. From the viewpoint of the subject, the test is simple; he is merely required to sit inside the counter. But interpretation of the data is more difficult. It is necessary to assume an arbitrary relationship between potassium and lean mass, commonly 68.1 mEq/l (Myhre & Kessler, 1966; Roessler & Dunavant, 1967). Several factors depress the potassium/lean mass ratio in the elderly, leading to an underestimation of lean tissue and an overestimation of body fat. The true potassium content of the body may be underestimated because a thick layer of subcutaneous fat prevents a full registration of radiation by the counter. The potassium-rich muscle also makes up a smaller proportion of the total lean mass. Lastly, poorer function of the sodium pump (Chapter 2) leads to some replacement of potassium by sodium ions within the muscle fibres. A number of authors (Forbes *et al.*, 1961; Myhre & Kessler, 1966; Novak, 1972; Leusink, 1974; Sidney *et al.*, 1977) have commented on the resultant discrepancies between body potassium and hydrostatic estimates of body fat.

A third possible method of estimating body composition is to determine the total body water from the dilution of a marker such as deuterated or tritiated water (Shephard *et al.*, 1973). For this procedure, the subject does no more than furnish samples of urine three or four hours after drinking a small volume of 'heavy' water. Nevertheless, it is necessary to assume an arbitrary water content for the lean tissue (73.2 per cent). Uncertainties regarding the tissue hydration of elderly subjects were stressed in the previous chapter.

Reported percentages of body fat (Table 3.3) generally average about 26 per cent in elderly men and 38 per cent in women, but are 6-10 per cent higher if based on determinations of total body potassium. If the equations of Durnin and his associates are applied to the 'ideal' skinfold readings of Table 3.2, figures of 17.1 per cent and 21.4 per cent are obtained for young men and women respectively. Published series average 19.8 per cent for six groups of sedentary young men, and 28.4 per cent for six groups of sedentary young women (Sidney, 1976). It would thus seem that aging is associated with rather similar increases of subcutaneous and deep body fat.

It remains uncertain how far the increase of body fat is a necessary accompaniment of aging, and how far it is a secondary consequence of culturally imposed decrements of habitual activity. In parts of the world where food is in short supply, aging does not lead to any increase in either body weight (Frisch & Revelle, 1969) or skinfold thicknesses (Shephard, 1978). Equally, studies of Masters' class athletes have shown no more than 14 per cent body fat in men from the seventh, eighth and ninth decades of life (Shephard & Kavanagh, 1978).

Lean Body Mass

The lean body mass is given by the product of total body weight and $(100 - F)/100$, where F is the percentage of body fat. The results obtained thus vary with the method of estimation of body fat, as

Table 3.3 The percentage of body fat in elderly subjects

	Male subjects %	Female subjects %	Author
	27.9	36.3	Olesun (1963)
	–	44.6	Young *et al.* (1963)
	24.3-31.6	–	Norris *et al.* (1963)
	23.4	–	Myhre & Kessler (1966)
	36.2*	–	Myhre & Kessler (1966)
	26.0*	49.0*	Forbes & Reina (1970)
	29.9*	43.5*	Novak (1972)
	28.4	–	Adams *et al.* (1972)
	20.2	32.0	Sidney *et al.* (1977)
	36.6*	48.7*	Sidney *et al.* (1977)
Average data:			
Body potassium*	32.2*	47.1*	
Other methods	25.6	37.6	

discussed above.

One would anticipate a lesser lean mass in the elderly, partly because they are smaller than younger subjects, and partly because there is muscle wasting. Korenchevsky (1961) weighed individual organs of the body and noted that wasting began between the fifth and seventh decades of life. The main loss was in the muscle, liver, kidneys and adrenal glands, but there was also a significant decrease of brain weight. Some bones such as the ribs became lighter, but others (for example the sternum) increased in weight (Timiras, 1972).

Available data refers mainly to 'young' old people, before tissue wasting is far advanced. In the men, the lean mass is 47-53 kg (Olesun, 1963; Forbes & Reina, 1970; Novak, 1972; Sidney *et al.*, 1977), compared with 56-59 kg in young adults. In the women, the weight of lean tissue is 31-41 kg (Young *et al.*, 1963; Olesun, 1963; Forbes & Reina, 1970; Novak, 1972; Sidney *et al.*, 1977), compared with 38-42 kg in young adults. Corresponding values for total body potassium can be summarised as follows:

Men	Women	Author
135g	88g	Allen *et al.* (1960)
124-141g	92-93g	Novak (1972)
129g	85g	Sidney *et al.* (1977)

The average for four series of young men (Sidney, 1976) is 155g, while three studies of young women yield an average of 96g.

Body Circumference

Changes in body circumference reflect the resultant of muscle wasting and the accumulation of subcutaneous fat (Table 3.4). In most regions of the body (chest, buttocks, thigh, calf and upper arm) there is little net change of girth, although the body contours of the elderly have a less firm and 'muscular' appearance. The main exception is the abdominal girth, which shows a 6-16 per cent increase in the men and a 25-35 per cent increase in the women.

Table 3.4   Body circumferences of old men and women (cm)

Variable	Men				Women		
	1	2	3	4	1	5	4
Height (cm)	179.3	169	173	173	165.6	163	158
Weight (kg)	73.5	70.7	76.6	74.7	57.5	62.0	61.2
Chest	96.0	94.8	99.6	96.7	82.3	80.9	87.5
Abdomen	82.1	87.5	95.5	92.4	70.8	95.9	88.3
Buttocks	93.4	—	—	98.5	95.0	99.1	97.1
Thigh	52.4	52.8	—	51.8	49.4	55.5	51.2
Calf	36.7	35.4	35.9	36.5	35.0	34.1	34.3
Upper arm	30.1	31.3	30.9	31.8[a] 29.1[b]	26.3	29.6	28.6[a] 27.6[b]

[a] Flexed arm
[b] Relaxed arm

References

1. Average data for young adults (Sidney, 1976)
2. Párizková & Eiselt (1966)
3. Damon *et al.* (1972)
4. Sidney & Shephard (unpublished data)
5. Young *et al.* (1963)

Bone Loss

Senescence is associated with a progressive loss of both minerals and matrix from the bones of the body. Some authors have distinguished osteomalacia (where there is a pathological deficiency of calcification but a normal matrix) and osteoporosis (where the amount of bone is reduced but its characteristics are unchanged). However, the distinction between aging and pathological change is far from clear-cut. Often, osteoporosis is proclaimed as pathological on the day a fracture is incurred, but from the viewpoint of the patient it would have been more useful to learn this fact several days previously!

The phenomenon of bone loss was first described in sawn sections of long bones studied at post-mortem (Minot, 1908). It has subsequently been confirmed by a wide variety of techniques, including the weighing and ashing of dry, defatted skeletons (Trotter & Peterson, 1955), density determinations on cubes cut from the vertebrae of cadavers (Arnold, 1960), caliper measurements of bone shadows on radiographs (Garn, 1975), estimates of the density of radiographic bone shadows (Gershon-Cohen *et al.*, 1955), absorption of photons emitted from a low energy source such as ^{125}iodine (Sorenson & Cameron, 1967), and neutron activation (Sidney *et al.*, 1977). Substance is lost from the interior of the bone, but at the same time smaller quantities of new bone may be laid down exteriorly.

Garn (1975) studied the phenomenon extensively in terms of the cortical (D) and medullary (d) widths at the mid-shaft of the second metacarpal. Cortical thickness $(D - d)$ began to decrease at about 35 years of age (Figure 3.1), and the cumulative loss among those surviving to 90 years was about 20 per cent in men and 30 per cent in women. Curves were similar for most racial groups except US negro women,

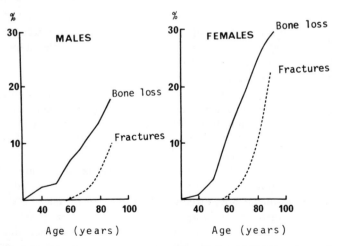

Figure 3.1   Relationship between bone loss (USA, 1968-70) and cumulative probability of bone fracture (Malmo, Sweden, 1951-60) (after Garn, 1975).

who lost less bone than their 'white' counterparts; however, there were substantial inter-individual differences, and some 80-year-old people still had more bone than others aged thirty.

The metacarpal data seems surprisingly representative of changes in other parts of the body. We have used the neutron activation method (McNeill *et al.*, 1973, 1978) to measure bone calcium from the shoulder to the middle of the thigh. An appropriate small dose of irradiation (0.4 r.e.m.) converts normal ^{48}calcium to ^{49}calcium with a half-life of nine minutes. During the decay process, gamma rays are emitted and detected by a whole-body counter. Our results for 65-year-old subjects show an 8.8 per cent loss in men and a 13.8 per cent loss in women relative to young and middle-aged subjects (Sidney *et al.*, 1977). These figures are very comparable with the results reported by Garn (1975). Further confirmation of the generality of the findings is provided by measurements of vertebral density (Arnold *et al.*, 1966) and by photon absorption data (Smith, 1971; Mazess & Cameron, 1973).

At present, there is no completely satisfactory explanation of why the bone loss occurs. Extreme protein deprivation, calcium lack, and an adverse calcium/phosphorus ratio could all theoretically cause the phenomenon, but the average senior citizen does not suffer the required degree of malnutrition; measurements of serum calcium, inorganic phosphate and alkaline phosphatase are all typically within normal limits (Exton-Smith, 1973). The sex difference might suggest an hormonal influence such as oestrogen withdrawal or androgen lack, and in support of this view osteoporosis is marked in ovarian agenesis and eunuchoid males, while osteoblast activity can be stimulated by administration of oestrogens (Timiras, 1972). However, if lack of sex hormones can be blamed, it is puzzling that the bone loss commences so far before the menopause. A third possible contributing factor is the low level of habitual activity in the elderly. Bone loss is well-recognised as a complication of bed rest (Rodahl *et al.*, 1967), immobilisation of a limb, or the loss of normal gravitational stimuli due to space travel (Sawin *et al.*, 1975). Appropriate forms of exercise can also protect the astronaut against this hazard (Sawin *et al.*, 1975). It is less certain the smaller reductions of activity associated with aging can influence bone structure. Montoye (1975) made questionnaire estimates of daily activity in the US community of Tecumseh; unfortunately, few of this population were really active, but nevertheless he found no relationship between his indices of activity and radiographic estimates of bone loss.

The potential contribution of bone loss to vertebral collapse and senile kyphosis has been noted. The other serious functional consequence is an increased risk of bone fracture. Garn (1975) related the reduction of cortical thickness in his US population with the cumulative probability of sustaining a fracture as established some years earlier for the Swedish community of Malmo (Figure 3.1). The two curves ran roughly parallel, with a time lag of some ten years from the commencement of bone loss to the corresponding appearance of fractures.

Cardio-Respiratory Function

The sustained physical performance of the young adult depends upon the rate at which oxygen can be moved from the atmosphere to the working tissues, the maximum oxygen intake (Shephard, 1977d). The maximum arterio-venous oxygen difference of the elderly is smaller than that of a young adult (Niinimaa & Shephard, 1978). Nevertheless, peripheral oxygen extraction remains relatively complete, and it is plain that cardio-respiratory function rather than the activity of cellular and sub-cellular mechanisms still limits sustained energy usage.

Cardiac output is by far the most important single determinant of oxygen transport in the young adult (Shephard, 1977d). However, in an older individual it is necessary to consider possible additional limitations imposed by pulmonary function, the interaction of pulmonary blood flow with ventilation and diffusion, and the peripheral distribution of blood flow. We shall also look at the resultant of these various factors, in terms of the maximum oxygen intake that is actually achieved.

Lung Function

1. Anatomical changes Aging is associated with several anatomical changes that have adverse mechanical consequences for the chest wall and lungs (Richards, 1965; Mithoefer & Karetzky, 1968; Freeman, 1973). The work required to modify thoracic volume is increased by kyphosis (Edge *et al.*, 1964), a flattening or a barrel deformity of the rib cage, and stiffening or even ankylosis of the joints about which the ribs rotate. At the same time there is a wasting of the respiratory muscles.

Microscopic observations show a thinning of the alveolar wall and a reduction in the number of pulmonary capillaries (Reid, 1967). The alveoli and the alveolar ducts are also enlarged and there is an increase in the number of window-like communications between adjacent alveoli. The number and thickness of the radial elastic fibres that maintain the patency of the small airways is reduced, but the dimensions of the larger air passages remain unaltered. The pulmonary arteries and venules are marked by increasing intimal fibrosis (Wagenvoort & Wagenvoort, 1965), while the walls of the smaller vessels show collagen deposition and hyalinisation (Simons & Reid, 1969).

2. *Pulmonary gas volumes*   The loss of elastic tissue leads to an increase of residual gas volume and a roughly parallel decrease of vital capacity, without much change of total lung capacity (Table 3.5). The extent of such changes varies substantially from one study to another, depending on both the method of sample selection and the cumulative insults to which the subjects' lungs have been exposed. Some authors have been content to examine patients hospitalised for non-respiratory disease; Niinimaa & Shephard (1978) found much less functional loss with aging, since their subjects were healthy volunteers for an exercise class, most of whom were non-smokers.

We have already noted (Chapter 1) the large influence of a history of previous respiratory disease upon the results of simple spirometry. Exposure to cigarette smoke and air pollutants are also variables of possible importance. Anderson *et al.* (1968) noted a correlation between smoking habits and vital capacity ($P < 0.05$), but the addition of a 'smoking' term did not improve the prediction of vital capacity if the multiple regression equation already made allowance for a history of respiratory disease. Others (for example Wilson *et al.*, 1960) have shown large differences of vital capacity between smokers and non-smokers, but have not tested how far such differences are attributable to that segment of the smokers who develop chronic obstructive lung disease.

Most large series of lung function data are cross-sectional in type and include both smokers and non-smokers. Shephard (1978) collected age regression coefficients for many world populations. In six series of urban men, the average loss of vital capacity was 24.4 ml/yr, while in thirteen assorted ethnic groups it was 25.4 ml/yr. Mainly because of their smaller body size, the women showed a lesser loss, 18.3 ml/yr in five studies from developed countries, and 12.7 ml/yr in three groups living under less 'privileged' conditions. Several authors have used their data to develop 'prediction equations'; in terms of the actual status of healthy non-smoking senior citizens, those proposed by Anderson *et al.* (1968) seem to give the most

Table 3.5 Pulmonary gas volumes. Comparison of reported data for elderly subjects with (a) typical values for a healthy 25-year-old of comparable size, and (b) values predicted from published multiple regression equations for 65-year-old subjects of specified height and weight

Variable	Men							Women				
	Typical 25 years	1	2	3	4	5	6	Typical 25 years	1	2	4	6
Sample size	25	9	11	29	18	8	10		10	15	20	8
Age (yrs)	25	64.4	61.5	63.2	65.0	64.0	64.2	25	66.8	60.4	64.0	64.6
Height (cm)	175	175.4	169	172	174.3	–	172	162	162.2	157	163.9	159.0
Weight (kg)	72	71.7	65.9	78	71.8	–	67	60	60.3	66.8	68.0	61.5
Vital capacity (l)[a]	5.05	4.44	3.48	4.32	4.30	3.43	3.28	3.35	2.86	2.34	2.90	2.34
Functional residual capacity (l)[a]	2.30	3.33	3.44	2.52	3.50	–	3.56	2.40	2.26	2.22	2.32	2.34
Expiratory reserve volume (l)[a]	0.60	1.31	1.01	0.77	–	0.46	–	0.85	0.76	0.44	–	–
Residual volume (l)[a]	1.70	2.02	2.43	1.75	2.46	1.58	2.70	1.55	1.51	1.78	1.81	1.82
Total lung capacity (l)[a]	6.70	6.45	5.92	6.07	6.50	5.01	5.97	5.25	4.36	4.14	4.56	4.00
Residual volume/ total lung capacity (%)	25.3	31.3	40.9	28.1	37.8	–	–	29.5	34.3	41.9	39.5	–

[a] All volumes expressed at body temperature and pressure, saturated with water vapour (BTPS)

References

1. Niinimaa & Shephard (1978)
2. Greifenstein *et al.* (1952)
3. Boren *et al.* (1966)
4. Ericsson & Irnell (1969a, b)
5. Kaltreider *et al.* (1938)
6. Needham *et al.* (1954)

Prediction equation values for vital capacity: Anderson *et al.* (1968) 4.34, 2.84 l BTPS; Miller *et al.* (1959) 3.96, 3.03 l BTPS; Schmidt *et al.* (1973) 3.90, 2.38 l BTPS.

realistic answers (Table 3.5). One problem with the majority of prediction formulae is that they assume aging to proceed in a linear fashion. Longitudinal data (Cole, 1974) do not altogether support this idea, and it seems likely that the functional loss accelerates beyond the age of 65.

The increase of residual gas volume and functional residual capacity probably has little consequence for steady gas exchange. It has the advantage of reducing oscillations in alveolar gas composition over the breathing cycle, but it slows the rate of increase of alveolar oxygen concentration when the exercise load is suddenly increased.

A young person finds difficulty in using more than 50 per cent of his vital capacity during maximum effort, and on occasion this ceiling may be reached. The loss of vital capacity with senescence thus reduces the potential tidal volume that can be developed during vigorous activity.

3. Pulmonary dynamics   The loss of elastic tissue and the partial breakdown of alveolar structure inevitably has marked effects upon pulmonary dynamics. While the resistance of the major airways may show little change (Frank *et al.*, 1957), the smaller air passages become more liable to collapse during expiration. There is thus a greater likelihood that a person who is exercising will reach the effort-independent portion of his expiratory flow/volume curve (Hyatt, 1972), where added expiratory force increases collapse of the small airways rather than promoting airflow. This situation is reflected by a progressive decrease in various indices of dynamic function such as the maximum voluntary ventilation, the peak expiratory flow rate, the maximum mid-expiratory flow rate, and the one-second forced expiratory volume. Data for the one-second forced expiratory volume, for example, show a faster relative deterioration than the forced vital capacity (Table 3.6), so that the proportion of the vital capacity expelled in one second drops from about 82 per cent to the mid-seventies in men, and from about 86 per cent to the high seventies in women. As with vital capacity, the rate of functional deterioration depends partly on the type of sample selected, and on any history of smoking and respiratory infection. Nevertheless, non-smokers living in an area with little air pollution still show an annual loss of $FEV_{1.0}$ amounting to about 32 ml in men and 25 ml in women (Morris *et al.*, 1971). The loss of ability to make rapid expirations compounds the ventilatory problem posed by the diminution of vital capacity, but nevertheless a healthy 65-year-old person still has a fair ventilatory reserve. If dyspnoea arises at 50 per cent of $FEV_{1.0}$, and a respiratory rate of 50 breaths/min can be developed, shortness of breath will be noted at a ventilation of about 75 l/min BTPS (62.5 l/min STPD) in men and 50 l/min BTPS (47.7 l/min STPD) in women.

Table 3.6   Forced expiratory volumes of elderly subjects. Comparison with typical values for healthy young adults

Height (cm)	Males $FEV_{1.0}$ (l BTPS)	$FEV_{1.0}/FVC$ (%)	Height (cm	Females $FEV_{1.0}$ (l BTPS)	$FEV_{1.0}/FVC$ (%)	Reference
175	4.15	82	162	2.88	86	Typical 25 yr old
174	2.50	72.2	160	1.97	79.1	1
—	—	—	—	1.95	74.3	2
173	2.96	75.7	158	1.93	74.4	3
171	3.00[a]	71.4	158	2.00[a]	76.9	4/5
173	3.21[b]	80.3[b]	161	2.59[b]	80.5[b]	6
172	2.91	73.7	—	—	—	7
175	2.97	71.4	160	2.25	79.8	8
—	2.18	68.6	—	1.63	80.5	9

[a] Volume measured at atmospheric temperature — about 6 per cent larger under BTPS conditions

[b] Subjects 50-59 rather than 60-69 years old

References

1. Sidney & Shephard, unpublished data
2. Brown & Shephard (1967)
3. Schmidt *et al.* (1973)
4. Berglund *et al.* (1963)
5. Birath *et al.* (1963)
6. Miller *et al.* (1959)
7. Schlesinger *et al.* (1973)
8. Ericsson & Irnell (1969a,b)
9. Matarazzo *et al.* (1961)

A related consequence of the loss of elastic tissue is an increase in the lung volume at which airway collapse becomes inevitable (the 'closing volume', Anthonisen *et al.*, 1969/70). By the age of 65, at least a quarter of the vital capacity range is affected by airway closure, mainly in the dependent parts of the lung (LeBlanc *et al.*, 1970):

| Closing volume (% of vital capacity) | | Author |
Men	Women	
24.5	29.2	Niinimaa & Shephard (1978)
23.0	23.0	Buist & Ross (1973)
24.9	26.6	Begin *et al.* (1975)

Partly because of airway closure, gas distribution is less uniform in the elderly than in younger subjects; thus Cohn & Donoso (1963) found the single breath nitrogen index to increase from 1.34 per cent at 33 to 2.3 per cent at 66 years. Fortunately, exercise is associated with an increase of mean lung volume. In maximum effort, typical usage is from 40 to 90 per cent of vital capacity, and most individuals no longer operate over that part of the vital capacity range where airway closure is likely. Laboratory studies (Edelman *et al.*, 1968) have confirmed that deep breathing corrects the non-uniformity of gas distribution.

The compliance of the lungs (the change of volume per unit of applied pressure) increases as elastic tissue is lost, more consistently in men (Cohn & Donoso, 1963) than in women (Frank *et al.*, 1957). A reduction in the elastic work of breathing might be anticipated, but in practice any benefit from this source is counteracted by an increase in the rigidity of the chest wall (Turner *et al.*, 1968). Because of stiffness in the rib cage, an increased proportion of respiration is undertaken by diaphragmatic movement (Rizzato & Marrazini, 1970).

During exhausting work, a young person may divert 5 to 10 per cent of his maximum oxygen intake to the respiratory muscles (Shephard, 1966b). Given that there is little change of elastic work with aging, but that there is some increase of airflow resistance in the small airways together with an increased resistance in the rib cage, it is inevitable that an older person will have a higher respiratory work-load for a given external effort. In severe emphysema, the oxygen cost of breathing may be 10 to 20 times greater than in a young person, and even in a healthy elderly subject a substantial part of the diminishing maximum oxygen intake is consumed in respiratory work.

4. External ventilation   The resting respiratory minute volume, and its components (tidal volume and respiratory rate) remain unchanged with advancing age (Norris *et al.*, 1956, 1963; Shock, 1961; Fischer *et al.*, 1965; Mithoefer & Karetzky, 1968; Hollmann *et al.*, 1970; Rose *et al.*, 1970). However, the ventilation associated with performance of a given external task increases progressively with age. This is partly a question of reduced mechanical efficiency. Joint stiffness, poor motor co-ordination and lack of recent familiarity with most types of laboratory exercise all increase the oxygen cost of effort. Thus, bicycle ergometer work has an efficiency of 21.5 per cent compared with 23 per cent in a healthy young adult (Sidney & Shephard, 1977). Ventilation must also be augmented to allow for any increase of physiological dead space. Lastly, a poor peripheral circulation and a sluggish response of the heart to effort lead to a greater accumulation of lactic acid in sub-maximum work, with resultant hyperventilation (see section on integration of cardio-respiratory responses).

Nevertheless, the aged lung functions quite well under the stress of moderate exercise (Robinson, 1938; Greifenstein *et al.*, 1952; Richards, 1965; Mithoefer & Karetzky, 1968). One commonly used index is the ventilatory equivalent, the number of litres of ventilation required to transport a litre of oxygen. Sidney & Shephard (1977) found relatively normal values for treadmill effort (25.2 l per l in men and 27.4 l per l in women), but there was some increase in the ventilatory cost of bicycle ergometer work (34.0 l per l in the men and 33.9 l per l in the women). This reflects difficulty in perfusing the quadriceps muscles of elderly subjects during vigorous effort (see section on tissue oxygen extraction).

Men Ventilation l/min STPD	Author	Women Ventilation l/min STPD	Author
67.3[a]	Robinson (1938)	57.9[a,b]	I Åstrand (1960)
42.0	Fischer *et al.* (1965)	34.5[c]	Julius *et al.* (1967)
58.3[a]	Benestad (1965)	46.2	Sidney & Shephard
66.5[a]	I Åstrand (1960)		(1977)
58.9[a]	Adams *et al.* (1972)		
72.5	I Åstrand *et al.* (1959)		
73.8	Sidney & Shephard (1977a)		
62.7	Average, men	47.3	Average, women

[a] Data converted from BTPS reading assuming 1 l/min STPD = 1.2 l/min BTPS
[b] Only three subjects over 60 years
[c] Mixture of male and female subjects

When the treadmill data are plotted to show the relationship
between ventilation and oxygen consumption expressed as a percentage
of maximum oxygen intake, the form of the curves is similar in young
and in elderly subjects (Figure 3.2), although there is a slight suggestion
that the breakpoint where lactate begins to accumulate is displaced
towards the left in the older groups.

5. Alveolar ventilation   Most authors agree there is some increase of
the respiratory dead space with aging. The characteristic dimensions
of the larger airways may be increased due to a greater mean expansion
of the chest, but the main responsibility for the enlarged dead space
lies in the finer structure of the lungs. Expansion of the alveolar ducts
and alveoli leads to a less complete diffusional mixing between inspired
and alveolar gas. Airway closure and patchy bronchial disease cause
impaired ventilation of some alveoli, and a reduction of the pulmonary
capillary bed leaves a larger number of the alveolar spaces poorly
perfused. There is thus a decrease in the number of alveolar units with
a normal ventilation/perfusion ratio, and an increase of units that are
over-ventilated relative to their perfusion. The physiological dead space
takes account not only of the size of the airways, but also of their
effectiveness from the viewpoint of gas exchange; under resting

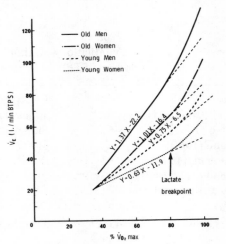

Figure 3.2   Relationship between minute expired volume ($\dot{V}_E$) and percentage of
aerobic power (% $\dot{V}_{O_2}$max) during progressive (5 min/grade) treadmill walking in
elderly persons. Comparison with young adults. Unpublished data, Sidney &
Shephard.

conditions, dead space increases by about 1 ml per year of adult life (Cotes, 1965). Vigorous exercise leads to a substantial increase of pulmonary arterial pressure in the elderly (Emirgil *et al.*, 1967), and this tends to improve the matching of perfusion with ventilation. However, missing pulmonary capillaries are not replaced, and even during exercise alveolar ventilation thus remains a smaller fraction of external ventilation than in a young subject — perhaps 70 per cent rather than 75 or 80 per cent of the respiratory minute volume.

Taking into account the fact that it is the STPD ventilation (standard temperature and pressure, dry gas) which is important from the viewpoint of oxygen exchange, we may conclude that alveolar ventilation reaches a maximum value of about 44 l/min in a 65-year-old man, and 29 l/min in a woman of the same age.

Interactions with Pulmonary Blood Flow

In the young adult, there is virtually no gradient of oxygen pressure between alveolar gas and blood leaving the lungs, showing that the pulmonary diffusing capacity and its interactions with ventilation and blood flow offer no appreciable barriers to oxygen transport (Shephard, 1977d). The pulmonary diffusing capacity falls with aging, due to poorer gas mixing, a decrease in the proportion of the alveolar surface covered by capillaries and a decrease of the capillary blood volume. Data obtained by Niinimaa & Shephard (1978) are for 65-year-old adults:

	Men			Women		
Oxygen intake (l/min STPD)	0.30	0.93	1.44	0.25	0.73	1.01
Diffusing capacity (mM/min/kPa)	3.8	7.6	12.5	2.8	5.7	9.1

Each of the new standard international units (mM/min/kPa) is equal to approximately three of the traditional units (ml/min/mm Hg). The resting values are smaller than reported by Sundström (1975), but in line with a larger sample studied by Turino *et al.* (1959). They could be explained if the pulmonary diffusing capacity decreased by 0.07 to 0.08 mM/min/kPa annually between the ages of 25 and 65 years (Donevan *et al.*, 1955; Ogilvie *et al.*, 1957; Anderson & Shephard, 1968a,b).

As in younger subjects, Niinimaa & Shephard (1978) did not find a plateau of pulmonary diffusing capacity over the range of oxygen intakes examined. Nevertheless, heart rates exceeded the range where Patsch (1973) had previously reported a plateau of diffusing capacity, and there seems some doubt whether the latter author stressed his subjects sufficiently to realise their physiological potential. Our exercise data, as reported above, agrees quite well with the findings of Hanson & Tabakin (1960) and Turino *et al.* (1959) for elderly subjects. In young adults, the pulmonary diffusing capacity increases by about 4 mM/min/kPa for each litre/min increase of oxygen intake. The slope of the relationship is almost twice as steep in the 65-year-old age group, presumably because exercise helps to correct both uneven ventilation and a poor distribution of blood flow.

There is some widening of the alveolar-arterial oxygen pressure gradient with aging (Tenney & Miller, 1956; Cotes, 1965), and the resting arterial oxygen saturation drops from about 97 per cent to around 94 per cent. However, it is difficult to distinguish the relative contributions of a poor pulmonary diffusing capacity and an increased admixture of venous blood to the drop in arterial oxygen content. Assuming that the diffusing capacity continues to increase in linear fashion to maximum oxygen intake, the maximum diffusing capacity would have been 18.7 mM/min/kPa for the men and 13.8 mM/min/kPa for the women of Niinimaa & Shephard's study, almost as great as the

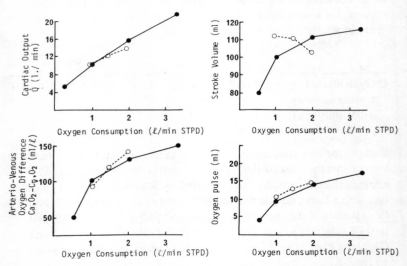

Figure 3.3 Cardiac response to exercise in the elderly subject - comparison of values for 65-year-old men o —o (Niinimaa & Shephard, 1978) and typical values for sedentary young men • —•.

value anticipated in young adults. There thus seems no reason to suppose that the lung is offering a major barrier to gas exchange in the healthy older adult.

Table 3.7   Resting heart rate and blood pressure of elderly subjects

Heart rate	Systolic blood pressure		Diastolic pressure		Reference
(min)	(mm Hg)	(kPa)	(mm Hg)	(kPa)	
MEN					
79	136	18.1	82	10.9	Cumming *et al.* (1972)
–	143	19.1	83	11.1	Master *et al.* (1958)
–	153	20.4	86	11.5	Anderson & Cowan (1972)
70	–	–	–	–	Fischer *et al.* (1965)
71	135	18.0	–	–	Asmussen & Mathiasen (1962)[a]
76	126	16.8	–	–	DeVries & Adams (1972a)
68	143[b]	18.6[b]	83[b]	11.1[b]	Adams *et al.* (1972)
77	–	–	–	–	Granath *et al.* (1961)
73.1	139	18.6	83.5	11.1	Average – elderly subjects
72.6	120	16.0	71	9.5	Sidney (1976) – young normals
WOMEN					
75	131	17.5	76	10.1	Adams & DeVries (1973)
73	137	18.3	79	10.5	Brown & Shephard (1967)
–	154	20.5	85	11.3	Anderson & Cowan (1972)
74	130	17.3	–	–	Asmussen & Mathiasen (1962)[a]
74	142	19.0	81.5	10.9	Average – elderly subjects
77.3	119	15.9	74	9.9	Sidney (1976) – young normals

[a] Former physical education students
[b] Data obtained with subjects supine

Cardiac Output

Aging has a number of adverse effects upon cardiac performance both at rest and in sub-maximum and maximum work (Figure 3.3, Tables 3.7-3.10). In particular, there are decreases of peak heart rate, maximum stroke volume, cardiac contractility and maximum arterio-venous oxygen difference.

1. Heart rate   The resting heart rate changes but little with age
(Table 12, Robinson, 1938; Granath *et al.*, 1961; Strandell, 1964d;
Fischer *et al.*, 1965; Hollmann *et al.*, 1970; W.F. Anderson & Cowan,
1972).

Equally, during sub-maximal work the relationship between heart
rate and oxygen consumption is much as found in younger subjects of
comparable fitness (Figure 3.3, Tables 3.8, 3.9; I. Åstrand, 1960;
Rode & Shephard, 1971). This finding is reflected in the constancy of
such indices as the oxygen pulse (oxygen consumption/heart rate,
Table 3.9) and the heart rate at a fixed oxygen consumption
($f_{h,1.0}$: the heart rate at an oxygen consumption of 1 l/min, 22.4
mM/min).*

Some early reports indicated quite a steep decline of maximum
heart rate, from the young adult value of about 195/min to 155-160/
min at the age of 65 years (Robinson, 1938; Asmussen & Molbech,
1959; I. Åstrand, 1960). Thus, one easily remembered formula
estimated the maximum heart rate as 220 minus the individual's age
in years. More recent investigations have shown substantially higher
heart rates in the elderly. Lester *et al.* (1968) found an average of
177/min at age 65, and the men studied by Sidney & Shephard
(ages 60 to 83 years) also reached a maximum averaging 170/min.
It is still unclear how far the lower heart rates of the earlier series
were due to a high level of fitness in the subjects examined, and how
far they reflect a less complete stressing of the cardio-respiratory
system.

The reasons underlying the decline of maximum heart rate with age
have yet to be resolved. Since a similar response is observed at high
altitudes, it is tempting to blame the change on myocardial oxygen
lack. Pathological impairment of blood flow to the cardiac pacemaker
can indeed lead to a slow heart rate in maximum exercise (the 'sick
sinus' syndrome), but the phenomenon is by no means common even
in patients with severe coronary arterial disease. A strong argument
against a 'hypoxic' explanation is that the slow heart rate of the average
older person cannot be increased to a youthful level by the administration of oxygen during vigorous work. Greater stiffness (a reduced
compliance) of the heart wall is a second possibility; this could increase the time required for filling of the ventricles, and modify the
'feedback' of information on venous filling to the cardio-regulatory

---

*   From the viewpoint of oxygen conductance (Shephard, 1977d), it remains
convenient to consider the oxygen consumption as litres of gas measured
under standard conditions of temperature and pressure dry gas (STPD).

Table 3.8 Effects of aging upon the cardio-respiratory response to
sub-maximal levels of work (based largely on data collected by Sidney,
1976): ↑ increase ↓ decrease →no change

Variable	Direction of change with age	Reference (numbers refer to bibliography)
Oxygen consumption[a]	→	7, 23, 58, 65, 91, 277, 304, 426, 427, 440, 468, 482, 521, 826, 997, 1026
	↑	8, 54, 61, 304, 415, 427, 446, 723, 736, 935, 1081, 1082, 1084
	↓	468
Heart rate	→	8, 23, 53, 65, 91, 238, 256, 277, 283, 416, 427, 468, 482, 521, 689, 723, 826, 866, 935, 993, 997, 1026
	↑	52, 61, 304
	↓	91, 135, 231, 277
Cardiac output	↓	143, 415, 416, 440, 521, 561, 723
	↑	91, 440
External ventilation	→	8, 54, 231, 521
	↑	100, 256, 278, 304, 446, 482, 736, 935, 1026, 1084
Systolic blood pressure	↑	56, 65, 161, 277, 415, 416, 440, 482, 582, 735, 811, 894, 993, 935, 993
Arterial blood lactic acid conc.	↑	53, 256, 426, 624, 826, 866, 997

[a] Since there is little change of basal metabolism with aging (20, 246, 349, 482, 825), any increase of oxygen consumption implies a decrease of mechanical efficiency

Table 3.9 Cardiovascular response to exercise in elderly subjects

Age (yrs)	N	Heart rate (/min)	Oxygen cons. (l/min)	Cardiac output (l/min)	Stroke volume (ml)	Oxygen pulse (ml)	Art-venous ox. diff. (ml/l)	Reference
MEN								
40-49	25	108	1.11	13.5	126	10.3	9.1	Hanson et al. (1968a)
		121	1.56	15.1	125	12.9	10.3	
		151	2.07	18.9	126	13.7	10.9	
51	9	171	3.56	26.8	158	10.7	13.3	Grimby et al. (1966) – active ex-athletes
47	13	182	2.68	18.7	103	14.7	14.4	Hartley et al. (1969)
70	8	126				9.7		Barry et al. (1966) – includes three women
63	7	96	0.87	12.8	140	9.9	7.1	Becklake et al. (1965)
	5	122	1.42	15.8	131	12.6	9.6	
	3	156	1.83	20.6	133	12.1	9.1	
64	8	92	0.95	10.2	113	10.6	9.4	Niinimaa & Shephard (1978)
		111	1.43	12.2	110	12.9	11.9	
		137	1.97	14.1	103	14.4	14.1	
WOMEN								
64	6	110	0.75	9.6	90	11.2	8.0	Becklake et al. (1965)
	5	133	1.20	14.1	109	9.5	8.7	
55	4	110	0.90	7.0	65	8.2	13.0	Kilböm & Åstrand (1971)
		137	1.18	8.4	63	8.6	14.1	
		155	1.56	10.3	66	10.1	15.3	
67	7	103	0.80	9.4	91	8.2	8.7	Niinimaa & Shephard (1978)
		115	1.00	10.2	91	8.8	9.9	
		136	1.28	11.7	87	9.6	11.2	

Table 3.10   Anaemia in the elderly — reports collected by Hyams (1973), based on hospital surveys

Number of subjects	Criterion (g Hb/100 ml)	Percentage of sample anaemic	Authors
7,916	< 10.4	17.5	Monroe (1951)
156	< 11.7	41	Bedford & Wollner (1958)
319	< 11.9	37	Lawson (1960)
400	< 12	32	Davison (1967)
100	< 11.7	33	Batata *et al.* (1967)
?	< 12	22	W.F. Anderson (1967)
333	< 11.7	29	Powell *et al.* (1968)
2,700	< 10	6.4	Evans *et al.* (1968)
500F	< 11.7	16	Griffiths *et al.* (1970)
229	< 11	21	Bose *et al.* (1970)
1,367	< 12	33	DHSS (1970)

centres of the medulla. Lastly, the sympathetic drive to the cardiac pacemaker may diminish with age.

2. Stroke volume   Except in extreme old age, the heart volume is well maintained — indeed, in some instances it is even increased (Strandell, 1964a; Durusoy *et al.*, 1968; P.O. Åstrand, 1968; C.T.M. Davies, 1972). Nevertheless, the resting stroke volume is diminished (Brandfonbrener *et al.*, 1955; Granath *et al.*, 1961, 1964; Strandell, 1964a).

In many young subjects, the stroke volume increases progressively with work load, until maximum effort is attained. It is rare to find an appreciable decrease of stroke volume as the external work is augmented. Depending upon the fitness of the subject and the type of work performed, a maximum stroke volume as large as 150 ml may be realised. In sedentary subjects, values are 20 to 30 ml smaller, and figures are also 10 to 15 ml lower on the bicycle ergometer than on the treadmill (Shephard, 1977d). Elderly subjects develop almost the same stroke volume (110-120 ml) at light work loads, but as the effort is increased the stroke output diminishes (Granath *et al.*, 1964; Becklake *et al.*, 1965; Grimby *et al.*, 1966; Hanson *et al.*, 1968a; Niinimaa & Shephard, 1978). During exhausting work, the stroke volume is thus 10 to 20 per cent smaller than in a young adult (Simonson, 1957; Strandell, 1964a; Grimby & Saltin, 1966; P.O. Åstrand, 1968; Kilböm,

& Åstrand, 1971). This may reflect poorer myocardial perfusion, lesser cardiac compliance or poorer contractility.

3. Cardiac contractility   The force exerted by the left ventricle is such that little perfusion of its wall is possible during the contraction phase of the cardiac cycle. The coronary blood flow to the left side of the heart thus depends on the duration of systole. The contractility of the heart may influence both the duration of systole and the volume of blood that is expelled from the ventricle.

Because of practical difficulties in making more direct measurements, the timing of the cardiac cycle is commonly deduced from simultaneous recordings of the electrocardiogram, heart sounds (phonocardiogram) and the carotid pulse wave (Blumberger & Sigisbert, 1959; Raab, 1966). Measurements include the total period of ventricular systole (from the Q wave of the electrocardiogram to the second heart sound, QS_2), the ejection period (from the beginning of the carotid pulse wave to its dicrotic notch, LVET) and the pre-ejection period (PEP = QS_2 − LVET). Data can be expressed directly in milliseconds, but since the results then vary with heart rate, there is some virtue in calculating an index that allows for heart rate-related changes of contractility (Montoye *et al.*, 1971).

The resting pre-ejection period increases from about 80 msec at age 25 to 95-100 msec in a 65-year-old person (Gabbato & Media, 1956; Harrison *et al.*, 1964; Montoye *et al.*, 1971). According to Montoye *et al.* (1971), an age difference of at least 10 per cent persists even when the PEP is corrected for heart rate. The LVET is essentially independent of age, so that a small increase of QS_2 is observed as a subject becomes older (Montoye *et al.*, 1971, but not Lombard & Cope, 1926).

Interpretation of the changes in PEP is complicated, since the duration of this phase of the cardiac cycle reflects both electrical and mechanical events within the ventricle. There have been suggestions (Raab, 1966, but not Montoye, 1975) that a high level of physical activity lengthens the pre-ejection period. If so, this would presumably be attributable to a decrease of resting sympathetic tone and there would be a greater potential for increase of contractility. The age-related lengthening of the PEP is more likely to be due to a mechanical slowing of tension development in the cardiac muscle fibres (Albert *et al.*, 1967) and a general loss of co-ordination of the contractile process (Starr, 1964); one contributing factor is a diminution in the ATP^{ase} activity of the myofibrils (Albert *et al.*, 1967). Unfortunately, it is difficult to measure the carotid pulse wave accurately during effort. However, it seems unlikely that the effects of age upon the rate of muscle contraction can be reversed by exercise.

4. Cardiac output   Cardiac output is given by the product of stroke volume and heart rate. During rest, an unchanged heart rate (Table 3.7) and a reduced stroke volume inevitably give the older person a low cardiac output (Brandfonbrener *et al.*, 1955; Granath *et al.*, 1961, 1964; Shock, 1964; Strandell, 1964a; Kilböm, 1971; Toscani, 1971). The decrease from young adult values is substantially larger than could be explained by any associated decreases of resting metabolism (Chapter 2).

Remarkably few measurements of exercise cardiac output have been reported for elderly subjects (Table 3.9). Becklake *et al.* (1965) studied a group of men and women aged over 60 years, and Kilböm & Åstrand (1971) examined some 55-year-old women. Most of the remaining information is for the middle aged rather than the elderly — Hanson *et al.* (1968a) studied 40- to 49-year-old men, Hartley *et al.* tested 47-year-old men, Grimby *et al.* (1966) examined athletes aged 45-55 years, and Barry *et al.* (1966) recorded some oxygen pulses in elderly subjects.

The cardiac outputs of the men tested by Niinimaa & Shephard (1978) are 2 to 4 l/min lower than those reported by Becklake *et al.* (1965) and Hanson *et al.* (1968a). In the case of Becklake *et al.* (1965), a systematic error in their nitrous oxide method of measuring cardiac output may have been responsible, while the subjects tested by Hanson *et al.* (1968a) were substantially younger than our sample. The values for female subjects obtained by Niinimaa & Shephard (1978) seem fairly representative, lying between those obtained by Kilböm & Åstrand (1971) and Becklake *et al.* (1965).

During light exercise, neither stroke volume nor heart rate are greatly affected by age. A 65-year-old person thus develops almost the same cardiac output as a young adult who is working at a comparable rate. However, the elderly reach their peak cardiac output at a substantially lower work load (Figure 3.3). The maximum cardiac output of a 65-year-old is typically 17 to 20 l/min (100 to 120 ml $\times$ 170/min), some 20 to 30 per cent less than in a young adult.

5. Arterio-venous oxygen difference   The oxygen transport accomplished by a given cardiac output depends on the magnitude of the arterio-venous oxygen difference. At rest and at any given sub-maximum effort, the arterio-venous oxygen difference is greater in the elderly than in young adults (Granath *et al.*, 1964; Strandell, 1964a; Toscani, 1971; Wahren *et al.*, 1974; Niinimaa & Shephard, 1978). This reflects some decrease of stroke volume, particularly at the higher work-loads, together with a poorer mechanical efficiency of effort. Values reported by Niinimaa & Shephard (1978) were 23-50 ml/l larger than those reported by Becklake *et al.* (1965), but the latter authors used the fallible nitrous oxide method to measure their cardiac outputs. Results from our laboratory were also somewhat higher than in the series of Hanson *et al.* (1968a) and Hartley *et al.* (1969). We have already noted that the subjects tested by these latter authors were middle-aged rather than elderly; Hartley *et al.* (1969) also used a bicycle ergometer rather than a treadmill as the source of exercise. Among the data for women, Kilböm & Åstrand (1971) found quite wide arterio-venous oxygen differences, perhaps due to the use of relatively athletic subjects. Niinimaa & Shephard (1978) also obtained somewhat larger figures than those yielded by the nitrous oxide method (Becklake *et al.*, 1965).

The maximum arterio-venous oxygen difference tends to diminish with age. Contributory factors include (1) a reduction of physical fitness levels, (2) a reduction of arterial oxygen saturation, (3) a lowered haemoglobin level, (4) a poorer peripheral blood distribution, (5) a loss of activity in tissue enzyme systems, and (6) a greater relative blood flow to the skin. We will look further at several of these issues in subsequent sections. However, for the present we may note that despite these various problems, a healthy 65-year-old person can still develop an arterio-venous oxygen difference of 140-150 ml/l.

6. *Anaemia*   The oxygen carrying capacity of the blood is almost directly proportional to its haemoglobin content. Unfortunately, a number of factors predispose to the development of anaemia in an older person. Red marrow tends to be replaced by fatty marrow, particularly in the long bones. One study of elderly rats (Roylance *et al.*, 1969) observed some slowing of red cell formation relative to younger animals, but most human studies have suggested that the elderly retain their capacity to react to a challenge such as sudden haemorrhage by a rapid increase in the rate of erythropoiesis. Again, there have been reports that the red cells of older people are vulnerable to destruction in terms of their osmotic fragility (Lodenkamper & Steinen, 1954), although other investigators have found the average longevity of an erythrocyte to be much the same

as in a young person (Hurdle & Rosin, 1962; Williams *et al.*, 1962). Occasionally, gastro-intestinal atrophy may hamper the absorption of iron or vitamin B_{12}. More commonly, there may be chronic unrecognised gastro-intestinal bleeding. However, the most important reasons for a low haemoglobin level are sociological rather than medical — income is insufficient to buy adequate food, or there is a loss of interest in cooking and eating adequate meals.

Anaemia is a frequent finding among patients admitted to geriatric wards (Table 3.10). Evans (1971) noted that the frequency of severe anaemias doubled from the seventh to the ninth decades of life, and Williams *et al.* (1962) commented on a significant reduction of red cell mass, haematocrit and blood volume in patients over the age of 80 years. Nevertheless, Elwood (1971) has stressed that anaemia is not an inevitable accompaniment of aging. In two community surveys of subjects over the age of 65 years, he found average haemoglobin readings of 14.5 and 14.9 g per 100 ml in the men and 13.3 and 12.9 g per 100 ml in the women, much as would have been anticipated in young adults.

Peripheral Factors

In this section, we shall consider the influence of age upon the distribution of the available cardiac output between muscle, skin and viscera, changes in the peripheral vasculature and associated effects on blood pressure, and the efficiency of oxygen extraction within the active tissues.

1. Distribution of blood flow There have been no specific studies on the distribution of the blood flow in elderly subjects during exercise, but certain inferences can be drawn from general principles.

At least 75 per cent of the maximum cardiac output is normally directed to the active muscles (Shephard, 1968b). If the work to be performed is dispersed over a number of large muscle groups, there is no problem in accommodating the resultant blood flow. On the other hand, if the task is carried out mainly by a single relatively small muscle mass (as in bicycle ergometry, and more obviously in short-crank arm ergometry), the heart has difficulty in pumping blood through the strongly contracting muscles. Blood flow is first impeded when the active muscles exert more than 15 per cent of their maximum force (Royce, 1959), and studies with radio-isotopes suggest that during bicycle ergometry the blood flow to the quadriceps muscle plateaus at some 70 per cent of maximum oxygen intake (Clausen,

1973). The older person is at particular risk of this type of peripheral flow limitation, since (1) the heart muscle has more difficulty in developing a sufficient systolic pressure to overcome the local muscle force, and (2) weakening of skeletal muscle implies that the remaining tissue must contract at a higher percentage of its maximum voluntary force.

Under resting conditions, the skin blood flow of the elderly may be quite poor, leaving them vulnerable to chilblains and a variety of ulcers and pressure sores. However, during exercise the skin blood flow is likely to be larger than in a young person, since (1) direct conduction of body heat to the skin surface is impeded by a thick layer of subcutaneous fat, and (2) sweating is induced less readily on account of a lower level of physical fitness. Because of the low maximum cardiac output, a given increase in the absolute skin flow also produces a larger change of relative skin flow than in a young person.

The absolute blood flow requirements of the viscera are likely to be at least as great in the elderly as in a younger person. Again, because of the 20 to 30 per cent decrease of maximum cardiac output, the relative visceral flow during maximum exercise is thus at least 20 to 30 per cent larger than that of a young adult.

2. Peripheral vasculature and systemic blood pressure   It has been recognised for many years that the elasticity of the major blood vessels declines with age (Roy, 1880; Wilens, 1937). This reflects an atrophy of the elastic lamellae, with both diffuse and focal increases of collagen in the vessel walls (Hass, 1943). The aorta becomes progressively larger, as can be seen on angiography (Dotter & Steinberg, 1949) and at post-mortem (Suter, 1897). The pulse wave has a more rapid upstroke and a faster peripheral propagation (Bramwell, 1924).

The more rigid arteries accept the cardiac stroke volume less readily. There is thus an increase in the resting pulse pressure and the systolic blood pressure (Table 3.7), with much smaller changes in diastolic readings. Interestingly, the rise of blood pressures seems to cease around 65 years of age, and Master *et al.* (1958) have observed little change in subsequent decades:

Men

| Age | Syst. Pressure | | Diast. Pressure | |
(yrs)	(mm Hg)	(kPa)	(mm Hg)	(kPa)
65 – 69	143	19.1	83	11.1
85 – 89	145	19.3	79	10.5
95 – 106	145	19.3	78	10.4

Women

| Age | Syst. Pressure | | Diast. Pressure | |
(yrs)	(mm Hg)	(kPa)	(mm Hg)	(kPa)
65 – 69	154	20.5	85	11.3
85 – 89	154	20.5	82	10.9
95 – 106	149	19.9	81	10.8

As with many systems of the body, there is a reduced tolerance of change. On moving suddenly from a horizontal to a vertical position there may be a marked drop of systemic blood pressure (postural hypotension), with symptoms of dizziness, confusion, weakness and fainting. Rodstein & Zeman (1957) found a fall of 20 mm Hg (2.7 kPa) in 11 per cent of 'reasonably healthy' old people, while 4 per cent of their sample showed a fall of 40 mm Hg (5.3 kPa) or more.

Since the maximum stroke volume and cardiac output become smaller with aging, one might have anticipated a lower maximum systolic blood pressure in an old person. However, most authors are agreed that the pressure reached in maximum effort is somewhat higher than in a younger individual (Granath *et al.*, 1964; I. Åstrand, 1965b; Julius *et al.*, 1967; Kasser & Bruce, 1969; Sheffield & Roitman, 1973). Using a standard blood pressure cuff, Sidney & Shephard (unpublished data) found average maxima of 217 ± 38 mm Hg (28.9 ± 5.1 kPa) in elderly men and 206 ± 32 mm Hg (27.5 ± 4.3 kPa) in elderly women; the corresponding heart rates were 175 ± 11 and 163 ± 9. A maximum of 180 mm Hg (24.0 kPa) would be more usual in a young adult; however, because of the associated differences in heart rate and stroke volume, the amount of work performed by the heart may be no greater in the older person.

3. Tissue oxygen extraction   A proportion of elderly subjects develop frank oxygen want in their muscles during physical activity. For example, acute pain ('intermittent claudication') may occur in the calves while walking. However, this is due to arterial disease (arterio-sclerosis or thrombo-angiitis obliterans) rather than to any difficulty of oxygen extraction within the tissues.

There may be some reduction in the number of tissue capillaries with aging (Pářizková *et al.*, 1971), but because of associated wasting of the muscle fibres, the diffusion pathway from the blood vessels to the metabolic sites within the mitochondria remains relatively constant. A second reason for poorer oxygen extraction might be loss of enzyme activity in an older person. Many enzyme systems do show reduced activity, although it is unclear whether this reflects lack of physical fitness or aging *per se* (Kraus, 1971; Björntorp *et al.*, 1971).

As in a young person, the main argument against a significant peripheral limitation of oxygen consumption is the very low oxygen content of blood leaving the active muscles (Shephard, 1977d). While there have been no femoral vein cannulations, approximate figures for muscle vein oxygen content can be calculated as suggested by Shephard (1968b). Let us suppose a maximum cardiac output of 17 l/min, an arterial oxygen content of 190 ml/l, an overall arterio-venous oxygen difference of 124 ml/l, and a maximum oxygen intake of 2.10 l/min. Approximately 10 per cent of the cardiac output will be directed to the viscera, and a further 10 per cent to skin. A balance sheet may then be written as follows:

Tissue	Oxygen consumption (l/min)	Total blood flow (l/min)	Arterio-venous oxygen difference (ml/l)
Viscera	0.138	1.7	69
Skin	0.012	1.7	6
Muscle	1.959	13.6	143
Overall	2.100	17.0	124

In this example, the oxygen content of blood leaving the active muscle is 47 ml/l, corresponding to an oxygen partial pressure of about 18 mm Hg (2.4 kPa). Some of the men tested by Niinimaa & Shephard (1978) had an overall arterio-venous oxygen difference of 140-150 ml/l, and in their case the muscle arterio-venous oxygen difference must have been 160-170 ml/l. The corresponding oxygen pressure in venous blood leaving the active muscles would have been 10-12 mm Hg

(1.3-1.6 kPa). Evidently, the main oxygen pressure gradient and thus the main impedance to oxygen transport remains in the cardio-respiratory system rather than within the contracting muscles (Shephard, 1977d).

Integration of Cardio-Respiratory Responses

To this point, we have considered only steady state values of the various variables involved in gas exchange. However, a further consequence of advancing age is that a longer time is required for the heart rate, blood pressure and ventilation to attain equilibrium at any given work load (Robinson, 1938; Harris & Thomson, 1958; Shock, 1961; Skinner, 1970).

The maximum working capacity and the maximum oxygen intake decline with increasing age (see following section). Thus, for a specific intensity of effort, each element of the cardio-respiratory transport system must operate closer to its maximum value, with a diminution of reserve capacity (Simonson, 1958; Shock, 1961, 1964). One practical consequence of this is that anaerobic metabolism begins at a lower rate of working in the elderly than in a young person (Tlusty, 1969a,b; Wasserman *et al.*, 1973).

Finally, the recovery period following effort is prolonged (Robinson, 1938; Norris *et al.*, 1953, 1955; Andersen, 1959; Norris & Shock, 1960; Shock, 1961; Granath *et al.*, 1964; Wessel *et al.*, 1966, 1968; Montoye *et al.*, 1968; Tlusty, 1969b). Among other factors, this reflects a greater relative work load, an increased proportion of anaerobic metabolism, a slower heat elimination, and a lower level of physical fitness.

Resultant Maximum Oxygen Intake

A conductance theorem (Shephard, 1977d) provides a convenient method to analyse the respective effects of the several cardio-respiratory variables upon oxygen transport. Conductance is the reciprocal of resistance. The overall oxygen conductance $\dot{G}_{O_2}$ is related to the maximum oxygen intake $\dot{V}_{O_2 (max)}$ by an equation of the type:

$$\dot{V}_{O_2 (max)} = \dot{G}_{O_2} (C_{I,O_2} - C_{t,O_2})$$

where C_{I,O_2} is the concentration of oxygen in the inspired air and C_{t,O_2} is the corresponding gas phase concentration within the active tissues. The overall conductance is related to the conductance of individual series elements G_1, G_2, G_3 and G_4 as follows:

$$\frac{1}{\dot{G}} = \frac{1}{\dot{G}_1} + \frac{1}{\dot{G}_2} + \frac{1}{\dot{G}_3} + \frac{1}{\dot{G}_4}$$

The four individual elements are alveolar ventilation $\dot{V}_A$, the interaction between pulmonary diffusion and blood transport, blood transport $\lambda\dot{Q}$ (the product of the slope of the blood oxygen dissociation curve λ and the cardiac output $\dot{Q}$), and the interaction between tissue diffusion and blood transport (Shephard, 1977d).

Published information regarding the aging of individual elements is summarised in Table 3.11. In the young adult, the second and the fourth terms are usually so small that they can be neglected. From our discussion of pulmonary diffusion and tissue oxygen extraction (above), the same is probably true of a healthy older person. We may thus simplify the conductance equation to

$$\frac{1}{\dot{G}_{O_2}} = \frac{1}{\dot{V}_A} + \frac{1}{\lambda\dot{Q}}$$

Substituting real values of $\dot{V}_A$ (44 l/min in the men, 29 l/min in the women), λ (1.2) and $\dot{Q}$ (17 l/min in the men, 15 l/min in the women), we find that $\dot{G}_{O_2}$ is 13.9 l/min in the men and 11.1 l/min in the women. Given an oxygen concentration of 28 ml/l in the venous blood, the concentration gradient from inspired gas to the tissues is approximately 181 ml/l. The maximum oxygen intake should then be about 2.5 l/min in the men, and 2.0 l/min in the women. As we shall see in the next section, actual values are a little smaller than this, due to inefficiencies in the temporal and spatial matching of alveolar ventilation and pulmonary blood flow.

Maximum Oxygen Intake

The maximum oxygen intake or aerobic power provides a valuable index of the overall performance of the cardio-respiratory system in a given environment. However, not all of the measured oxygen intake is available to muscles performing 'useful' external work; indeed, a substantial proportion of this oxygen can be consumed in work performed by respiratory and cardiac muscle.

Measurement of the maximum oxygen intake may be made directly, as a subject works to exhaustion. It may be predicted from his responses to sub-maximum exercise. The status of the individual may be reported in terms of his performance of sub-maximum work (for example, the physical working capacity at a heart rate of 170/min or 150/min, the PWC_{170} and PWC_{150}; the heart rate at an oxygen

Table 3.11   A summary of the effect of aging upon individual
components of the oxygen transfer process (based largely on data of
Sidney, 1976): ↑ increase ↓ decrease → no change

Process variable	Direction of change with age	Reference
Ventilation		
1. Dimensional		
Vital capacity	↓	8, 23, 54, 110, 256, 349, 421, 674, 723, 733, 826
	→	60
TLC	→	680, 723, 734
	↓	826
	↑	60
FRC	↑	421, 680, 723, 734
	→	826
2. Functional		
$FEV_{1.0}$	↓	54, 102, 256, 349, 68, 723
MVV	↓	349, 421, 661, 667, 694
$\dot{V}_{E(max)}$	↓	3, 5, 24, 349, 826, 935, 1026
	→	60, 256
$\dot{V}_{E(max)}/\dot{V}_{O_2(max)}$	↑	53, 304, 427, 521, 736, 826
	→	8, 54
$\dot{V}_{A(max)}$	↓	54
$f_{R(max)}$	↓	54, 826, 1026
	→	8, 349
$V_{T(max)}$	↓	349, 826
	→	54
V_T/FVC	↑	54
Diffusion		
$\dot{D}_{L(max)}$	↓	30, 65, 210, 935
$\dot{D}_t$	↓	757
Circulation		
1. Dimensional		
THb, Hb, BV	→	256, 331, 993, 997, 1113
HV	↑	256, 995
	→	308, 482
$f_{h(max)}$	↓	8, 24, 54, 61, 237, 256, 283, 349, 534, 605, 606, 794, 935, 996, 1026

/cont.

Table 3.11—cont.

Process	Variable	Direction of change with age	Reference
2.	Functional		
	$\dot{Q}_{(max)}$	↓	65, 516, 521, 723, 957
	$SV_{(max)}$	↓	57, 65, 416, 723, 957
		→	630
	$a - \bar{v}\, O_2$ diff	↓	52, 630, 723
	$SBP_{(max)}$	↑	416, 521, 634, 894
		→	8
	$f_h \times SBP_{(max)}$	→	894
Anaerobic metabolism			
	$LA_{(max)}$	↓	8, 53, 54, 65, 826,
		→	61, 256, 1027
	$R_{(max)}$	→	8, 349, 1027
	O_2 (debt)	↓	349, 1027

consumption of 1.5 or 1.0 l/min, the $f_{h,1.5}$ and $f_{h,1.0}$; the heart rate at an estimated 75 per cent of maximum oxygen intake). Lastly, the subject may be required to carry out maximum effort in the field, running as far as possible in a fixed time such as fifteen or twelve minutes.

Directly Measured Maximum Oxygen Intake

In a young adult, there is little question that the most satisfactory approach to measurement of the maximum oxygen intake is to make a direct determination during uphill treadmill running. However, many investigators have been hesitant about using this approach in the elderly, questioning both the safety and the practicality of maximum testing.

1. Safety   Accidents during any type of exercise test are rare events, and for this reason it is difficult to estimate the relative risks of maximum and sub-maximum procedures. Cumming (1976) collected reports from seven laboratories, covering 49,035 exercise tests (both maximal and sub-maximal). Subjects were of all ages, and the sample included some individuals with coronary vascular disease. There was one death, and four episodes of ventricular fibrillation would also have been fatal but for prompt therapy, implying a total risk of about 1 in

10,000 tests. In one of the series cited, McDonough & Bruce (1969) distinguished maximum and sub-maximum tests, reporting the relative risks of cardiac arrest as 1 in 3,000 and 1 in 15,000 tests respectively. Rochmis & Blackburn (1971) collected the experience of 74 laboratories across North America; in 170,000 tests, there were 16 fatalities, 40 immediate and 10 subsequent admissions to hospital (mainly for chest pain or abnormalities of heart rhythm). In their series, no difference of risk was found between sub-maximum and maximum testing; further, all except one of the individuals affected had known cardio-vascular disease, and it is possible that some would have been judged as unsuitable candidates for testing by modern criteria (Andersen *et al.*, 1971).

How far can these risks be attributed to chance (Shephard, 1977a)? The main problem in answering such a question is to establish a suitable time base for comparison. In order not to miss any untoward events, Rochmis & Blackburn (1971) requested details of all complications for one week following testing. However, if there is to be an emergency, it usually begins during a test or shortly afterwards. Thirteen of the sixteen fatal episodes collected by Rochmis & Blackburn appear to have commenced within one hour of exercise, an attack rate of almost 700 per 1,000 man years, some twenty times the anticipated rate for a population all of whom had known cardio-vascular disease. One important variable is anxiety, particularly when a physician is to report on the condition of the heart. Other more pleasurable types of physical activity carry a lower risk, probably only three or four times that of sitting at rest (Shephard, 1977a).

There are no statistics on how risks change with aging. On the other hand, there is good evidence that the incidence of severe myocardial oxygen lack and abnormalities of cardiac rhythm rises progressively as a person becomes older (see next section); thus, at the age of 65 years, as many as 30 per cent of a 'normal' population are showing an abnormal exercise electrocardiogram. On the most pessimistic assumption, this group should fare no worse than younger patients with known cardio-vascular disease, implying a risk of one episode of ventricular fibrillation in 30,000 tests, and (with efficient treatment) a mortality of about 1 in 150,000 tests. Sidney & Shephard (1977) carried out 55 maximum tests on subjects aged 60 to 83 years. There were no injuries, but one lady did develop a ventricular tachycardia when a blood sample was taken two minutes after exercise. The abnormal rhythm was a frequent occurrence in the individual concerned and on the test day there was a spontaneous reversion to normal rhythm within a few minutes.

2. *Practicality*   In a young adult, the maximum oxygen intake is
identified fairly readily as the point where a further increase in the
external work load produces an increase of oxygen consumption less
than a specified and arbitrary criterion (for example, 150 ml/min,
6.7 mM/min; 2 ml/kg min, 89 μM/kg min). Such a criterion
necessarily has less precision in an older person, since it represents a
larger proportion of his total maximum oxygen intake. A more
serious objection is that the old person may cease the exercise test
before the oxygen plateau has been defined (I. Åstrand, 1960, 1967a;
Shephard, 1971; Nagle, 1973). In such circumstances, effort is
limited not by the maximum power of the cardio-respiratory system,
but by shortness of breath (Von Döbeln *et al.*, 1967; Grimby *et al.*,
1972), fear of over-exertion (Julius *et al.*, 1967; Lester *et al.*, 1968),
muscular weakness and lack of recent experience of exhausting exercise
(I. Åstrand *et al.*, 1959; Barry *et al.*, 1966; Von Döbeln *et al.*, 1967;
I. Åstrand *et al.*, 1967a; Grimby *et al.*, 1972), poor motivation (Von
Döbeln *et al.*, 1967) or the appearance of electrocardiographic
abnormalities (Barry *et al.*, 1966; Daly *et al.*, 1968).

   I. Åstrand *et al.* (1959) were able to reach 'definite' oxygen plateaus
in all nine of a group of men aged 56 to 68 years who were well trained
and accustomed to heavy exercise. In contrast, oxygen consumption
'levelled off' in only 20 of 44 middle-aged housewives enrolled in a
calisthenics programme. Cumming & Borysyk (1972) blamed such
problems on use of a bicycle ergometer rather than a treadmill. Sidney
& Shephard (1977) carried out treadmill tests on 55 subjects aged 60
to 83 years. Despite preliminary medical screening, sufficient
enthusiasm to volunteer for an exercise programme, and a good rapport
with the investigators, only about three quarters of the sample
realised the plateau criterion proposed for younger subjects at their
first test; however, about a half of the unsuccessful candidates were
able to reach a plateau when the test was repeated after a few weeks
of conditioning.

   Cumming & Borysyk (1972) have argued it may be dangerous to
push older subjects to a plateau where a substantial proportion of the
work is being performed anaerobically. However, our data do not
support the view that valid information can be obtained without
working the subjects to exhaustion. We had an observer rate each
subject's effort as 'fair' or 'good'; those making a 'good' attempt
naturally had higher lactate readings than those making only a 'fair'

Table 3.12 Direct measurements of maximum oxygen intake in 55 elderly men and women (Sidney & Shephard, 1977)

All data are mean ± SD

	Directly measured maximum O_2 intake				Error of Åstrand prediction	Heart rate	Resp. min. volume	Resp. gas exchange ratio	Arterial lactate	Plateau $\Delta \dot{V}_{O_2}$	Syst. blood pressure
	(l/min) STPD	(mM/min)	(ml/kg min) STPD	(mM/kg min)	(l/min) STPD	(/min)	(l/min) BTPS		(mM/l)	(ml/kg min)	(kPa)
MEN											
'Fair' effort (n = 7)	2.06 ±0.39	92 ±17.4	27.2 ±5.3	1.21 ±0.24	+0.04 ±0.32	154 ±14	83.0 ±18.2	1.05 ±0.04	6.6 ±2.2	2.0 ±1.7	26.5 ±3.7
'Good' effort (n = 19)	2.35 ±0.33	105 ±14.7	31.4 ±4.4	1.40 ±0.20	−0.23 ±0.35	172 ±12	90.6 ±14.4	1.11 ±0.08	11.1 ±3.3	0.5 ±1.8	28.0 ±4.1
All men (n = 26)	2.27 ±0.36	101 ±16.1	30.2 ±4.9	1.35 ±0.22	−0.16 ±0.35	167 ±15	88.6 ±15.5	1.09 ±0.07	10.3 ±3.6	0.9 ±1.8	27.6 ±4.0
WOMEN											
'Fair' effort (n = 9)	1.50 ±0.21	69 ±9.4	25.5 ±4.4	1.14 ±0.20	+0.15 ±0.20	155 ±10	52.8 ±10.1	1.01 ±0.09	5.4 ±3.0	1.8 ±1.7	25.5 ±2.1
'Good' effort (n = 20)	1.64 ±0.21	73 ±9.4	26.8 ±2.9	1.20 ±0.13	+0.28 ±0.47	161 ±12	62.5 ±9.2	1.07 ±0.09	9.1 ±2.0	0.8 ±1.4	25.6 ±3.6
All women (n = 29)	1.60 ±0.22	71 ±9.8	26.4 ±3.4	1.18 ±0.15	+0.23 ±0.41	159 ±11	59.5 ±10.4	1.05 ±0.09	8.1 ±2.9	1.1 ±1.5	25.6 ±3.2

Table 3.13   Criteria for the attainment of maximum oxygen intake in elderly subjects. Based largely on Sidney (1976)

Author	Age of subjects (years)	Criteria
Weiner & Lourie (1969)	—	Oxygen intake for the last three loads must agree to within 5%
Andersen *et al.* (1971)	—	Plateau of oxygen intake with increasing work (difference unspecified), blood lactate over 100mg/100ml, resp. gas exchange ratio over 1.15, heart rate greater than predicted max. for age
Robinson (1938)	6 – 91	Run/walk on 8% grade at a speed that exhausts subjects in 2 to 5 minutes
I. Åstrand (1960)	20 – 65	Plateau of oxygen intake despite unspecified increase of work load, blood lactate over 90mg/100ml (the latter criterion was not met by the older subjects)
Hollmann (1964)	6 – 80	No further increase of oxygen intake, heart rate over 180/min, systolic blood pressure over 250 mm Hg, blood lactate over 80mg/100ml
Benestad (1965)	70 – 81	Plateau of oxygen intake (unspecified)
Fischer *et al.* (1965)	50 – 90	Transition to anaerobic work (no details) or heart rate within 2 SDs of max. for age
Barry *et al.* (1966)	55 – 83	Highest work-load sustained for 6 min. (effort limited by ecg abnormalities in some subjects)
Brown & Shephard (1967)	40 – 70	Plateau of oxygen intake to within 0.15 l/min, observed maximum exceeds predicted maximum
Von Döbeln *et al.* (1967)	30 – 70	Oxygen intake 10% less than predicted from work-load, blood lactate over 50mg/100ml
Cumming *et al.* (1972)	40 – 65	Heart rate within 5 beats of predicted max. Oxygen intake 10% less than predicted from work-

/cont.

Table 3.13—cont.

Author	Age of. subjects (years)	Criteria
		load, resp. gas exchange ratio over 1.12, blood lactate over 72mg/100ml
Dehn & Bruce (1972)	40 - 72	Oxygen intake plateau to within 0.15 l/min, resp. gas exchange ratio over 1.15
Profant *et al.* (1972)	29 — 70	Highest observed oxygen intake, with self-determined limits of fatigue
Adams *et al.* (1972)	60 — 69	Tendency to plateau, with mean increase of 2.3 ml/kg min oxygen intake for 2% increase of tread-mill slope

effort, but they also developed a higher maximum oxygen intake (Table 3.12). It would seem that in order to demonstrate an individual s potential, it is necessary for him to build up a substantial oxygen debt.*

Is it possible to apply any secondary criteria of maximum effort when the oxygen plateau is not well defined (Table 3.13)? In a young person, it is possible to look for an arterial blood lactate of 100-120 mg/100ml (11-13 mM/l), a heart rate of close to 195/min, and a respiratory gas exchange ratio of near 1.15 (Shephard, 1977d). However, none of these variables are very helpful in the old person (Table 3.14). While the blood lactate was generally greater in those making a 'good' effort, a quarter of the men and a half of the women rated as making 'good' efforts failed to attain blood levels of 8.8 mM/l. Classification on the basis of maximum heart rate, Δ heart rate at the plateau, respiratory gas exchange ratio, or maximum systolic blood pressure was even less reliable. It would seem that if a satisfactory oxygen plateau is not attained, the test must be repeated, or some alternative procedure must be chosen to assess the individual's working capacity.

* The proof is not categoric. It is conceivable that subjects making a 'good' effort were able to do so because they were more fit.

Table 3.14   Percentages of elderly subjects satisfying commonly employed criteria for attainment of maximum oxygen intake (total sample = 26 men, 29 women). Based on data of Sidney & Shephard (1977)

	Δ Plateau oxygen intake		Δ Plateau heart rate	Respiratory gas exchange ratio		Arterial blood lactate	Peak heart rate		Systolic blood pressure
	≤1 ml/ kg min	≤2 ml/ kg min	≤5 beats/min	≥1.15	≥1.00	≥8.8 mM/l	≥160/min	≥165/min	≥200 mm Hg (26.7 kPa)
	%	%	%	%	%	%	%	%	%
MEN									
'Fair' effort (n = 7)	14.2	42.8	28.6	0	85.7	25.0	42.8	14.2	57.1
'Good' effort (n = 19)	63.2	78.9	63.2	36.8	100.0	77.8	84.2	68.4	57.9
All male subjects (n = 26)	50.0	69.2	65.5	26.9	96.2	68.2[a]	73.1	53.8	57.7
WOMEN									
'Fair' effort (n = 9)	33.3	44.4	33.3	0	55.6	11.1	44.4	22.2	33.3
'Good' effort (n = 20)	55.0	75.0	75.0	20.0	80.0	50.0	60.0	35.0	35.0
All female subjects (n = 29)	48.3	65.5	62.1	13.8	72.4	37.9	55.2	31.0	34.5

a   22 subjects only

Despite occasional difficulties in reaching a plateau, the reproducibility of the maximum test data is good. In young adults, the coefficient of variation for repeated measures of maximum oxygen intake is 4 to 6 per cent (Wright *et al.*, 1978). Direct measurements were repeated on fifteen of our elderly subjects one week after their initial test. The results showed at least as good a correspondence as in younger people:

		Correlation between first and second measurements	Difference between first and second measurements	Coefficient of variation %
Men	7	r = 0.96	− 0.04 ± 0.05	2.2
Women	8	r = 0.86	0.01 ± 0.04	2.5

There was no systematic change in the readings from the first to the second series of measurements, but five of the fifteen subjects who had not reached an oxygen plateau at their first attempt did so on the second occasion.

3. Characteristics of maxima   Many authors have held that the maximum arterial blood lactate of an older person is as low as 60mg/100ml, 7 mM/l. However, it has been less clear whether the limited accumulation of lactate is due to a lesser intramuscular breakdown of glycogen, a reduction of the ratio of muscle mass to blood volume, a slower diffusion of lactic acid out of the active fibres, or poorer motivation. Our blood lactate readings (Sidney & Shephard, 1977) for men making a 'good' effort averaged 11.1 mM/l, less than the 12-14 mM/l anticipated in a young person, but higher than in most previous series of data. We were careful to check our lactate estimations for systematic errors by both the use of standard preparations and determinations on young adults. We should thus conclude that a fair part of the previously reported deficit in lactate production is due to a lack of motivation and/or the caution of investigators when subjecting older people to anaerobic stress.

In keeping with this view, our maximum heart rates were higher than some authors have found. One 64-year-old desk worker sustained a cardiac frequency of 190-192/min for several minutes, and among those making a 'good' effort the average maxima were 172/min in the men and 161/min in the women.

The female subjects scored almost as well as the men in terms of observer ratings of effort, and this verdict seems borne out by a comparison of average $\Delta \dot{V}_{O_2}$ values at the oxygen plateau. However, a smaller proportion of the women satisfied the various secondary criteria of a centrally limited maximum oxygen intake (Table 3.13). Despite the observer ratings, we may thus suspect that the women were slightly less well motivated than our male subjects.

Sub-Maximum Tests

1. The predicted maximum oxygen intake   The Åstrand nomogram (I. Åstrand, 1960) and similar procedures for the prediction of maximum oxygen intake from responses to sub-maximum effort all assume a linear relationship between heart rate and oxygen consumption or the equivalent work load, from 50 to 100 per cent of maximum oxygen intake. This requirement is scarcely fulfilled in a young person, where predictions have an accuracy of 10 to 15 per cent (Shephard, 1977d). Precision is insufficient for scientific examination of an individual subject, but since a large part of the error is randomly distributed the technique can be used in field studies of entire populations. Furthermore, systematic errors in predictions for any given individual remain relatively constant over many months, so that this type of procedure can be used to monitor changes in the fitness of a subject over a season of training (Wright *et al.*, 1978).

There are reasons to suppose that prediction techniques might work less well in an older person. Inter-individual differences of maximum heart rate are exaggerated by aging, so that there is uncertainty regarding the values to be used in extrapolation; even in those of our subjects making a 'good' maximum effort (Table 3.12), the variation of peak heart rate was ± 12 beats/min, 7.0 per cent in the men and 7.5 per cent in the women. Further, failure to sustain stroke volume at high work loads (Figure 3.3) leads to a non-linearity of the heart rate/oxygen consumption relationship. At near maximum loads, the elderly show an increase of heart rate that is disproportionate to oxygen intake (Table 3.15). This is in contrast with most (Wyndham *et al.*, 1959; C.T.M. Davies, 1968; Cumming & Borysyk, 1972) but not all (Karlsson *et al.*, 1967; P.O. Åstrand, 1967) observations on younger subjects. Indeed, some studies of young adults (Shephard, 1969a; C.T.M. Davies *et al.*, 1970) have shown a plateauing of heart rate, although this disappears as subjects become habituated to the test procedure.

How accurate are predicted values when compared with actual measurements of maximum oxygen intake? With both bicycle and treadmill methods, individual predicted maxima for elderly subjects

Table 3.15   Deviations of directly measured maximum heart rate from values predicted by linear extrapolation of regression equations relating heart rate to oxygen consumption in progressive sub-maximal treadmill exercise (three minutes at each of three sub-maximum work-loads). Based on data of Sidney & Shephard (1977)

Subjects		Deviation (beats/min)	Chance probability
Elderly men	(n = 26)	− 8.1 ± 7.2	< 0.001
Elderly women	(n = 29)	− 11.5 ± 9.7	< 0.05
Young men	(n = 8)	+ 3.2 ± 7.3	not significant
Young women	(n = 5)	+ 7.2 ± 14.3	not significant

Table 3.16   Errors in the prediction of maximum oxygen intake by the Åstrand nomogram. Based on data of Sidney & Shephard (1977) for elderly subjects

Test method	Sex and N	Predicted $\dot{V}_{O_2}$ (max) (l/min) STPD	Measured $\dot{V}_{O_2}$ (max) (l/min) STPD	Discrepancy $\dot{V}_{O_2}$ (max) (l/min) STPD	Percentage error
Bicycle erg.,	13M	1.72 ± 0.36	2.27 ± 0.42	−0.56 ± 0.33	−24.7 ± 14.5
4 min/load	17F	1.37 ± 0.36	1.62 ± 0.17	−0.25 ± 0.26	−15.4 ± 16.0
Treadmill,	26M	2.11 ± 0.38	2.27 ± 0.36	−0.16 ± 0.35	− 7.0 ± 15.4
3 min/load	29F	1.83 ± 0.43	1.60 ± 0.22	0.23 ± 0.41	14.3 ± 25.6

show a scatter of at least 15 per cent, relative to direct determinations, the discrepancies being even larger for women exercising on the treadmill (Table 3.16). The bicycle ergometer data systematically underestimate the true maximum oxygen intake, a finding foreshadowed by a previous large-scale comparison of step test and bicycle ergometer data in 65-year-old adults (Bailey *et al.*, 1974). The probable explanation is that excessive reliance is placed upon the quadriceps muscle during bicycle ergometry (Shephard, 1977d). In an attempt to sustain quadriceps perfusion, the subject develops an increase of systemic blood pressure and a tachycardia reminiscent of that seen in isometric effort (Lind & McNicol, 1967). From the practical point of view, it would seem that if prediction methods are to be used in older subjects, it is better to use the treadmill or the step test than the bicycle ergometer.

Some field tests (for example, the work scale of the Åstrand nomogram and the step test of Margaria *et al.*, 1965) relate heart rate to the work performed rather than to the oxygen consumed. Errors can then arise from a reduction of mechanical efficiency with aging. Certain protagonists of the bicycle ergometer have claimed that this is always operated with a mechanical efficiency of 23 per cent. In fact, variations from the 'constant' figure can be discerned in a number of populations (Shephard, 1978). The elderly seem particularly liable to a poor mechanical efficiency, since they lack recent familiarity with bicycle exercise and are handicapped by stiffer joints, less ready relaxation of antagonistic muscles, and a need to support a greater mass of body fat. Furthermore, a high blood pressure and aging airways add to the oxygen demands of cardiac and respiratory muscles. Although Denolin *et al.* (1970) observed no change in subjects aged 45 to 64 years, other published reports show that the mechanical efficiency of bicycle ergometry is reduced in the elderly:

Subjects	Load	Efficiency %	Author
Men	600 kg-m/min	21.8	I. Åstrand *et al.*, 1959
Men	PWC_{130}	21.1	Sidney & Shephard, 1977
Women	450 kg-m/min	21.4	I. Åstrand, 1960
Women	PWC_{130}	21.8	Sidney & Shephard, 1977

We may conclude that if a bicycle ergometer is used without measurement of oxygen consumption, a mechanical efficiency of 21.5 rather than 23 per cent should be presumed for an elderly subject. It is likely that there are at least parallel changes in the efficiency of running and stepping (Robinson, 1938; Molina & Giorgi, 1951; Ryhming, 1953; Norris *et al.*, 1953, 1955; Hellon *et al.*, 1956; Durnin & Mikulic, 1956).

2. *Interpolated values*   The main advantage that can be claimed for interpolated values such as the PWC_{170}, the PWC_{150}, the $f_{h,1.5}$ and the $f_{h,1.0}$ is that they avoid the uncertainties of extrapolation — particularly doubts concerning the influence of age on the maximum heart rate and the linearity of the heart rate/oxygen consumption relationship.

On the other hand, scores for the PWC_{170} and PWC_{150} are affected by the decrease of mechanical efficiency with aging. A second and more important source of difficulty is that the relative stress imposed by a given heart rate or a given oxygen consumption increases with age. Thus, the PWC_{170} is a relatively light load for a young man, but it may exceed the maximum capacity of an old person. Because the PWC_{170} becomes an excessive load, it is necessary to make recourse to a PWC_{150}, or even a PWC_{130} in an aged subject. On the other hand, the heart rate/oxygen consumption line is displaced but little as an individual becomes older. The interpolated indices may thus show no age-related trend, although the working capacity of the subject is plainly declining as he becomes older.

In elderly North American populations (Sidney & Shephard, 1977) the problem of quadriceps weakness already discussed leads to substantial differences between the interpolated indices for bicycle ergometer and treadmill tests:

		Men	Women
Treadmill	$f_{h,1.0}$ (beats/min)	101.2	118.8
Bicycle erg.	$f_{h,1.0}$ (beats/min)	114.8	145.5
	PWC_{130} (Watts)	84.0 ± 33.5	54.9 ± 19.5
	PWC_{150} (Watts)	118.5 ± 32.0	80.9 ± 32.9

Perhaps for this reason, the PWC_{130} values for the men are substantially inferior to data reported for elderly Scandinavians (I. Åstrand *et al.*, 1959; Von Döbeln *et al.*, 1967; Borg & Linderholm, 1967; Grimby *et al.*, 1972), although results for the female subjects are comparable with those reported by Ericsson & Irnell (1969b). The treadmill data at an oxygen intake of 1 l/min coincide well with Scandinavian estimates for bicycle ergometer work (see, for example, P.O. Åstrand, 1952; I. Åstrand, 1960).

An alternative treatment of the interpolated data is to report the work accomplished or the oxygen consumption developed at an age-specific 'target' heart rate corresponding to a fixed proportion such as 75 per cent of maximum oxygen intake (Shephard, 1971). The main difficulty with this approach is again an uncertainty regarding the heart rate of the elderly person during exercise. A simple descending series of 'target' rates (160 at age 25 years, 150 at 35, 140 at 45 and 130 at 55) was suggested initially. The series was based largely on Scandinavian reports concerning the maximum heart rate of the elderly; more recent experience has shown that a 65-year-old North American can develop

Table 3.17 Canadian Home Fitness Test. Rates of ascent and descent of a double eight inch step, fitness ratings based on test duration and the immediate post-exercise ten-second pulse count, with percentages of the Saskatoon population attaining the several fitness ratings (Bailey *et al.*, 1976)

| Age (yrs) | Rate of ascent per minute | | Fitness rating, pulse count and per cent of population attaining rating | | | | | |
	Men	Women	Very good (9 min)	Good (9 min)	Average fit (9 min)	Average unfit (6 min)	Poor (6 min)	Very poor (3 min)
20 – 30	24	19	23 1%M , 0%F	24 – 25 1%M , 1%F	26 7%M , 4%F	26 – 28 24%M , 27%F	29 52%M , 27%F	29 16%M , 41%F
30 – 40	22	19	22 0%M , 0%F	23 – 24 5%M , 3%F	25 17%M , 8%F	25 – 27 36%M , 36%F	28 34%M , 35%F	28 8%M , 19%F
40 – 50	19	17	21 3%M , 0%F	22 – 23 2%M , 3%F	24 26%M , 14%F	24 – 25 41%M , 30%F	26 23%M , 35%F	26 4%M , 18%F
50 – 60	16	14	20 5%M , 3%F	21 – 22 11%M , 7%F	23 43%M , 32%F	23 – 24 29%M , 43%F	25 11%M , 18%F	25 1%M , 7%F
60 – 70	13	11	—	19 (M) 20 (F) 38%M , 27%F	20 – 21 (M) 21 – 22 (F) 43%M , 33%F	22 – 23 (M) 23 – 24 (F) 10%M , 28%F	24 (M) 25 (F) 18%M , 23%F	24 (M) 24 (F) 3%M , 9%F

a faster heart rate at 75 per cent of maximum oxygen intake, averaging 136/min in men, and 131/min in women (Sidney & Shephard, 1977).

A final variant of the interpolated sub-maximum test is to choose a load that is a fixed percentage of maximum oxygen intake for the average sedentary individual of a given age and sex, and to observe the exercise reponse at this level of effort (for example the duration of work and/or the resultant heart rate). This is the plan adopted in the Canadian Home Fitness Test (Table 3.17, Bailey *et al.*, 1976). Subjects are required to climb and descend the bottom two steps of a domestic staircase at a pace set by a long-playing record. Fitness is classed on the test duration (3, 6 or 9 minutes of a progressive rhythm) and the immediate post-exercise pulse count. During initial validation of the test, an attempt was made to recruit a randomly selected sample of the Saskatoon population. Over 2,800 names were taken from the telephone directory, but unfortunately only about a third of those contacted agreed to participate; it was thus necessary to supplement the sample from such sources as the local police and fire departments. Particular difficulty was encountered in recruiting older subjects, and this may have biased our results towards an overestimation of average levels of fitness in the elderly.

Field Tests

The original field test run was of fifteen minutes duration (Balke, 1954), but the twelve minute all-out run of Cooper (1968a,b) is better known. In young adults, results of the latter test are closely correlated with the maximum oxygen intake (r = 0.90); those capable of covering 1½ miles (2.4 km) in twelve minutes have an aerobic power of 42.6 ml/kg min (1.9 mM/kg min).

It has been suggested that correlations are poorer in the elderly, due to lack of recent familiarity with all-out running, a poor choice of pace and lesser motivation. Sidney & Shephard (1977) reported correlation coefficients of 0.83 for 65-year-old men, and 0.51 for women of the same age. Equations for the prediction of maximum oxygen intake from the number of kilometers covered in twelve minutes were as follows:

Men   = 12.4 (km) + 21.5 ml/kg min   (coefficient of variation 10%)
Women = 11.4 (km) + 11.9 ml/kg min   (coefficient of variation 16%)

These equations are at least as precise as other procedures for the prediction of maximum oxygen intake; however, the field tests require movement at top speed for twelve minutes, and this may have some danger for an elderly subject who is badly out of condition.

From the regression lines, our men needed an aerobic power of 51.4 ml/kg min (2.29 mM/kg min) and our women 39.4 ml/kg min (1.76 mM/kg min) to cover the 2.4 km distance in twelve minutes. The implication is that the old men (but not the old women) moved inefficiently relative to the sample studied by Cooper (1968a). Some of the reasons for a poor mechanical efficiency have been discussed above. A further consideration in the Cooper test is that some older subjects walk rather than run over at least a part of the required distance; at the speeds under consideration (8-12 km/hr), walking is generally much less economical than running (Durnin & Passmore, 1967; Shephard, 1971).

Test Strategy in the Elderly

Having reviewed the various options, what test strategy should be recommended for the elderly subject? The present author's experience suggests that about three quarters of the usual test population (those interested in exercise training and passing a preliminary medical examination) can attain a plateau of maximum oxygen intake with a single maximum test. Perhaps as many as a half of the remaining subjects also reach a plateau in a second test with a more appropriate choice of work loads. This leaves only a small minority to be assessed from some type of sub-maximal procedure.

Immediate medical supervision may not be available in some laboratories, and in such circumstances it is necessary to rely on the results of sub-maximal tests. Note must be taken of potentially interfering phenomena, such as lack of habituation, a low mechanical efficiency, and possible effects of quadriceps weakness. A declining stroke volume gives non-linearity of the heart rate/oxygen consumption relationship, and for this reason it is often preferable to report sub-maximal data at a target heart rate rather than attempt extrapolation to a predicted maximum oxygen intake.

Population Data for Maximum Oxygen Intake

The maximal oxygen intake declines with age, irrespective of whether it is expressed in absolute units (l/min, mM/min) or relative to body weight (ml/kg min, mM/kg min). However, because of fat accumulation in an older person, the relative change is usually greater than the absolute variation. The rate of decline has been studied in both cross-sectional (Robinson, 1938; I. Åstrand, 1960; Hollmann, 1964; Fischer

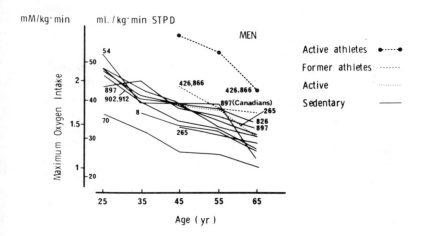

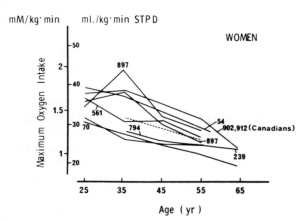

Figure 3.4   The decline of aerobic power with age. Based largely on data collected by Sidney (1976).

et al., 1965; Malhotra *et al.*, 1966; Shephard, 1966a; Brown & Shephard, 1967; Cumming, 1967; Von Döbeln *et al.*, 1967; P.O. Åstrand, 1968; Shephard, 1969b; Tlusty, 1969a; Hollmann *et al.*, 1970; Rode & Shephard, 1971; Cumming *et al.*, 1972; Profrant *et al.*, 1972; Coleman *et al.*, 1973; Bailey *et al.*, 1974; Shephard, 1977d, 1978) and longitudinal (Asmussen & Mathiasen, 1962; Robinson, 1964; Hollmann, 1966; P.O. Åstrand, 1972; Dehn & Bruce, 1972; Robinson *et al.*, 1972; I. Åstrand *et al.*, 1973) experiments. Although mean levels of aerobic power differ substantially between the various populations examined (Figure 3.4), there is good general agreement on the course of aging. Maximum oxygen intake begins to decline at about twenty years of age in men, perhaps rather later in women. By the 65th year it is 30 to 40 per cent smaller than in a young adult.

Various factors bias the apparent rate of aging in both cross-sectional and longitudinal studies. With the cross-sectional approach, there is a selective attenuation of the sample in older age groups. However, the problem of selective death has perhaps been overstated, at least to the age of 65, for while there is a progressive elimination of the very sick members of the population, at the same time the very fit show a disproportionate number of deaths from accidents and violence. On the other hand, there is little question that older people who volunteer for fitness testing represent a health-conscious and relatively fit sub-sample of the total elderly population. A longitudinal protocol does not necessarily avoid such problems. It is very likely that those recruited for a longitudinal study of exercise tolerance will be both health conscious and relatively fit. Again, there will be a selective attenuation of the sample, with a progressive loss of the sick and the poorly motivated. Lastly, there may be a decline of habitual activity over the period of observation, so that effects due to a loss of fitness become confounded with the true effects of aging.

In cross-sectional studies, men generally lose aerobic power at a rate of 0.42-0.52 ml/kg min per year (18.8-23.2 μM/kg min per year); the women maintain a relatively constant aerobic power to about thirty-five years of age, but thereafter show a loss of 0.5-0.7 ml/kg min per year (22.3-31.2 μM/kg min per year). Some longitudinal studies have reported a more rapid deterioration of maximum oxygen intake. Dehn & Bruce (1972), for example, cited a loss of 0.56 ml/kg min per year for active men, and 1.62 ml/kg min per year for inactive men. It seems improbable that inactive men could sustain such a heavy loss for more than a few years, and it must be suspected that these estimates have been distorted by a change in the habitual activity of the subjects studied.

Typical values for the sedentary 65-year-old are summarised in Table 3.18. Excluding the rather low bicycle ergometer readings obtained by Bailey *et al.* (1974), the average for the men is about 2.14 l/min (96 mM/min), or 28.5 ml/kg min (1.27 mM/kg min); corresponding figures for the women are 1.68 l/min (75 mM/min) and 25.5 ml/kg min (1.14 mM/kg min). It seems generally agreed (I. Åstrand, 1967b; Bonjer, 1968; Hughes & Goldman, 1970;

Shephard, 1974b) that the average work load of a young person should not exceed 40 per cent of aerobic power for an eight-hour day. On this basis, the average 65-year-old man would tolerate a loading of 4.28 kcal/min (19.0 kJ/min), while the average 65-year-old woman would be capable of 3.36 kcal/min (14.1 kJ/min). Furthermore, the standard deviation of aerobic power is about 20 per cent. Thus the 40 per cent ceiling would amount to only 2.57 kcal/min (10.8 kJ/min) for one man in forty, and 2.02 kcal/min (8.5 kJ/min) for one woman in forty. Such standards may still prove excessive for some elderly subjects, since their lactate production is enhanced by slow adaptation to an increased rate of working and by local muscular weakness.

Typical figures for the metabolic costs of light industrial work are summarised in Table 3.19. The data were collected some years ago, and in many industries costs have subsequently been reduced by modern technology. However, the results cited refer to a 65 kg man and a 55 kg woman; since most 65-year-old subjects are substantially heavier than these figures, the energy expenditures remain reasonably realistic for the present day. Many of the occupational categories include at least one task with a fairly high rate of energy expenditure; this usually involves lifting either of raw materials or of finished products. Brown & Crowden (1963) distinguished four categories of employment: light work (2.0-3.3 kcal/min, 8.4-13.9 kJ/min), moderate work (3.3-5.4 kcal/min, 13.9-22.7 kJ/min), heavy work (5.4-9.0 kcal/min, 22.7-37.8 kJ/min) and very heavy work (> 9.0 kcal/min, 37.8 kJ/min). Plainly, the majority of older workers would encounter some difficulty with heavy and very heavy work. However, those who have spent a life-time in such employment may have kept their fitness levels above the population average. It is also conceivable that accumulated skills reduce the energy costs somewhat for experienced workers, and finally adjustment to many tasks is possible through a slowing of the rate of working. In light industry, almost all occupations have some tasks that remain within the competence of the average 65 year old, and many categories of employment could accommodate even those individuals who are at the lower end of the fitness distribution curve.

By virtue of seniority or the sympathy of management and colleagues, many older employees are allocated the lighter tasks within their occupational category. Those whose work has undergone rapid technological change are less fortunate. They lack the skills needed to operate the new machines and so are left to carry out the heavier activities in a factory, such as general labouring and stockroom work.

Table 3.18 Maximum oxygen intake of elderly men and women

	Men				Women				Reference
	Absolute		Relative		Absolute		Relative		
	(l/min) STPD	(mM/min)	(ml/kg min) STPD	(mM/kg min)	(l/min) STPD	(mM/min)	(ml/kg min) STPD	(mM/kg min)	
	2.04	91	26.9	1.20	1.85	83	28.4	1.27	Adams et al. (1972)
	2.23	100	31.4	1.40	1.19	53	19.0	0.85	I. Åstrand (1960)
	1.75	78	22.8	1.02					Bailey et al. (1974)[a,b]
	2.39	107	30.7	1.37	1.90	85	30.2	1.35	Bailey et al. (1974)[a]
	1.97	88	23.9	1.07	1.61	72	25.6	1.14	Cumming et al. (1972)
									Cumming et al. (1973a)
	2.25	100	30.7	1.37					Dehn & Bruce (1972)
	2.35	105	34.5	1.54					Robinson (1938)
	1.91	85	25.1	1.12	1.66	74	25.5	1.14	Shephard (1966a)
			26.8	1.20			24.1	1.06	Shephard (1977d)[a]
	1.87	83	25.4	1.13					Tlusty (1969)
	2.29	102	29.2	1.30	1.40	63	19.2	0.86	Von Döbeln et al. (1967)

a Predicted maximum oxygen intake
b Bicycle ergometer test

Table 3.19   Energy costs of light industrial activity (based on data collected by Durnin & Passmore, 1967, for men of 65 kg and women of 55 kg). Upper and lower limits indicate mean values for different tasks within a given occupational category

Occupational category	kcal/min	kJ/min
MEN		
Watch repairing	1.6	6.7
Draughting	1.9	8.0
Printing	2.2–2.5	9.2–10.5
Tailoring	2.1–4.0	8.8–16.8
Furrier	5.4	22.6
Shoemaking	2.6–3.3	10.9–13.8
Locksmith	3.1–4.3	13.0–18.0
Garage work	3.5–4.1	14.7–17.2
Woodwork factory	2.9–5.6	12.2–23.5
Electrical factory	2.2–5.4	9.2–22.6
Machine tool and motor industry	3.1–5.7	13.0–23.9
Paint factory	3.6–6.3	15.1–26.4
WOMEN		
Baking	1.6–2.7	6.7–11.3
Book-binding	2.5	10.5
Brewing	1.6–3.0	6.7–12.6
Canteen staff	2.4–4.9	10.1–20.5
Paint factory	2.7–2.9	11.3–12.2
Vehicle cleaning	3.4–4.2	14.2–17.6
Electrical factory	1.4–2.6	5.9–10.9
Furniture factory	2.4–4.8	10.1–20.1
Laundry	2.9–4.0	12.2–16.8
Machine tool	1.3–4.4	5.4–18.4

Electrocardiographic Findings

Aging leads to an increase in the proportion of the population who cannot increase their coronary blood flow sufficiently to meet the demands of physical or emotional strain. The problem is one expression of the more general condition of atherosclerosis, with rigidity and narrowing or occlusion of the coronary vessels.

The majority of authors have regarded atherosclerosis as a pathological rather than a normal consequence of aging. Nevertheless, by the age of 65 years the majority of the population have at least mild vascular changes, and as many as 30 per cent develop some myocardial ischaemia during vigorous exercise. Silver & Landowne (1953) have commented that population distribution curves shade imperceptibly into an ischaemic response, without the discontinuity that would be anticipated with a pathological process. Blumenthal (1975) has also argued strongly that atherosclerosis should be studied within the context of gerontology rather than vascular pathology.

Several potential mechanisms for the production of atheromatous plaques can be postulated from general aging theory (Chapter 2):

(1)   With the general loss of enzyme activity, the cardiovascular tissues lose their ability to handle lipids, so that fat accumulates in the sub-intimal zone. Some support for this concept is seen in the age-related decrease of serum lipoprotein lipase activity.

(2)   Basic mechanisms of structural homeostasis maintain a constant ratio of arterial wall thickness and internal diameter. However, with aging, the artery dilates and the mechanism of homeostasis may fail, with formation of an aneurysmal swelling or an excessive intimal proliferation that encroaches on the lumen of the vessel.

(3)   Feedback mechanisms that normally restrict multiplication of the intimal cells may no longer function in the elderly (Martin & Sprague, 1973).

(4)   The plaques may represent benign tumours, formed from repeated reproduction of abnormal intimal smooth muscle cells (Benditt & Benditt, 1973).

(5)   The intimal proliferation may be a vascular expression of auto-immunity (Blumenthal, 1968).

(6)   The progressive failure of insulin secretion (maturity onset diabetes) and the development of hypothyroidism both aggravate the condition.

The condition of the vasculature can be studied at post-mortem, or (at some risk to the individual) by the intra-arterial injection of a radio opaque dye. However, in the first instance the ischaemia is usually inferred from an abnormal electrocardiogram. Some authors (for example, I. Åstrand, 1960, 1967c; Punsar *et al.*, 1968; Elgrishi *et al.*, 1970) have proposed detailed codes for classification of the resting and the exercise electrocardiogram. However, the two items currently accepted as good evidence of myocardial oxygen lack are (1) the development of a horizontal or downward sloping ST segment (negative voltage > 0.1 mV at the commencement of the T wave) and (2) the appearance of frequent ventricular extra-systoles (Chiang *et al.*, 1970; Vedin *et al.*, 1972). The latter commonly appear in parallel with the ST change, and are regarded as harbingers of sudden death; they carry a particularly adverse prognosis if they arise at several sites (as shown by differences of waveform) or occur soon after the T wave of the preceding ECG complex.

Resting Electrocardiogram

The standard resting electrocardiogram shows relatively little change with age. Emphysema may reduce all voltages in the standard limb leads, and the electrical axis of the heart is usually more horizontal than in a younger subject (Larsen & Skulason, 1941; Mazer & Reisinger, 1944). Some authors have found an increase of PR interval (Harlan *et al.*, 1967). Declining physical fitness and a low stroke volume may be responsible for low amplitude T waves (Mazer & Reisinger, 1944; Silver & Landowne, 1953). An increased proportion of subjects show a saddle-shaped rather than a flat and iso-electric ST segment. Finally, sinus arrhythmia is less frequent than in a young adult (Mazer & Reisinger, 1944).

If observations are made over a longer period (for example, using a 24-hour tape recorder, Lopez *et al.*, 1975), changes can be seen much as in the exercise record. As a person ages, there is an increased likelihood of detecting dysrhythmias and ST segmental depression. Opinions are divided on the relative merits of 24-hour tapes and exercise tests as a means of detecting early ischaemic heart disease (Coronary Drug Research Group, 1973; Jelinek & Lown, 1974). One recent study (Wolf *et al.*, 1974) examined 47 subjects over the age of forty years. Twenty-one of the group showed ST segmental changes on both types of record, and nineteen subjects had normal tracings on both tests. The findings were discordant in the remaining seven cases. Four showed ST changes during bicycle ergometry, and three during 24-hour monitoring. It would seem that both approaches have a rather similar sensitivity to myocardial ischaemia, but that the total yield of positive diagnoses can be increased if both techniques are employed on the same person. Further study is needed to determine whether the additional positive records represent true or false diagnoses of myocardial ischaemia.

Exercise Electrocardiogram

The percentage of abnormal electrocardiograms that are discovered in a given population depends upon the intensity of effort that is

developed (Bruce, 1967; Westura & Ronan, 1969; Cumming, 1972)
and upon the rigour of the diagnostic criteria that are applied to
the resultant records. Early investigators used a fairly light sub-maximal
work load. For example, Rumball & Acheson (1963) walked their
subjects up a flight of stairs, and Master (1969) used an age, weight and
sex adjusted rate of stepping that produced a final heart rate of
about 120/min (Master *et al.*, 1942). In both of these tests, the
electrocardiogram was studied only during the recovery from exercise.
More recently, the load has been standardised to 75 per cent
(Shephard, 1971) or 85 per cent (I. Åstrand, 1967c) of maximum
oxygen intake, or the test has been pursued to a 'symptom-limited'
maximum (Bruce, 1967; Bruce *et al.*, 1969). Furthermore, improvements in electrocardiographic technique have allowed measurements
to be made during as well as following exercise. Since some abnormal
records are seen only during exercise, and a few appear only during
recovery, the examination of records from both test phases inevitably
increases the diagnostic yield:

Author	Occurrence of abnormal electrocardiogram		
	Exercise only %	Recovery only %	Both phases %
Cumming (1972)	41.5	12.1	46.4
Sidney & Shephard (1977d)	46.2	15.4	38.4

An ST depression of 0.5 mm (0.05 mV) was regarded as abnormal in
some of the early, low intensity recovery tests (for example, Mattingly,
1962). Currently, the usual criterion is a horizontal or downward sloping depression of more than 1 mm (0.1 mV). Correlation of
electrocardiographic findings with the results of intra-arterial coronary
arteriography has shown that the 1 mm criterion strikes an optimum
balance between the proportion of false negative and false positive
diagnoses (Mason *et al.*, 1969).

  Abnormal records are first seen at about 40 years of age, and the
proportion of the apparently healthy population with ST changes
increases steadily with a further advance in years (Figure 3.5). At
least 30 per cent of both men and women in the 65-year-old age group
are affected (Table 3.20). For the men, there is a strong statistical
association between the ST abnormality and the risk of subsequent
ischaemic heart disease (Rumball & Acheson, 1963; Blomqvist, 1965;
Robb & Marks, 1964, 1967; Most *et al.*, 1968; Blackburn, 1969a,b;

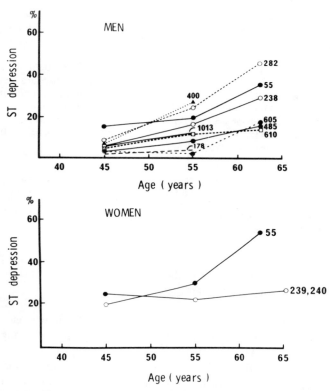

Figure 3.5   The percentage of subjects showing depression of the ST segment of the electrocardiogram during or following maximum or near maximum exercise. Published reports for middle and old age.

Kasser & Bruce, 1969; Bruce *et al.*, 1969; Andersen *et al.*, 1971). Subjects showing ST abnormalities have a 4-14 fold increase in the likelihood of developing ischaemic heart disease over the next five to ten years. Furthermore, the added risk for a given ST segmental displacement is closely comparable in subjects aged 41-50 and 51-99 years (Ellerstad, 1975).

The elderly women show the paradox of at least equally frequent abnormal records, despite a much lower risk of ischaemic heart disease than that seen in the men (I. Åstrand, 1965a; Ostrander *et al.*, 1965; Blackburn, 1969a,b; Profant *et al.*, 1972; Cumming *et al.*,

Table 3.20   Frequency of 'positive' exercise electrocardiograms in elderly subjects

MEN %	Reference	WOMEN %	Reference
35	I. Åstrand (1969)	55	I. Åstrand (1969)
37	Cumming *et al.* (1972)	36	Brown & Shephard (1967)
46	Doan *et al.* (1965)	33[a]	Cumming *et al.* (1973a)
25	Kasser & Bruce (1969)	100	Profant *et al.* (1972)
17[b]	Kavanagh & Shephard (1977b)	21	Riley *et al.* (1970)
32	Riley *et al.* (1970)	36	Sidney & Shephard (1977d)
29	Sidney & Shephard (1977d)		

[a]   Although the authors cite a frequency of 33 per cent, their figures appear to show 9 of 33 cases (27 per cent) with ST depression; a subsequent report (Cumming *et al.*, 1973b) shows 27 per cent having A1, A2 or A4 ST depression on the criteria of Punsar *et al.* (1968)

[b]   Masters' Class athletes

1973a,b). Several hypotheses have been advanced to explain this phenomenon (Sidney & Shephard, 1977d):

(1)   Because of the rarity of ischaemic heart disease in women, doctors may order an exercise ECG only if clinical symptoms of angina are present (Lepeschkin, 1969). This could perhaps explain a high incidence of abnormal records where the test sample is derived from a cardiology clinic, but it can hardly explain the findings of our laboratory when examining healthy volunteers for an exercise programme (Sidney & Shephard, 1977d).

(2)   Women have a more horizontal ST segment and a smaller T wave than men. A given amount of ST depression is thus more obvious in a woman than in a man (Lepeschkin, 1969). This could conceivably influence the proportion of reported anomalies in some of the early 'eyeball' studies (Profant *et al.*, 1972), but could hardly account for the findings where records have been measured objectively.

(3)   It has been suggested that sympathetic activity is greater in women than in men at a given level of exercise. Any difference must be small, since the heart rate at a given percentage of maximum effort is only a little higher in the women (P.O. Åstrand & Rhyming, 1954). Furthermore, there is no strong evidence that vaso-regulatory asthenia, hyperventilation, postural effects and related ST artefacts are more

prevalent in women than in men.

(4)   Abnormal ST responses are more common in the obese (Blackburn, 1969a). The higher percentage of body fat in the female might thus contribute to the elevated frequency of abnormal electro-cardiograms.

(5)   There are suggestions that women have as much atheroma as men, yet escape the fatal consequences of the disease process (Dawber *et al.*, 1957; I. Åstrand, 1965a; Kannel & Fanlieb, 1972). Hormonal factors and differences in mineral reserves possibly make the female myocardium less vulnerable for a given amount of coronary vascular disease (W.F. Andersen, 1973). However, the hormonal advantage is surely waning at the age of 65 years, and coronary angiograms often fail to demonstrate vascular abnormalities in women with apparently ischaemic electrocardiograms (Likoff *et al.*, 1966).

(6)   Constitutional and cultural factors may keep an older woman from the sudden physical effort and resultant increase of cardiac work-load that could precipitate ventricular fibrillation. It is arguable that an exercise test that requires an equal relative stress of men and woman is culturally unrealistic.

(7)   Kasser & Bruce (1969) have pointed out that if the heart of an elderly person is sufficiently stressed, ST segmental depression may arise in the absence of significant coronary disease. Since the quadriceps muscles are generally weaker in a woman, it could be that bicycle ergometry gives rise to a greater tachycardia, a greater increase of systolic blood pressure, and a greater increase in cardiac work-load than in men. Sidney & Shephard (1977d) found a marginally higher blood pressure in the women (194 versus 191 mm Hg, 25.9 versus 25.5 kPa), but at the same time the heart rate was slightly lower, so that the total cardiac work-load at 75 per cent of maximum oxygen intake was approximately the same in both sexes.

(8)   Problems may also arise from weakness of the cardiac muscle. Since women generally have smaller hearts than men, the same absolute cardiac work-load throws a greater strain on unit volume of the cardiac tissue. It is most unlikely that there is a compensatory increase in the capillary supply per unit mass of cardiac tissue, so that at a given rate of working, a woman's heart is inevitably more liable to ischaemia.

From the practical point of view, the detection of electrocardio-graphic abnormalities is an indication for caution when prescribing exercise. Work loads should be held below an intensity that provokes frequent ventricular extra-systoles or > 2 mm of ST segmental depression. If the subject is intelligent and not unduly neurotic, it is useful to teach him not only to monitor the prescribed exercise ceiling by counting his heart rate, but also to detect any extra-systoles ('thumps') in the chest or mild anginal symptoms (tightness in the chest or throat) that may accompany ST depression.

Musculo-Skeletal Changes

Information on changes in musculo-skeletal function with aging is rather sketchy. We have considered previously decreases of lean body mass, anaerobic capacity, anaerobic power and bone density. In this section we will make specific review of changes in muscle strength and co-ordination, joint structure and tendon strength.

Muscle Strength

Muscle strength diminishes progressively with age (Figures 3.6 and 3.7). Some studies such as the early data of Quetelet (1835) have shown a loss of up to 40 per cent of maximum force by the age of 65 years. Other and more recent material such as that of Fisher & Birren (1947), Asmussen (1964) and Shephard (1977d) indicated a loss of 18 to 20 per cent (Table 3.21), while Shock & Norris (1970) found no significant deterioration prior to the age of 60 (Figure 3.7).

Presumably, the peak values attained and thus the subsequent rate of loss depend upon the demands of occupation and leisure; this may explain why many authors have found a rather slower loss in women than in men. The scores also depend upon habitual activity in later life and upon the willingness of the subjects to make a maximal effort. Nevertheless, several surveys of 65-year-old subjects show remarkably uniform figures for grip strength at this age (Table 3.21). Shock & Norris (1970) have drawn attention to the discrepancy between maximum power output, as measured in a brief cranking test, and the loss of muscle strength. In their 80-year-old subjects, power output was reduced by 45 per cent, whereas strength had declined by only 28 per cent relative to its middle-aged peak; the investigators attributed this difference to a reduced co-ordinating ability in the later years of life, although other factors such as a reduction of myosin ATP^{ase} activity may have been involved.

Joint Structure

The integrity of the synovial joints is affected by general changes in the structure of collagen (Grahame, 1973). In particular, the chondroitin content of the cartilage is reduced, and this leads to a loss

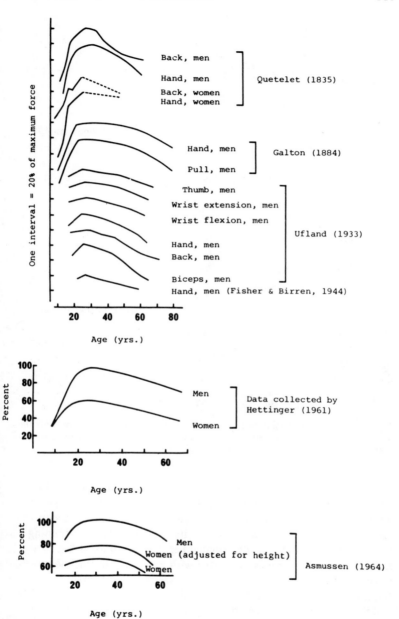

Figure 3.6 Some published cross-sectional data on changes in muscle force with age. Based in part on data collected by Fisher & Birren (1947).

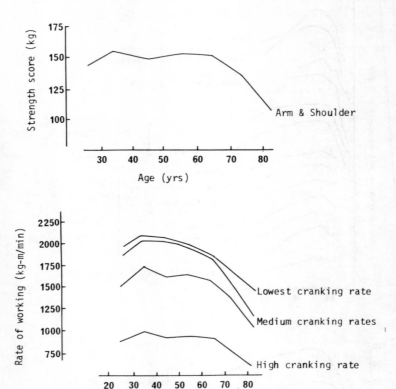

Figure 3.7   Longitudinal data on the aging of composite strength scores for the arm and shoulder muscles, and the maximum rate of working at various speeds of cranking. Based on data of Shock & Norris (1970).

of resilience, a change in staining properties, and an increased liability to degenerative change (G.M. Hass, 1943). The articular cartilage of a young child is glistening and translucent, but with aging it assumes an opaque, yellowish colour and loses its elasticity. Whereas training increases the thickness of the articular cartilage (Holmdahl & Ingelmark, 1948), aging is associated with a decrease in thickness and the appearance of frank defects over the weight-bearing areas. Degenerative changes can first be detected in the second decade of life, and their frequency and severity increase progressively as a person becomes older (Chung, 1966a). There may also be some calcification, for example in the cartilages of the knee. Related changes in the

Table 3.21   Published values for handgrip strength and leg extension force of elderly subjects (kg).* Based in part on data collected by Sidney (1976)

| MEN | | WOMEN | | |
Grip[a]	Leg extension	Grip[a]	Leg extension	Authors
46.4		32.7		Asmussen & Heebøll-Nielsen (1961)
45.0				Barry *et al.* (1966)
44.3		30.7		Bookwalter (1950)
47.0				Damon *et al.* (1972)
48.0				Fisher & Birren (1947)
43.7	25.1			Kutal *et al.* (1970)
44.1		27.5		Shephard (1977d)
44.2	71.7	25.9	43.9	Sidney & Shephard (unpublished)
45.3		29.2		Average, all studies
56.4	70.3	32.6	53.4	Young normal
80.3%		89.6%		Elderly, per cent of young normals

*   Data would be approximately 9.8 times larger if expressed in Newtons
[a]   Usually for dominant hand

synovial lining of the joint include an increase in the number of villi, a decrease in the vascularity of the underlying stroma (possibly secondary to a local atherosclerosis), and the occasional development of cartilaginous areas in the synovial membrane (Bennett *et al.*, 1942; Chung, 1966b).

Heredity, previous joint disease, trauma and metabolic diseases all accelerate the speed of joint degeneration. Nevertheless, aging of a joint can be distinguished from a pathological osteo-arthrosis only in terms of the severity of the changes that are observed. Kellgren & Lawrence (1957) found that 87 per cent of females and 83 per cent of males aged 55-64 years had radiographic changes that would be interpreted as osteo-arthrosis, although only 22 per cent of the women and 15 per cent of the men complained of any symptoms. The common features of the aging joint are loss of mobility and instability. Allman (1974) commented that the loss of flexibility was

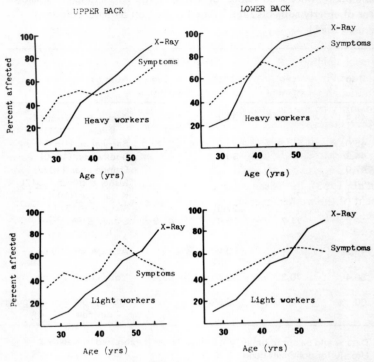

Figure 3.8   Symptoms and radiographic signs of vertebral disc degeneration in light and heavy workers. Based on the data of Hult (1954). Note (1) there is a progressive increase in the frequency of radiographic lesions with age, (2) the increase in radiographic lesions occurs somewhat earlier in the heavy workers, and they also experience a greater increase of symptoms with aging.

so consistent that its measurement provided one useful index of physiological age. Osteo-arthrosis of the upper limb leads to a painful restriction of movement, without much deformity. If the lower limbs are affected, there may be a serious impairment of gait. A lesion of the hip causes limping, with difficulty in climbing stairs, getting out of a bath and rising from a low chair. Involvement of the knee joint also causes difficulty in stair-climbing; the joint may stiffen after a period of immobility ('articular gelling'), and if full extension of the knee is lost it becomes impossible to lock the joint, with a resultant loss of stability.

Degenerative changes are also frequently encountered in the spine of an older person. Hult (1954) found a progressive increase in both the symptoms and radiographic signs of upper and lower back disorders over the span of working life (Figure 3.8). Spira (1970) studied 20 men with an average age of 69 years. X-ray examinations revealed a limitation of spinal movements in all of the group. Six of the men had scoliosis (curvature of the spine) and three kyphosis (hunchback), all with associated osteo-arthritic changes. The majority of the sample also had arthritic changes in the knee joint. Nevertheless, none of the group was complaining of back ache or of static pain in the knee joints. A third survey of men and women aged 65-74 years showed 87 per cent of males and 74 per cent of females with radiographic evidence of cervical disc degeneration (Lawrence *et al.*, 1963). In the same survey, 60 per cent of the men and 44 per cent of the women over the age of 35 years showed degeneration of the lumbar discs, the condition being particularly common in manual workers.

Tendons

Sprains, strains and muscle and tendon rupture are all too common complications of physical activity programmes for the elderly. In some studies, as many as 50 per cent of participants have been incapacitated by problems of this type (Kilböm *et al.*, 1969; Mann *et al.*, 1969). We encountered no more than one or two minor tendon pulls when we initiated a programme of progressive endurance training for a group of 42 men and women ranging in age from 60 to 83 years; these were readily resolved by a week or two of rest from the prescribed activity (Sidney & Shephard, 1977a). Our favourable experience reflects (1) a gradual progression of the required training, (2) the use of well-groomed natural turf as an exercise surface, and (3) an emphasis upon walking rather than jogging as the mode of conditioning. Nevertheless, we would agree with previous authors that the tendons of an older person are much more vulnerable to injury than those of a young adult.

Specific problems of the aging musculo-skeletal system include (1) greater muscle stiffness due to greater fatigue, (2) a less rapid relaxation of antagonist muscles, (3) loss of elastic tissue and alterations in the structure of the collagen molecule (Chapter 2), (4) loss of flexibility of the joints (Allman, 1974), and (5) a progressive decrease in the capillary blood supply to the tendon (Rothman & Parke, 1965). The last change is hard to distinguish from a parallel response to a reduction in habitual activity (Rothman & Slogoff, 1967);

it inevitably slows the healing of any micro-traumata.

Some authors have argued that the major tendons of the body do not rupture while they remain healthy. The tendo achilles, for example, can withstand a force of 1,000 kg (Burry, 1975). Nevertheless, it does rupture, typically in an older and heavier person (Ryan, 1974) who is in poor physical condition and suddenly resumes intensive training or takes up a vigorous sport such as squash (Klasen & Swiersta, 1971; S.W. Clarke, 1973). The lesion most commonly occurs in that part of the tendon where the blood flow is poorest, suggesting that the underlying pathology may be a subclinical ischaemic degeneration.

Aging may modify not only the tendon proper, but also its insertion into the bone. The cortex of the bone becomes thinner, and the marrow extends into the tendon through small fissures; subsequently, bone formation may occur in the proximal part of the tendon (Schaer, 1936; Schneider, 1959). It remains unclear whether the primary process in ossification is a pH change that favours the deposition of calcium salts (Schneider, 1959), or whether deposition of calcium salts leads to a secondary necrosis of the tendon (Selye, 1962). As with changes in the tendon proper, it is difficult to distinguish the intrinsic consequences of aging from the results of reduced activity and intercurrent disease. A careful study of tendon insertions at the lateral epicondyle of the elbow joint (Goldie, 1964) was unable to show either degenerative changes or calcification in those subjects under the age of 50 years who had never complained of painful elbows.

Cerebral Function

There is a vast literature on age-related changes in the function of the central nervous system (Walford & Birren, 1965; Burr, 1971; Brocklehurst, 1973). This section can do no more than highlight a few issues that are important to physical activity, including a deterioration of the sensory receptors, an alteration in the central processing of information, a loss of balance and an impairment in the performance of psychomotor tasks. We shall leave largely unanswered the question whether the observed loss of function is due to an intrinsic change of neural activity, or whether it is a secondary consequence of pathological processes such as atherosclerosis of the cerebral blood vessels.

Special Senses

1. Vision   Visual problems of the elderly include a progressive
reduction in the field of vision, a difficulty in focusing upon near
objects (lack of 'accommodation'), and a steady diminution in visual
acuity. A substantial minority of the total population reach the legal
definition of blindness; some 60 per cent of the blind are over the
age of 65 years.

Shrinkage of the visual field is partly mechanical in origin.
Drooping of the eyelid (senile ptosis) restricts vision in an upward
direction, while loss of fat from the socket (retro-orbital fat) gives
a sunken eyeball with limitation of vision in all directions. These
changes may be compounded by a pathological distortion and
injury of the retina associated with an increase of intra-ocular
pressure. An increase in the antero-posterior diameter of the lens
and a shrinkage in the dimensions of the anterior chamber of the
eye hamper the normal intra-ocular circulation of fluid. Pressures
within the eye capsule reach the high end of the normal range in an
increased proportion of supposedly normal individuals, and the
distinction between aging and the onset of a frankly pathological
'glaucoma' becomes difficult (Armaly, 1965).

The 'near point' at which print can first be brought into focus
increases from 10 cm at the age of 20 years to 18 cm at 40 years, 50
cm at 50 years and 100 cm at 70 years. Some (but not all) authors
have found a corresponding slowing in the rate of accommodation of
the eye (Weale, 1965). Loss of accommodation is due in part to
general changes in the structure of connective tissue; the capsule
of the lens suffers a loss of elasticity and it becomes set in a flat and
unaccommodated form (R.F. Fisher, 1969). At the same time, the
rigidity of the lens is increased by the continuous formation of new
fibres on its exterior. Recent studies with ultra-sound (Leighton, 1973)
have confirmed the increase in antero-posterior diameter, average
values rising from 3.8 mm at age 20 to 4.7 mm at age 60, and 5.2 mm
at age 80 years. Difficulties of refraction are compounded by (1) a
yellowing of the lens, with the progressive exclusion of blue light,
(2) the development of corneal astigmatism associated with the loss
of retro-orbital fat (Leighton, 1973) and (3) an increased scattering of
light within both the lens and the vitreous field of the eye.

The diameter of the pupil is greatly reduced in an old person, due
to rigidity and atrophy of the iris (Figure 3.7). Unfortunately, the
decrease in the amount of light admitted to the eye is proportional to
the square of any change in pupillary diameter. A second major reason

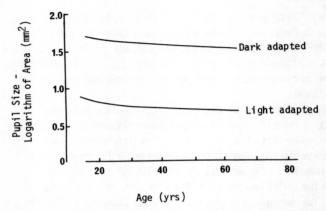

Figure 3.9   Influence of aging upon the area of the dark-adapted and the light-adapted pupil. Based on data of Leinhos (1959).

for deterioration in visual acuity is the change in optical properties of the crystalline lens. Increasing opacity is related to a reduction in its content of low molecular weight protein, due to either leakage through the capsule (Charlton & Van Heyningen, 1968) or conversion to an insoluble compound (Pirie, 1968). Opacities may also develop in the vitreous fluid, these being noted as misty floating objects ('floaters'). By the age of 60, the retina receives only one third as much white light as at the age of 20 years (Figure 3.10), while the penetration of blue light is reduced to a ninth of that in the young adult. Some authors have described a deterioration in function of the sensitive macular region of the retina, but most workers believe that the sensitivity of the retina is well preserved (Weale, 1965); certainly, the usual changes of visual acuity can be explained adequately in terms of changes in the pupil and lens.

Blindness naturally restricts movement, with loss of endurance fitness. The more minor visual problems also have practical consequences for the active individual. The need to wear glasses and the reduction of visual field are substantial handicaps for any older person who wishes to participate in sport. There may be difficulty in distinguishing colours, especially in poor light. Dark adaptation is slow, due to the reduction of retinal illumination rather than impairment in the resynthesis of the pigment visual purple; any activity thus becomes more difficult and more hazardous when performed in failing light. Weakness of one eye, a deterioration in function of the position-

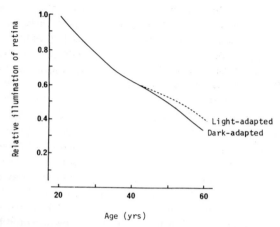

Figure 3.10   Influence of aging upon the relative amounts of light reaching the light-adapted and the dark-adapted retina. Based on data of Weale (1961).

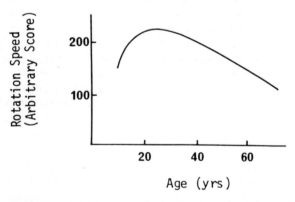

Figure 3.11   Changes in the speed of rotation of the 'blink-test' apparatus at which patterns can be recognised. Based on data of Fukui & Morioka (1971) for workers living in 'good conditions'.

sensing proprioceptors in the eye muscles and poor retinal focusing may give a loss of stereoscopic vision, with difficulty in judging the speed of moving objects. Above all, there is a loss of ability to distinguish fine detail.

One measure of overall perception and pattern recognition is provided by the 'blink' test of Fukui & Morioka (1971). Subjects attempt to recognise a rotating pattern by repeated rapid blinking. The speed of rotation of the display is slowed until recognition becomes possible; the score, measured in arbitrary units, is halved between 20 and 70 years of age (Figure 3.11).

2. *Hearing*   A multiplicity of changes conspire to reduce the auditory acuity of an older person. There is some loss of receptor nerve cells in the 'Organ of Corti', perhaps secondary to an atrophy of the associated vascular stria. The vibrating partition within the cochlea shows a progressive diminution in its elasticity, and there may also be some loss of neurons from the cochlea. A narrowing of the internal auditory canal may cause pressure on the main auditory nerve. The central processing of information may be impaired by a deterioration of function in the auditory (temporal) lobe of the cerebral cortex. Finally, the peripheral conduction of sound is hampered by a thickening and loss of elasticity in the ear drum (tympanic membrane), with a reduced efficiency of articulation in the small ossicles of the middle ear. The resultant changes of hearing include not only a loss of acuity, but also a derangement of loudness perception, a decline in discrimination, and a loss of time-related processing abilities (Fisch, 1973).

There is a progressive deterioration in the ability to detect pure tones at the upper end of the frequency spectrum (Figure 3.12). While it has been argued that much of the observed loss is due to excessive noise exposure over the life span, Hinchcliffe (1959a) has demonstrated that the changes occur in rural populations who presumably have been spared much of the noisy environment of the city dweller.

Under quiet conditions, an older person may have little difficulty in interpreting speech, but background noise or distortion of a voice by reverberation lead to frequent misinterpretation of words and sentences (Bergman, 1971). Difficulties might be anticipated when the pure tone loss affects the frequency band 1,000-3,000 Hz, but in practice older subjects show increasing discrepancies between their pure tone loss as measured on an audiometer and their capacity to understand normal conversation (Pestalozza & Shore, 1955). This may reflect a lengthening of the time needed for the central processing of information and a missing of some of the brief cues associated with the articulation of consonants. Auditory time

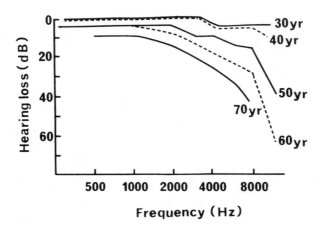

Figure 3.12   Increase of hearing loss with aging (after Hinchcliffe, 1959b).

discrimination (Weiss, 1959) and auditory reaction time (Feldman & Roger, 1967) show parallel impairment.

Many older people also develop a hypersensitivity to sound; attempts to communicate with them through an increase in the loudness of a conversation thus cause annoyance and even pain. There is increasing difficulty in detecting the direction from which a sound originates. This seems due to a deranged processing of time differences in the cues detected by the two ears (Matzker & Springborn, 1958) and a reduction of hearing (particularly if the latter is assymetric). Lastly, confusion may arise because of internally generated noise (tinnitus); complaints of this nature are seen in only 3 per cent of young adults, but in 11 per cent of those aged 65 to 74 years (US Dept. of Health, Education & Welfare, 1965).

Hinchcliffe (1959a) has set the prevalence of a pure tone loss $\geqslant$ 25 dB at 21 per cent of the rural population aged 65 to 74 years. The US HEW study (1965) found a 15 dB loss in 28 per cent of those aged 65 to 74 years, and 48 per cent of those aged 75 to 79 years. From the viewpoint of activity, the main consequence of such changes is a withdrawal of the older person from all types of social event. The crucial statistic is thus the prevalence of hearing difficulty. In the young adult, as few as 1.6 per cent of the population encounter problems (Wilkins, 1947). Estimates for the age of retirement are 12.2 per cent (Wilkins, 1947), 31 per cent (Sheldon, 1948), 39.5 per cent (Hobson

& Pemberton, 1955), and 31.5 per cent (A. Harris, 1962). At the age of 80 and above, more than 50 per cent of the population have hearing difficulties (Lempert, 1958).

Central Processing and Psychomotor Performance

Elderly people perform most tasks less quickly than a young adult. In theory, the delay could arise at any point between the detection of the signal by the receptor and execution of an appropriate response by the peripheral muscle, but most authors believe that the main responsibility for the slowing of response rests with mechanisms for the central processing of information (Botwinik, 1965).

We have noted already that diminished illumination of the retina in an old person does not usually influence the reaction time to a simple visual signal (although it could conceivably hamper recognition of a more complex visual cue, Welford, 1965). Likewise, changes in peripheral nerve conduction velocity are insufficient to account for more than a 4 per cent increase of reaction time (Norris *et al.*, 1953b; Birren & Botwinik, 1955) although the impact of a given stimulus upon the brain may be weakened through a greater temporal dispersion in the central presentation of the information (Welford, 1965).

1. Basis of altered brain function   The prime cause of the alteration in central processing is presumably a progressive death of neurons, although viable cells may also perform more poorly due to a loss of chromidial substance and an accumulation of pigment granules (Birren, 1965). The problem can be envisaged in terms of a deterioration in signal/noise ratio for the system. A reduction in the number of functional nerve cells attenuates the signal strength, and gives less 'smoothing' of occasional aberrant signals. At the same time, noise may be increased by random neural activity (the example of tinnitus has been discussed above), or the long persistence of signals within the brain. It is arguable that the slow response of the elderly is an attempt to compensate for the poor signal/noise ratio, freshly acquired information being melded with the persistent signal until its strength is sufficient to be distinguished from background noise.

The long-term memory of the aged may be better than in a young person. Thus Birren *et al.* (1963) found that men over the age of 65 years had higher scores than adults between the ages of 25 and 34 years on tests requiring a knowledge of words. On the other hand, the short-term memory deteriorates, so that the person over 65 years of age has difficulty in recalling six digits, compared with seven digits in the young adult (Birren *et al.*, 1963). The brain is also less adaptable than in a young person, and it finds difficulty in switching from one piece of information to another and back again (Broadbent & Heron, 1962).

Increase of noise and loss of neurons decreases the 'channel capacity' of the brain. It becomes difficult to handle several pieces of information simultaneously, and the system is more easily overloaded. The level of sensory input (degree of arousal) needed for optimum performance is thus lower in the elderly than in a young person. Unfortunately, there is lack of agreement on levels of arousal in the aged. Both York (1962) and Griew & Davies (1962) found no differences of vigilance between young and older subjects, although they suspected that the older subjects may have tried harder to perform well. Shmavonian *et al.* (1965) found that some peripheral indices of arousal (skin blood flow and galvanic resistance) were higher in young than in elderly subjects; however, it could be argued that the responses of the elderly were modified by secondary pathologies such as arteriosclerosis and a disruption of sweat gland function. On the other hand, the elderly produced more catecholamines than the young, both at rest and during exercise, while their fast electro-encephalographic (e.e.g.) activity was greater for a given task; if this evidence of greater arousal in the elderly, it may reflect the fact that they find most psychomotor tasks more difficult to perform. Some authors have suggested that the fast e.e.g. activity in fact reflects habituation to a task rather than arousal. Obrist (1965) remarked upon an association between the appearance of slow brain potentials and a slowing of the reaction time. The electrical activity of the brain in an older person is marked by a slowing of the dominant alpha rhythm, with an increase in both theta (4-7 Hz) and delta (1-3 Hz) activity. Nevertheless, if the old person is in good health, differences of e.e.g. relative to a younger adult are quite small.

In addition to the overall changes of cerebral function, more local cellular losses are found in such regions of the brain as the basal nuclei and the pallidum (Hassler, 1965). Disturbance of function in these regions of the brain can cause emotional problems, loss of co-ordination (ataxia) and various forms of tremor associated with over-activity of the extra-pyramidal nerve fibres.

2. Functional consequences   It is quite difficult to measure the functional consequences of any alterations in central processing

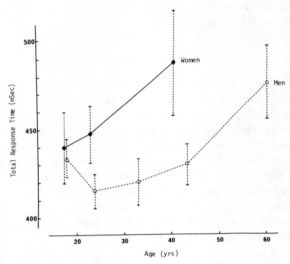

Figure 3.13   Total response time for operation of car brake in reaction to a red signal light (mean ± S.D.). Based on data of Weight & Shephard (1978).

capacity, since old people may have either a very high level of motivation or a wish to 'act' the part of a senior citizen. Some fail to make an all-out attempt at an experimental task, while others hide considerable disability by virtue of additional experience and effort (Murrell & Griew, 1965; Davies & Griew, 1965).

Problems of memory (Inglis, 1965) diminish the ability to develop new skills and concepts (Brinley, 1965); the capacity to tackle sequential tasks is impaired more than the ability to handle spatial problems (Talland, 1961). Perceptual tasks such as the identification of designs and patterns takes much longer in the aged (Wallace, 1956). Any errors tend to be made repeatedly (perseveration), due perhaps to the persistence of 'after-traces' of information in the brain.

Jalavisto (1965) carried out a factor analysis on data obtained from a wide variety of psychomotor tasks, including the memory for geometric figures, tapping rate, reaction time, critical flicker fusion, number reversing and abstracting ability. An 'age' factor was extracted, and tasks involving the element of speed showed the closest correlations with this factor.

Much of the published research has concerned reaction times and movement times (Figures 3.13, 3.14). These are substantially slower in older individuals (Stelmach & Diewert, 1977). Birren *et al.* (1963)

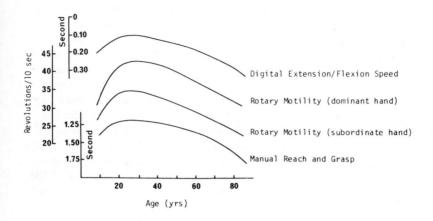

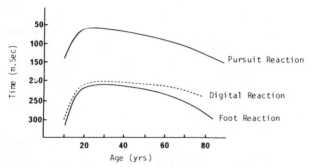

Figure 3.14   Changes in movement time (upper panel) and reaction time (lower panel) with aging. Based on data of Miles (1942).

found that the time needed to press a key in response to a musical note increased from 0.18 seconds in a young adult to 0.22 seconds in those over the age of 65 years. More complex responses, such as the movement of the foot from the accelerator to the brake pedal in response to a red signal light (Figure 3.13), show a greater deterioration. The time required for many simple sensory motor tasks increases 50 per cent between the ages of 20 and 65 years (Welford, 1965). Szafran (1965) suggested that the reaction time T_r was given by

$$T_r = a + b \log (n)$$

where a and b were constants, and n was the number of choices required of the subject. If the signal is brief, aging increases the intercept a; this seems an attempt to compensate for 'noise' in the system. Under conditions of information overload, the slope b may also be augmented; this reflects the restricted channel capacity of the elderly, and their difficulty in using short-term memory where necessary. The form of the aging curve for total reaction time differs between men and women (Henry, 1961; Hodgkins, 1963; Wright & Shephard, 1978). This has been attributed to the more strongly developed competitive sense of the male (Hodgkins, 1963), although in the specific instance of braking response (Figure 3.13) a greater experience in the operation of motor vehicles may also be a contributory factor (Wright & Shephard, 1978).

The effects of aging are particularly marked when the subject must discriminate, or choose between several alternatives. We have noted already the discrepancy between pure-tone hearing loss and the ability to understand conversation. Rabbit (1964) looked at card sorting ability, and found that the response of his subjects (aged 68-82 years) was sensitive to the number of types of card they had to separate; sorting into two piles took up to 50 per cent longer than in a young adult, but sorting into four piles took 100 per cent longer. Rabbit (1965) concluded the elderly (1) had difficulty learning which cues were critical to discrimination, and (2) were unable to ignore irrelevancy in a display. This implied problems in (1) forming and retaining sets, (2) integrating sensory information and (3) forming appropriate generalisations from the sensory input.

In an attempt to optimise their remaining capacities, the emphasis of the elderly typically shifts from speed to accuracy of performance (Welford, 1965). Less important details of the task are omitted, and there is an increased reliance on previously developed routines of problem solving. Difficulty is encountered particularly if the presentation of a given task does not conform to an existing 'set'.

In terms of overall athletic performance (Lehman, 1951; Shephard, 1977c), the optimum age varies with the relative importance of strength and skill. Events that make strenuous physical demands are performed best in the early twenties, but in competitions where experience plays a major role the top competitors are in their late twenties or early thirties. Probably because of economic pressures, the age of optimum attainment is also higher for professional than for amateur competitors.

Table 3.22   Median age of US Olympic contestants 1920-36
(collected by Lehman, 1951)

Event	Median age (yrs)
Swimming (women)	19.2
Swimming (men)	22.3
Boxing	21.2
Lacrosse	21.5
Cycling	21.6
Baseball	22.5
Handball	22.5
Hurdles	23.0
Rowing	23.4
Races up to 5,000 metres	23.5
Discus and throwing events	23.5
Wrestling	23.7
Field hockey	23.9
Weight-lifting	24.6
Steeple chase (3,000 metres)	25.0
Gymnastics	25.5
Ice hockey	25.5
Speed skating	26.0
Basketball	26.3
Association football	26.3
Figure skating	27.3
Yachting	27.8
Fencing	28.0
Skiing	28.2
10,000 metres & marathon	31.5
Bob-sledding	34.3
Equestrian events	36.4

3. Perception of effort   Despite low daily heart rates (Chapter 4)
and maximum oxygen intake readings, many old people regard
themselves as quite active (Sidney & Shephard, 1977a). One possible
explanation of this paradox might be an altered perception of
physical activity by the elderly, mild effort being sensed as vigorous
or even exhausting work. Borg (1962; 1971) developed a convenient
psycho-physical scale for the rating of perceived effort (RPE). When
this tool was applied to a mixed population, ranging in age from 18 to
79 years, the heart rate needed to attain a given RPE during bicycle
ergometer work showed a progressive decline from the young to the
elderly (Borg & Linderholm, 1967). The change ran parallel with the

decrease of maximum heart rate, so that the RPE maintained a rather constant relationship to relative stress (percentage of maximum oxygen intake). Sidney & Shephard (1977c) had similar findings during treadmill exercise. At any given work load, the RPE was greater in women than in men, and greater in the elderly than in the young. However, all data fell on very comparable regression lines when RPE was correlated with effort expressed as a percentage of maximum oxygen intake (Figure 3.16). The subjects of Sidney & Shephard (1977c) underwent a 34-week period of endurance training. This substantially reduced heart rates at a given treadmill speed and slope, but there was little change in the associated RPE.

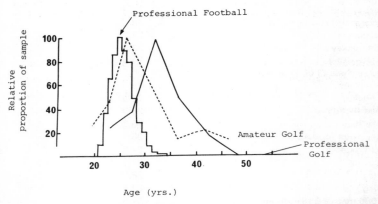

Figure 3.15   Age of 1,630 players of American football, and age on winning amateur and professional golf championships (after Lehman, 1951).

Suggested cues for the rating of exertion (Kay & Shephard, 1969; Ekblöm & Goldbarg, 1971; Kilböm, 1971; Noble *et al.*, 1973a,b) have included the respiratory minute volume, the breathing frequency, the skin temperature, the blood lactate level, and feelings of strain in the working muscles, tendons and joints. Mood state also has a marked effect on the RPE that is reported (W.P. Morgan, 1973). Many of these mechanisms would be expected to increase the perception of a given sub-maximum effort in the elderly. Ventilation is a larger fraction of the maximum voluntary ventilation, the breathing frequency is higher, blood lactate concentrations are greater, and the tension per unit cross-section is higher in the atrophied muscles. What is more surprising is the absence of change in the RPE when the elderly subjects

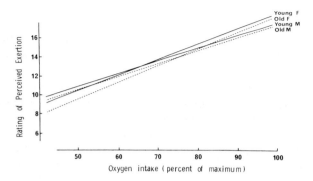

Figure 3.16   Rating of perceived exertion (Borg scale) and effort (expressed as a percentage of maximum oxygen intake). Based on data of Sidney & Shephard (1977b).

undergo conditioning, this despite evidence of improvements in mood (Sidney & Shephard, 1977a), an increase of aerobic power and muscle mass, and a loss of subcutaneous fat. One possible explanation is that with the loss of superficial fat, the skin temperature becomes higher, since it approximates more closely to core temperature; as the body senses the higher skin temperature, it concludes it is working harder. Certainly, in young adults physical training leads to a decrease of RPE at a given work load, although it does not alter perceived effort at a fixed percentage of maximum oxygen intake (Ekblöm & Goldbarg, 1971).

4. Prevention of central changes   As with other aspects of aging, there have been occasional unconfirmed reports claiming that changes in the central nervous system could be slowed or halted by specific forms of therapy. In the context of physical activity, Vogt & Vogt (1946) suggested that the involution of nerve cells could be delayed by a sufficient excess of activity to cause their hypertrophy. Retzlaff & Fontaine (1965) also reported that suitable controlled exercise could increase both the integrative activity of spinal motor neurons and nerve conduction velocity. Lastly, Inglis (1965) argued that the memory deficits of the elderly were due in part to overactivity of the enzyme ribonuclease; symptoms could thus be ameliorated by the oral or intravenous administration of ribonucleic acid. Despite such reports, it seems fair to conclude that no real cure has yet been discovered for age-related changes in the function of the central nervous system.

Balance and Falls

Older subjects not only fall rather frequently, but also suffer an appreciable morbidity and mortality as a result of such falls. In one random sample of the elderly, Sheldon (1948) found that 21 per cent of men and 43 per cent of women were affected. These figures have been confirmed in a recent survey of people aged 65 years and over who were living at home; 24 per cent of the men and 44 per cent of the women gave a history of falls, the proportion increasing with age (Exton-Smith, 1977).

The commonest cause of falling (Overstall *et al.*, 1977) is to trip over some obstacle (Table 3.23). While both young and old may stumble, the likelihood of a fall is increased in the elderly, because of poor eyesight, a reduced leg-lift when walking (Sheldon, 1960) and greater difficulty in restoring balance once stumbling has occurred. Loss of cells in the brain stem and the cerebellum plus a diminution of peripheral proprioceptor function limit the capacity for precise control of body movements, including the correction of externally imposed forces. One simple measure of balance is the postural sway that develops while standing with the feet comfortably apart looking at a distant object. Overstall *et al.* (1977) found that such sway reached a minimum in the teen years, and thereafter increased progressively (Figure 3.17). Women showed more body sway than men at all ages, certainly because of a poorer body weight/ muscle mass ratio, and possibly also because they obtained less ankle support from their shoes. Those subjects who had sustained five or more falls in the previous year had significantly more sway than those who reported none or one to four falls.

Causes other than tripping are responsible for an increased proportion of falls in those over 75 years of age (Exton-Smith, 1977). A variety of medications (night sedatives, anti-hypertensives, diuretics, phenothiazines and benzodiazepines) are likely to impair balance. Postural hypotension is seen in 15 to 24 per cent of elderly subjects (Caird *et al.*, 1973; Overstall *et al.*, 1977), although not all of those affected fall after rising. A proportion of the elderly are liable to 'drop attacks' (Sheldon, 1960), precipitated by turning or extension of the neck; the pathology in such cases seems a restriction of vertebral arterial flow, secondary to a kinking and tortuosity of the vertebral artery that follows degeneration of the intervertebral discs in the cervical region. In the 'subclavian steal' syndrome, flow in the vertebral artery is reversed to compensate for narrowing or occlusion of the first part of the subclavian artery; the problem may be initiated

Table 3.23   Cause of falls in 146 elderly subjects (Overstall *et al.*, 1977)

Tripping	81	(47.1%)
Drop attacks	21	(12.2%)
Giddiness	15	(8.7%)
Loss of balance	14	(8.2%)
After rising	11	(6.4%)
Turning head	9	(5.2%)
Miscellaneous	21	(12.2%)

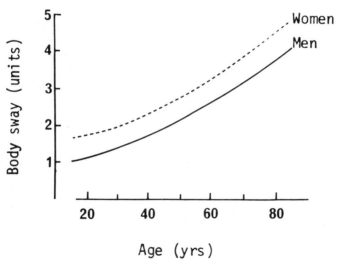

Figure 3.17   Influence of age upon body sway. Subjects standing with their feet comfortably apart looking at a distant object. Based on data of Overstall *et al.* (1977).

acutely by exercising the arm on the affected side of the body. Other causes of a brief loss of consciousness include syncope induced by a prolonged bout of coughing or urinary straining, various cardiac disorders (heart block, dysrhythmias, paroxysms of tachycardia and narrowing of the aortic orifice), epilepsy, anaemia and hypotension associated with Parkinson's disease.

Hormonal Function

Aging is marked by a deterioration not only in the function of individual cells and organs, but also by a failure of mechanisms for the co-ordination of function between various parts of the body. A weakening of both neural and hormonal controls reduces the ability of the body to adjust to external and internal stresses (Chapter 1). Some examples of central nervous impairment have already been noted, for instance the problems of postural hypotension and lack of balance. In this section, we shall review the scant evidence bearing on aging and the hormones concerned with adjustment to vigorous physical activity.

Among other responsibilities, the body hormones contribute to (1) regulation of circulating fluid volumes and cardio-vascular performance, (2) mobilisation of fuels for exercise (the breakdown of protein, gluconeogenesis; maintenance of blood glucose by breakdown of liver glycogen; liberation of depot fat) and (3) the synthesis of new protein (anabolism) in response to appropriate patterns of training.

Insulin Secretion

Anaerobic activity demands the availability of glucose. This is normally derived from intramuscular and hepatic glycogen, and insulin plays a key role in both the control of blood sugar and the promotion of glycogen storage. The biochemical mechanism involves a facilitation of the enzyme hexokinase:

$$\text{Glucose} \xrightarrow[\text{hexokinase}]{\text{Insulin}} \text{Glucose-6-phosphate} \longrightarrow \text{Glycogen}$$

Exercise apparently has no acute effect on the rate of insulin secretion (Nikkila *et al.*, 1970); however, the glucose disappearance rate is accelerated, probably because the blood flow to the muscles is increased by the activity.

Age is one of the most obvious factors predisposing to clinical diabetes (Figure 3.18), and by the age of 70 years some 20 per cent of men and 30 per cent of women show an abnormal glucose tolerance curve. Nevertheless, in the remainder of the population the secretory cells concerned (the Islets of Langerhans) maintain a normal functional capacity, with blood glucose readings of less than 120 mg/100 ml (6.7 mM/l) following a meal (Caird, 1972).

A poor glucose tolerance and frank diabetes are commonly

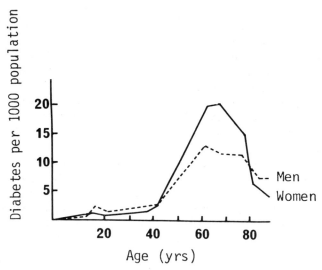

Figure 3.18 Relative incidence of newly diagnosed cases of diabetes. Based on data of Fitzgerald *et al.* (1961).

associated with obesity. Control of both problems by a low carbohydrate diet is not always very effective in the elderly, due to poverty and a lack of interest in alternative forms of food. If the obesity can be corrected through a combination of graded exercise and caloric restriction, then the need for insulin may be reduced or even avoided.

Thyroid Hormone

The thyroid hormone weakens the coupling between metabolic reactions and muscle contraction; for a given breakdown of foodstuffs, more energy is 'wasted', with a corresponding increase in body heat production. Other effects of the thyroid hormone are to increase the contractility of cardiac muscle (R.R. Taylor *et al.*, 1969), to enhance the utilisation of liver cholesterol and to mobilise free fatty acids from adipose tissue (Paul, 1971).

Studies in rats (Karenchevsky, 1961) and man (McGavak, 1951) have indicated an atrophy of the thyroid gland with age. A conflicting report (Mortensen *et al.*, 1955) has been criticised on the basis that the subjects concerned were drawn from an area of the United States where goitre was endemic (Irvine, 1973). Measurements of thyroxin turnover suggest that the production of thyroid hormone decreases by 50 per cent between the ages of 20 and 80 years (Gregerman *et al.*, 1962). Basal oxygen consumption also diminishes, but not if the data is expressed per gram of lean body mass (Chapter 2).

Androgenic Hormones

Androgenic hormones are secreted by the interstitial cells of the testes (in the male) and by the adrenal cortex (in both sexes). In addition to specific effects on growth of the secondary sex organs, the androgens have a general anabolic effect, bringing about an increase of protein synthesis, storage of glycogen and retention of water.

Sutton *et al.* (1973) found an increase of androgen levels 20-90 minutes following maximum activity, but Lamb (1975) observed no change when less well trained subjects were exercised to exhaustion. Sonka *et al.* (1972) noted that exercise nullified the fall of plasma androsterone that was seen in women who dieted but did not exercise; this would have obvious implications for the preservation of lean tissue during weight reduction.

Many of the published reports have been written in the context of the illegal use of testosterone analogues by top-level athletes (Lamb, 1975). The production of testosterone in the young adult is probably adequate for the needs of the body, and in view of pituitary feedback mechanisms that regulate the total level of androgens in the blood stream, it is very doubtful whether atheletes can increase either lean body mass or muscle strength by self-administration of androgenic drugs. In older subjects, a decline of testicular function provides more rationale for such treatment, and androgens are sometimes prescribed to correct muscle wasting and senile osteoporosis. Simonson *et al.* (1944) reported an increase of both strength and endurance when 48- to 67-year-old subjects were given a daily course of methyl testosterone, and Hettinger (1961) found significant increases of both strength and physical working capacity when 65- to 70-year-old men were given testosterone injections.

Sympatho-Adrenal Activity

Vigorous physical activity is associated with an increased output of epinephrine from the adrenal medulla, and of nor-epinephrine derived largely from the sympathetic nerves regulating the circulatory system (Von Euler, 1974). Specific functions of the catecholamines include (1) the maintenance of systemic blood pressure, (2) the mobilisation of muscle (and to a lesser extent liver) glycogen to sustain plasma glucose levels, (3) the liberation of fatty acids from depot fat,

(4) the stimulation of gluconeogenesis in the liver, (5) the stimulation of glucagon secretion and (6) the inhibition of insulin secretion. Little is known about the aging of these various mechanisms. Some early reports (M.R.P.Hall, 1973) indicated a decreased urinary excretion of catecholamines in the elderly. However, R.H. Fischer (1971) found no change in urinary excretion of the catecholamine metabolite 4-hydroxy 3-methoxy mandelic acid (vanil-mandelic acid) in 50 elderly men and women ranging in age from 69 to 96 years.

Adrenal Cortex

The adrenal cortex synthesises glucose and mineral regulating steroids, along with smaller quantities of several sex hormones (androgens, oestrogens and progesterone). Information relating to aging and physical activity is restricted largely to data on blood levels of the gluco-corticoid cortisol (hydrocortisone).

Cortisol increases the rate of tissue breakdown (catabolism). The bones show a reduction in their matrix and an increased calcium loss. In the muscles, glucose uptake is inhibited, carbohydrate utilisation is depressed, and there is an increased loss of amino acids. The lipolysis of depot fat is augmented, and the development of a general stress reaction is suggested by suppression of immune reactions, a decrease in the number of eosinophils in the blood and the involution of the thymus gland.

The influence of exercise on cortisol levels has been reviewed by Shephard & Sidney (1975). Brief periods of moderate exercise yield unchanged or reduced cortisol readings. However, exhausting exercise leads to an increase of plasma cortisol, particularly if the task is perceived as emotionally stressful. Endurance training modifies the response mainly in the sense that it makes a given work load less stressful. If exercise is performed at the same percentage of maximum oxygen intake, responses are essentially similar in young and elderly subjects (Figure 3.19); however, if a fixed work-load is adopted, the elderly may reach a level of stress where cortisol production is stimulated while younger individuals yet show no response.

Pituitary Gland

1. General considerations The pituitary gland plays an important part in metabolic regulation, not only through the secretion of its own active products such as growth hormone, but also by stimulating the secretions of other glands such as the thyroid and the adrenal cortex. Morphological changes with age include a diffuse fibrosis, a loss of

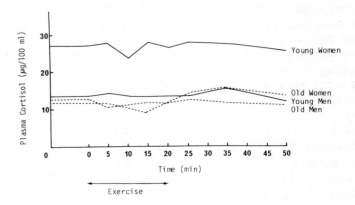

Figure 3.19   Responses of young and elderly subjects to treadmill exercise (four five minute stages of increasing intensity, final stage about 85 per cent of maximum oxygen intake). Data of Sidney & Shephard (1978b).

basophilic cells and an increased likelihood of adenoma formation (Fazekas & Jobba, 1970; Costello, 1936). Nevertheless, overall function seems well preserved, and a normal 17-hydroxycorticosteroid response to an insulin induced fall of blood sugar is seen in subjects aged 82 to 95 years (Cartlidge *et al.*, 1970).

2. Growth hormone secretion   The most important metabolic function of growth hormone is the regulation of tissue building (anabolism). The metabolic activity of the long bones is stimulated, and the muscles show an increased uptake of amino acids with an increased synthesis of protein. After a lag period of about one hour, fat is liberated from adipose tissue; the growth hormone promotes the synthesis of an inactive lipolytic enzyme, and this is subsequently activated by the compound cyclic adenosine monophosphate. The effects of insulin are counteracted, either directly or indirectly, and plasma levels of glucose and non-esterified fatty acids both rise. Liver glycogen stores are also increased, possibly through a stimulation of gluconeogenesis.

Brief moderate exercise may produce no increase of growth hormone levels in a healthy, well-trained young man (Shephard & Sidney, 1975). A response is more likely if the subject is (1) anxious, (2) unfit, or (3) a woman. Changes are also more marked if effort is sustained long enough to deplete muscle glycogen reserves, although very sustained effort may lead to a secondary decrease of growth hormone concentrations. Intense effort almost always increases growth hormone levels, although there is an initial lag period of at least ten minutes. If the intense activity is maintained, a secondary decrease of growth hormone concentrations can occur. Gains of fitness through an endurance training programme may reduce the growth hormone response to exercise, although at the same time eliminating the secondary decline in response associated with very prolonged activity.

Basal levels of growth hormone change very little from childhood to old age (Frantz & Rabkin, 1965; Glick *et al.*, 1965; Cartlidge *et al.*, 1970). Despite occasional contrary reports (Buckler, 1969; Laron *et al.*, 1970) most authors also find a normal response of the elderly hypothalamus and pituitary gland to a decrease of blood sugar (hypoglycaemia) or glucose loading (Danowski *et al.*, 1969; Root & Oski, 1969; Cartlidge *et al.*, 1970; Sacher *et al.*, 1971. Kalk *et al.*, 1973). Sidney & Shephard (1978b) observed an increase of plasma growth hormone concentrations in response to moderate exercise when elderly subjects of both sexes walked on the treadmill for twenty minutes (Figure 3.20). The response of the men was more marked than in their group of young adults, but was typical of many previously published reports for younger subjects (Shephard & Sidney, 1975). Interpretation of any age difference is complicated by the likelihood that younger subjects are fitter and have a higher level of habitual activity. It could be argued that because of lack of fitness, older subjects experience more stress, even when exercised at the same percentage of their maximum aerobic power. However, Sidney & Shephard (1978b) rejected differences of stress as an explanation of their findings, since no correlation was found between the maximum oxygen intake of the elderly subjects and the extent of their growth hormone response to a standard exercise test; further, the absence of any increase in cortisol secretion (Figure 3.19) suggests that the experience was not particularly stressful to them.

Contrary to findings in younger subjects, Sidney & Shephard (1978b) found that training augmented the exercise-induced increase of growth hormone concentrations in the elderly. The normal function of the hormone is to serve as a 'biochemical amplifier', enhancing the work-induced synthesis of muscle protein (A.L. Goldberg, 1967; A.L. Goldberg & Goldman, 1967). Larger quantities of growth hormone may be needed for this purpose in an older person. Not only is there an age-related decline in the availability of androgens, but small muscle glycogen reserves and a poor peripheral

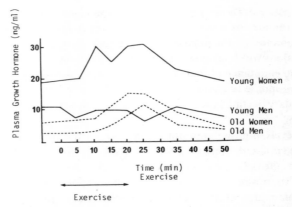

Figure 3.20   Plasma growth hormone levels of young and elderly subjects during four five minute stages of progressive treadmill exercise. Final loading approximately 85 per cent of maximum oxygen intake. Based on data of Sidney & Shephard, 1978b).

circulation may force the body to use protein as a fuel during exercise. By enhancing the release of depot fat, the growth hormone helps conserve glycogen and reduces protein breakdown during exercise. Practical support for these concepts can be found in the response of Sidney & Shephard's subjects to the conditioning programme. Over the year of endurance training, there was a substantial mobilisation of depot fat (skinfold readings decreased by an average of 3 mm) and at the same time there was a substantial increase of lean body mass (Chapter 5). A recent cross-sectional experiment of Szanto (1975) also supports the view that physical activity can alter the responsiveness of the pituitary. Szanto compared the response to glucose loading in active and sedentary old men; growth hormone concentrations were depressed in both groups immediately after the glucose had been administered, but the recovery of previous concentrations was much slower in the sedentary than in the active group.

Limitations of Data

In concluding our brief review of hormonal function, it must be stressed that almost all of the information cited refers to blood concentrations of the compounds concerned. Perplexing anomalies in existing reports may be resolved by studies that distinguish secretion from changes in excretion and breakdown of the hormone, that examine binding in the blood stream, differential delivery to the target organs and altered responsiveness at the receptor sites. Already, there are indications that the peripheral response to growth hormone may be reduced by aging (Root & Oski, 1969; Timiras, 1972), and many of the other variables we have just listed could upset the apparently simple relationship between hormone secretion, a rise of blood concentration and an effector response.

Sexual Activity

The sexual interest and potency of the male decline gradually from adolescence (Kinsey *et al.*, 1948; Stokes, 1951; Finckle, 1959; Newman & Nichols, 1960; Rubin, 1966; Post, 1967); however, as Kinsey has stressed, 'there is no point at which old age suddenly enters the picture'. Morning erections of the penis provide one indication of the preservation of physical potency; these still averaged 0.9 per week in the 75-year-old men studied by Kinsey *et al.* (1948), although in many instances intercourse had ceased. The same laboratory questioned 56 women over the age of 60 years, and found no evidence of a decline in sexual arousability (Kinsey *et al.*, 1953); if anything, responsiveness of the older women was increased. Newman & Nichols (1960) studied 250 subjects aged 60 to 93 years. Among the 149 who were still married and living with their spouses, 54 per cent claimed to be continuing a regular sexual relationship; 60 per cent of those under the age of 75 and 25 per cent of those over this age still engaged in intercourse. In contrast, only 7 per cent of the single, widowed or divorced subjects admitted finding opportunity for intercourse, although Dickinson & Beam (1931) noted that all of 11 widowed women aged 60 to 80 years engaged in regular masturbation. In the material of Kinsey *et al.* (1948, 1953), the oldest sexually active couple was a man aged 88 and his wife aged 90 years.

All studies agree that the early cessation of sexual activity is likely in persons with a low initial sex drive or high inhibitions. On the other hand, responsive and vigorous subjects may continue with sexual activity to an advanced age. Kinsey attributed waning function to both physiological and psychological factors: 'the decline in sexual activity of the older male is partly and perhaps primarily the result of a general decline in physical and physiologic capacity. It is undoubtedly affected by psychologic fatigue, a loss of interest in repetition of the same sort of experience . . .' In a young person, the physiological demands of sexual intercourse can be quite high; heart rates may reach 170/min, and blood pressures of 250/120 mm Hg (33/16 kPa) have been recorded (Boas & Goldschmidt, 1932; Klumbies & Kleinsorge,

1930; Bartlett & Bohr, 1956). However, in the senior citizen who has been married for many years, the response is much less dramatic, and the heart rate may only reach 120/min for 10 to 15 seconds (Hellerstein & Friedman, 1969; Zohman & Tobis, 1970; Kavanagh & Shephard, 1977a); it is hard to believe that such demands fall outside the capacity of the average older person. Nor can testicular atrophy offer a convincing explanation of functional loss. Stokes (1951), commenting on the uselessness of testosterone therapy, pointed out that only about one of twenty men castrated for prostatic carcinoma developed eunuchoid changes, and that in the majority of patients the adrenal cortex continued to produce sufficient androgens to maintain normal sexual function. Psychological factors are probably more important. Kinsey *et al.* (1948) remarked on older men whose frequency of orgasm had dropped materially 'until they met new partners, adopted new sexual techniques, or embraced new sources of outlet'. Stokes (1951) was intrigued by the discrepancy between morning erections and intercourse, and concluded that in many individuals unconscious fears caused them to abandon sexual activity long before their physiological potency had disappeared.

In many instances, the precipitating cause of a cessation of intercourse is widowing or ill health. Kavanagh & Shephard (1977a) examined the latter problem in the context of the patient with myocardial infarction. In about a half of their series of patients (81/161), the frequency of sexual intercourse was reduced after the 'heart attack'; 26 of the 161 also found less pleasure in the sex act, usually because it provoked extra systoles or anginal pain. Reasons cited for the diminished frequency of intercourse included personal apprehension (17/81), apprehension of the spouse (19/81), loss of desire (30/81) and a combination of these several factors (15/81). Interestingly, it did not seem an advantage to recommend an unfamiliar and physically less demanding sexual position such as side-lying; only 29 of the 161 patients had tried a more passive technique, and whether cause or effect, sexual activity had declined in all of these 29 subjects.

It is hard to assess the importance of continued sexual activity to the well-being of the elderly. However, Kavanagh & Shephard (1977a) questioned the wives of the 'post-coronary' patients, and found some evidence that loss of sexual capacity was associated with neuroticism, depression, unwillingness to assume responsibility and a deterioration in the overall quality of life. Unfortunately, it is difficult to determine from such a study whether the adverse findings are directly attributable to the loss of sexual function, or whether they are a consequence of failure to recover from the underlying 'heart attack'.

4   ACTIVITY PATTERNS OF THE ELDERLY

Many cultures decree that the habitual activity of a person should diminish as he becomes older. At retirement, Western man is expected to 'slow down' and 'enjoy a well-earned rest'. Equally, in many 'primitive' societies, young and middle-aged adults assume the responsibility of hunting and gathering not only for their children but also for aging parents. This chapter will make an objective assessment of activity patterns in the elderly. Findings will be correlated with attitudes towards physical activity. The impact of retirement, hospital admission and institutional care will be examined, and implications for diet and nutrition will be explored.

Current Levels of Physical Activity

Techniques of Measurement

Principles for the measurement of habitual activity are much as in a younger person (Shephard, 1977d). Information may be obtained by retrospective questionnaires and interviews, the subject may be observed, a prospective diary may be kept, heart rates may be measured for extended periods, oxygen consumption may be determined by a portable respirometer or the food intake may be recorded.

In practice, most techniques are more difficult to apply to the elderly than to a young adult. The use of a retrospective questionnaire is hampered by weakness of recent memory, poor eyesight, arthritic hands and often an intolerance of complex forms. The attempts of an interviewer to verify dubious entries may founder due to a faulty hearing aid or garrulous responses to simple questions. A prospective record of actual activities may be kept badly due to difficulty in understanding and remembering instructions, failing eyesight and deteriorating handwriting. Unless a group of subjects are living together in an institution, the cost of direct observation of movement patterns is usually prohibitive. Problems are also encountered if attempts are made to record physiological indices such as the heart rate. Pendulous skinfolds may cause electrodes to become detached long before the intended 24-hour record has been completed. Furthermore, the correlation between heart rate and

146

activity is less clear cut than in a younger person. Much of the day is
spent at very low rates of energy expenditure, where the relationship
between heart rate and oxygen consumption lacks linearity and can
be greatly distorted by extraneous factors such as anxiety and a high
room temperature. Other difficulties of interpretation include an
increase of heart rate at a given work-load due to weakness of the
musculature, an increase of heart rate at high work-loads due to a
decline of stroke volume (Figure 3.3 above), and in some instances a
frank dysrhythmia. Measurements of oxygen consumption by the
Kofranyi Michaelis respirometer cannot be generalised from one old
person to another, since there is a varying deterioration of mechanical
efficiency (Chapter 3), and often an increase of energy expenditure
due to specific disabilities. Dietary recall suffers from the same
difficulties as other forms of interview and retrospective questioning.

Energy Expenditures

Overall levels of energy expenditure are probably important to the
control of body weight, and may also have an impact on the risk of
subsequent coronary disease. Some factors such as an increase of
body weight and a decrease of mechanical efficiency increase the
energy expenditure of an old person for a given level of physical
activity. Added costs of movement are particularly likely where a
disease process such as arthritis, hemiplegia, limb deformity or amputation specifically handicaps movement (Bard, 1963; Hirschberg &
Ralston, 1965; Molbech, 1966; Müller & Hettinger, 1952). However,
these same handicaps generally make a person less active, and the
overall trend of energy expenditures is thus in a downward direction.
The World Health Organisation sets the average energy needs of 20- to
39-year-old subjects at 3,000 kcal/day for men and 2,200 kcal/day
for women; however, the corresponding figures for 60- to 69-year-
old individuals are 2,400 kcal/day for men and 1,700 kcal/day for
women (WHO, 1973). Immediately prior to retirement, energy
expenditures over the working day remain much as in younger subjects
(Asmussen & Poulsen, 1963; Cunningham *et al.*, 1969). In the city of
Tecumseh, Michigan, the ratio of working to basal metabolic rate
declined very slightly from about 3.1 in subjects aged 16 to 29 years
to about 2.9 in the 50-59 and 60-69 year old age groups (Cunningham
et al., 1968). Studies from both sides of the Atlantic have shown
much larger changes of leisure pursuits over the normal span of working
life. In the United States, the two commonest forms of voluntary
activity are walking and cycling (President's Council on Fitness, 1973);

such voluntary activity is most prevalent in the young, the better educated and the more affluent segments of the population. Statistics Canada (1972) has likewise found a progressive decrease in both sports participation and other forms of vigorous activity as the Canadian population becomes older; less than 9 per cent of those over the age of 55 years take any deliberate exercise, and those over 65 years of age lead the nation in spending more than four hours a day in watching television. In Tecumseh, Michigan (Cunningham *et al.*, 1968, 1969), aging led to a decrease of active leisure in all occupational categories, amounting to 35 minutes per day for blue-collar workers, and 15 minutes per day for those in 'white-collar' jobs. There was also a change in the nature of leisure pursuits (Figure 4.1), while the average intensity of active leisure diminished from 4.8 to 4.1 times the basal metabolic rate. In Glasgow, Durnin (1964, 1969) noted a 165 kcal (0.69 MJ) diminution in the daily energy usage of 51-year-old house-wives relative to their adult daughters. Neither the mothers nor their daughters were engaged in any strenuous recreation, and much of the change was attributable to a 45 minute reduction in the daily walking distance. Zabrowski *et al.* (1962) suggested that much of the change in leisure patterns was due to a change in cultural expectations. In their study, old people showed a significant decline in group activities, but no change in their individual pursuits.

The daily regimen of university staff approaching retirement is compared with that of elderly housewives in Table 4.1. In the Toronto data (Sidney & Shephard, 1977c), results were available for both working and weekend days. On a typical work day, the women allocated more time than the men to tasks demanding physical effort. This probably reflects the influence of traditional female domestic chores, a major item in the diaries of the Glasgow housewives studied by Durnin and his associates. The females also spent longer walking and less time sitting, sleeping and driving than the men. Over the weekend, the men sat less and spent more time in light and moderate effort. In contrast, the women did less moderate work at the weekend. Neither men nor women spent more than ten minutes per day at what they regarded as heavy physical work. It is interesting that the housewives apparently spent longer in bed than those who were working outside the home; they also engaged in more standing, but less walking. The World Health Organisation cal-culations of energy requirements are somewhat conservative in assuming four to six hours of sitting per day; seven to eight hours would be a more realistic figure for the Canadian senior citizen. Two

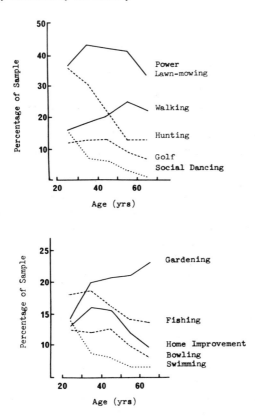

Figure 4.1 Influence of age upon participation in leisure activities. The graphs illustrate the percentage of the male population of Tecumseh (Michigan) who spent more than half an hour per week at the ten most popular leisure pursuits. Based on data of Montoye (1975).

hours of walking per day is not an excessive estimate for the employed group in Toronto, but again it seems incorrect for the Glasgow housewives.

Estimates of the total daily caloric expenditure are also influenced by changes in the basal metabolic rate. Because of loss of lean tissue, the total basal metabolism declines by some 2 per cent per decade (Chapter 2). Estimates of daily energy usage show a wide individual variability (Table 4.2). A person who was active in his youth tends to remain active (Zaborowski, 1962); such a person may even maintain

Table 4.1   Reported habitual activity of subjects as taken from diary records. Data for elderly men and women, minutes per day

Activity	MEN Ref (1)			WOMEN Ref (1)			Ref (2)	Ref (3)	Ref (4)
	Mon/ Fri	Sat/ Sun	Week	Mon/ Fri	Sat/ Sun	Week			
Lying	467	513	480	439	474	449	510	509	581
Sitting	535	397	495	458	447	455	420	405	436
Standing	96	80	92	160	145	155	420[a]	342[a]	305[a]
Walking	118	91	110	151	135	146	45	66	66
Shopping							15	26	23
Driving, riding	105	105	104	43	71	52			
Personal care	51	56	52	58	55	57	30	55	29
Light work	21	109	46	63	72	66			
Moderate work	41	79	52	57	33	50			
Heavy work	7	10	8	11	7	10			
Miscellaneous								37	

References:

(1)   Sidney & Shephard (1977c)
(2)   Durnin *et al.* (1960) — values estimated from graph
(3)   Durnin *et al.* (1961a)
(4)   Durnin *et al.* (1961c)

Notes

[a]   Total includes domestic duties

The subjects of series (1) were university staff approaching retirement. The subjects of series (2)-(4) were all housewives, with average ages of 51, 60 and 66 years respectively.

a higher daily energy usage than a relatively inactive young man who is employed in a 'heavy' industry. Durnin & Passmore (1967) cited examples of elderly farmers and forestry workers with daily expenditures as high as 4,500 to 5,000 kcal (18.9 to 20.9 MJ). By way of comparison, typical figures for young adults are as follows: office staff, 2,520 kcal, 10.6 MJ; construction workers, 3,000 kcal, 12.5 MJ; steel-workers, 3,280 kcal, 13.7 MJ; coal miners, 3,660 kcal, 15.3 MJ.

Intensity of Activity

The intensity of habitual activity is important from the viewpoint of maintaining cardio-respiratory fitness. In a recent study of the Saskatoon population, a substantial difference of predicted maximum oxygen intake was found between the most and the least active

Table 4.2   Daily energy expenditures of elderly men and women

Population	Mean energy expenditure		Reference
	kcal/day	MJ/day	
MEN			
Peasants	3,530	14.8	Durnin & Passmore (1967)
Crofters	2,800	11.7	Jerham *et al.* (1969)
Elderly Swiss			
< 70 yr	3,410	14.3	Wirths (1963)
71 − 75	2,990	12.5	
> 75 yr	2,650	11.1	
Heavy industry	3,276	13.7	Durnin *et al.* (1961b)
Light industry	2,990	12.5	Durnin *et al.* (1961b)
Light industry	2,684	11.2	Durnin *et al.* (1961b)
University staff	2,300	9.6	Sidney & Shephard (1977c)
Retired	2,330	9.8	Durnin & Passmore (1967)
Residents in institutions	2,116	8.9	Salvosa *et al.* (1971)
WOMEN			
Peasants	2,890	12.1	Durnin & Passmore (1967)
Elderly Swiss			
< 70 yr	2,960	12.4	Wirths (1963)
71 − 75	2,860	12.0	
> 75 yr	2,500	10.5	
University staff	2,050	8.6	Sidney & Shephard (1977c)
Housewives (with families)	2,113	8.9	Durnin (1966); Durnin *et al.* (1961a)
Housewives living alone	1,987	8.3	Durnin (1966); Durnin *et al.* (1961c)
Retired	1,700	7.1	Salvosa *et al.* (1971)
Residents in institutions	1,566	6.6	Salvosa *et al.* (1971)

members of the community (Table 4.3); however, differences in aerobic power showed more relationship to reported daily activity in young and middle-aged subjects than in the elderly.

Most authors are agreed that the intensity of effort required in modern daily work is insufficient to maintain fitness. High levels of energy expenditure are rare even in the traditional 'heavy' industries (Allen, 1966; Buskirk *et al.*, 1971), so that the maintainance of fitness is now dependent on the vigour of leisure pursuits. However, this has not always been the case. Durnin (1967) analysed relatively long-standing information for heavy workers, and found that a large part of the moderate and heavy work was encountered during the working

Table 4.3   Intensity and duration of activity at work in relation to whole day. Based on data of Durnin (1967) and Sidney & Shephard (1977c)

Subjects	At work (min)			Total day (min)		
	moderate	heavy	v. heavy	moderate	heavy	v. heavy
MEN						
17 − 45 yrs	49	14	0.3	91	17	2
> 45 yrs	84	5	1	110	7	2
~ 65 yrs	11	0	0	51	8	0
WOMEN						
17 − 45 yrs	30	0	0	59	2	0.6
> 45 yrs	46	0.3	0	59	1	0
~ 65 yrs	26	1.9	0	61	4	0

Note

In the two younger age groups, Durnin (1967) classed his energy expenditures as

moderate	5.0 − 7.4 kcal/min (M)	3.5 − 5.4 kcal/min (F)
heavy	7.5 − 9.9 kcal/min (M)	5.5 − 7.4 kcal/min (F)
very heavy	>10.0 kcal/min (M)	>7.5 kcal/min (F)

In the oldest age group, Sidney & Shephard (1977c) used the subject's rating of his or her effort.

day (Table 4.4). A more recent survey of Canadian university staff showed that more than two thirds of moderate and heavy activity was undertaken during leisure hours (Sidney & Shephard, 1977c).

Sidney & Shephard (1977c) used a portable tape recorder to demonstrate that the heart rates of their group of elderly university employees (Table 4.5) rarely reached the training threshold (at least 120 beats/min) except while they were participating in an exercise class. The average heart rates, although low, conformed with data from previous studies of younger individuals (page 154):

Table 4.4 Relationship between reported habitual activity and predicted maximum oxygen intake at different ages. Data for Saskatoon population (Bailey, Shephard & Mirwald, 1966), expressed in ml/kg min STPD and mM/kg min

Age and sex	1. None		2. Occasional		3. Regular		4. Very frequent or training		Difference 1 → 4
(yrs)	ml	mM	ml	mM	ml	mM	ml	mM	%
MEN									
20 − 29	41	1.83	39	1.74	40	1.79	52	2.32	26.8
30 − 39	35	1.56	36	1.61	38	1.70	45	2.01	28.5
40 − 49	33	1.47	34	1.52	34	1.52	41	1.83	24.2
50 − 59	30	1.33	32	1.43	32	1.43	37	1.65	23.3
60 − 69	26	1.16	33	1.47	30	1.33	29	1.29	11.5
WOMEN									
20 − 29	36	1.61	37	1.65	37	1.65	39	1.74	8.3
30 − 39	35	1.61	34	1.52	35	1.56	38	1.70	8.5
40 − 49	29	1.29	31	1.38	33	1.47	32	1.43	10.3
50 − 59	29	1.29	33	1.47	31	1.38	37	1.65	27.5
60 − 69	29	1.29	29	1.29	31	1.38	28	1.25	−3.5

Table 4.5 Frequency distribution of the heart rate of elderly subjects during specified portions of the day. Based on the data of Sidney & Shephard (1977c); mean and standard error of times in minutes

Period of day	100 beats/min		100 to 120 beats/min		120 beats/min	
	M	F	M	F	M	F
Afternoon work	175 ± 21	222 ± 10	35 ± 10	29 ± 9	15 ± 6	11 ± 6
Evening leisure	212 ± 31	262 ± 18	42 ± 16	27 ± 10	10 ± 2	9 ± 5
Exercise class	19 ± 7	9 ± 3	28 ± 5	17 ± 6	30 ± 5	8 ± 5

154   *Activity Patterns of the Elderly*

| | Heart rate (beats per minute) | | | |
Subjects	Work	Active leisure	Sleep	Reference
Middle-aged men	84	85	67	Richardson (1971)
Policemen	86–94	83–85	64–68	Goldsmith & Hale (1971)
Men aged 16-70	71–106	71–106	48–80	Glagov *et al.* (1970)
Men Type A	86	83	71	Friedman *et al.* (1963)
Men Type B	85	79	66	Friedman *et al.* (1963)
Elderly men	91	88	63[a]	Sidney & Shephard (1977c)
Elderly women	80	81	64[a]	Sidney & Shephard (1977c)

[a] Data obtained by SAMI heart rate integrator

Attitudes Towards Physical Activity

Although there have been frequent studies of attitudes towards physical activity in children and middle-aged men, much less is known about the attitudes of the senior citizen. Nevertheless, a marshalling of available information is vital to the design of an effective exercise programme for the older person. In this section we shall look at current perceptions of health and fitness, body image, perceived attitudes and motivation to participate in a regular exercise training class.

Current Perceptions of Health and Fitness

1. Health   Self-ratings of health bear only a limited relationship to data gleaned from medical records or clinical examination. Friedsam & Martin (1963) thus suggested that perceived health should be regarded as a 'barometer of self image'. Certainly, self image and morale influence reported health, although a more recent study by Tissue (1972) found a closer relationship of health ratings to clinical data than to self image.

Belloc *et al.* (1971) mailed a physical health questionnaire to a large probability-based sample of US adults. Depending on the number of reported symptoms and/or chronic conditions, health was classified on a continuum that ranged from marked disability to full physical vigour with an absence of complaints. Statistical analysis of the resultant data showed several trends: (1) the men were healthier than the women at all ages, (2) health diminished with increasing age, irrespective of income, (3) health improved with increasing family income, irrespective of age, and (4) those who were employed were healthier than those who were unemployed or retired. The design of the survey did not distinguish whether the fourth relationship was cause or effect. The same criticism applies to the observation that good health habits such as control of body weight and regular physical activity were positively correlated with physical health status (Belloc & Breslow, 1972).

One frequently employed measure of perceived health is the Cornell Medical Index (Table 4.6). With this tool, the subject is required to make a total of 195 yes/no responses to simple questions. Sections A-L of the questionnaire cover general health, and sections M-R refer specifically to behaviour, mood and feeling patterns. Total scores of over 30, or M-R sub-totals of over 10 are thought to reflect organic illness or emotional disturbance (Abramson *et al.*, 1965; Abramson, 1966; Brodman *et al.*, 1956). Average scores for the elderly show some increase relative to younger subjects (Abramson *et al.*, 1965; Brodman *et al.*, 1953; Cheraskin & Ringsdorf, 1973; Daly & Tyroler, 1972), due in part to a deterioration of physical health; nevertheless, average scores remain well below these limits. Sidney & Shephard (1977a) found that 28 of 124 elderly volunteers for an exercise class had scores of over 30. This is above the expectation for younger patients. The Cornell Medical Index manual (Brodman *et al.*, 1956) predicts abnormal scores in 5 per cent of normal women and 30 per cent of ostensibly healthy females; corresponding figures for men are 3 and 10 per cent. Abramson *et al.* (1965) summarised data from various surveys conducted in England and the US, and found scores indicative of emotional ill health in 14 per cent of ostensibly healthy women, and 10 per cent of ostensibly healthy men. In the study of Sidney & Shephard (1977a), seven of the subjects with high scores were rejected from the exercise class on medical grounds. They mainly had high scores on section C, dealing with cardio-vascular complaints, and an organic basis for their scores seems likely. The remaining 21 with high Cornell scores were accepted for the physical activity programme, but only three of them commenced training, and only one of these three progressed beyond irregular participation at a low intensity of effort. Classifying Cornell scores in terms of the self-selected pattern of training, those choosing a low frequency and low intensity of activity had significantly more complaints (26.7 ± 17.9) than the three other groups (low frequency, high

Table 4.6 Perceived health, as determined by the Cornell Medical Index. Scores for sections A-L of the questionnaire refer to general medical symptoms, and sections M-R explore mood and feeling patterns

Population	Section A-L	Section M-R	Total A-R	Author
MEN				
Young men			13.5	Brodman *et al.* (1953)
Daily exercisers <45 yr			12	Cheraskin & Ringsdorf
Inactive <45 yr			17	(1971)
Young men			5-12[a]	Daly & Tyroler (1972)
Daily exercisers >45 yr			15	Cheraskin & Ringsdorf
Inactive >45 yr			24	(1971)
Old men (employed)			9-19[a]	Daly & Tyroler (1972)
Old men[b]	13.7 ± 10.1	3.5	17.2 ± 15.4	Sidney & Shephard
Old men[c]	16.9 ± 8.7	4.7	21.6 ± 14.3	(1977a)
Old men (inst.)	11.8	3.7	14.3	Steinhardt *et al.* (1953)
Old men			19.5	Brodman *et al.* (1953)
WOMEN				
Young women			22.5	Brodman *et al.* (1953)
Old women			24.5	Brodman *et al.* (1953)
Old women[b]	17.1 ± 11.7	6.2	23.3 ± 16.8	Sidney & Shephard
Old women[c]	14.3 ± 6.0	4.4	18.7 ± 9.4	(1977a)
Old women (inst.)	21.1	6.0	27.1	Steinhardt *et al.* (1953)

[a] The range of scores is the middle tertile of the sample
[b] Subjects accepted for exercise programme on the basis of history and clinical examination
[c] Subjects rejected for exercise programme on the basis of history and clinical examination

intensity 11.8 ± 5.1; high frequency, low intensity 15.3 ± 8.6; high frequency, high intensity 15.0 ± 6.9). Since the examining physician had decided all subjects were capable of exercise, a large part of the added complaints probably reflects a poor perception of health rather than organic disability; however, it is also fair to comment that a substantial proportion of those volunteering for exercise had minor disabilities such as arthritis or bursitis, while 48 per cent of the women and 61 per cent of the men had some limitation of eyesight and/or hearing. Although participation in the programme was related to the Cornell score, neither Joseph (1967) nor Sidney & Shephard (1977a) found any relationship between the initial maximum oxygen intake and perceived health.

2. Anxiety and emotional health   It is necessary to distinguish state and trait anxiety (Martens, 1972). State anxiety is characterised by 'consciously perceived feelings of apprehension and tension, accompanied by arousal of the autonomic nervous system', while trait anxiety is 'an acquired behavioural disposition that predisposes an individual to perceive a wide range of objectively non-dangerous circumstances as threatening, and to respond with state anxiety reactions disproportionate in intensity to the magnitude of the objective danger'. Both trait and state anxiety can modify physical performance (Martens, 1972; Shephard, 1977c), each task having an optimum anxiety level for peak achievement. Conversely, physical activity can reduce state anxiety in overly anxious subjects, while increasing it in those who are less anxious (Gillet *et al.*, 1973); however, there is little evidence that trait anxiety can be modified either acutely or in the long term by an exercise programme.

Cheraskin & Ringsdorf (1971, 1973) used the M-R section of the Cornell Medical Index to assess emotional health, and noted that those who exercised daily had significantly lower scores than those who chose not to exercise. However, it remains unclear whether physical activity improved the psychological status of the exercise class, or whether those persons with some emotional disturbance could not or would not exercise.

A more specific measure of manifest anxiety is provided by the Taylor questionnaire (J.A. Taylor, 1953). In the material of Sidney & Shephard (1977a), scores for elderly exercise volunteers (7.8 ± 3.9 for the men, 13.0 ± 6.7 for the women) were quite low relative to previous studies of university students (Hammer, 1967; J.A. Taylor, 1953) and middle-aged exercise volunteers (Massie & Shephard, 1971).

3. Perception of activity needs   There is often a substantial discrepancy between actual and perceived exercise needs. In a 1973 sampling of 3,875 US citizens (National adult physical fitness survey, 1973), 46 per cent of those aged 20 to 29 and 71 per cent of those over the age of 60 years thought that they were getting enough exercise. Among the 55 per cent who were taking deliberate exercise, 46 per cent thought that their personal activity was insufficient. However, among the 45 per cent who were taking no deliberate exercise, 63 per cent nevertheless considered that their current activity level was adequate. Sidney & Shephard (1977a) had a similar experience with Canadian subjects. Among those volunteering for an exercise programme, all believed that at least moderate amounts of physical activity were necessary for optimum health, and only 25 per cent thought that they were engaging in sufficient activity at the time of recruitment. However, those who chose not to join the programme often said that they were already active enough, that their body weight was normal, and even that their fitness level was above average for their age. We may suspect that such faulty perceptions arise in part from a cultural expectation that the elderly will engage in very little physical activity. It is also likely that because of lack of fitness, non-participants became fatigued at an early stage of effort, and even minimal work was perceived as significant exercise. Concerns about the dangers of exercise were not voiced by either participants or non-participants; however, we suspect that such fears may also have modified the behaviour of some elderly subjects.

4. Perception of body build   The majority of those who participated in the exercise programme of Sidney & Shephard (1977a) realised that they were initially somewhat overweight. However, when asked to specify their ideal weight, they underestimated their excess relative to the actuarial 'ideal'.

	Actual excess weight kg	Perceived excess weight kg
Men	8.2	2.1
Women	7.1	4.3

Self-Concept

The self-concept of the body is potentially vulnerable to many of the stresses of aging — retirement, bereavement, institutionalisation, declining physical capabilities, specific disabilities and major diseases such as myocardial infarction. One approach to the assessment of body image is to ask subjects to place a dollar value on various parts (Plutchik *et al.*, 1973). This approach shows that women generally have a less secure body image than the men (Plutchik *et al.*, 1971, 1973), with more worries concerning their bodies. However, elderly subjects make a similar valuation of their bodies to young adults.

Other test instruments, such as those of Kenyon (1968) and

Table 4.7 Self-concept data for middle-aged men (Massie & Shephard, 1971) and elderly men and women (Sidney & Shephard, 1977a). Mean ± SD of scores, a high score indicating a good body image

| Group | Kenyon test ('my body') | | McPherson test |
	Perceived	Ideal	('real me')
Middle-aged	141.9 ± 10.2	118.1 ± 16.3	261 ± 29
Elderly men	138.6 ± 12.0	116.8 ± 8.6	259 ± 19
Elderly women	136.4 ± 10.2	109.8 ± 12.3	245 ± 30

McPherson & Yuhasz (1968), use a semantic differential scale that allows a rating of various body characteristics such as strong-weak. Scoring is arranged so that a high total indicates a favourable body image. As in Plutchik's study, average scores for elderly men (Table 4.7) are much as in middle-aged volunteers (Sidney & Shephard, 1977a). Again, the women have a more negative concept of their bodies than the men, with a larger discrepancy between the perceived and the desired body image.

In contrast to these reports, Kreitler & Kreitler (1970) suggested that the inactivity of old age distorted body image, old people perceiving their bodies as heavier and broader than they actually were, and physical tasks as harder to perform. Distortion of body image, fear of activity and feelings of clumsiness and insecurity augmented inactivity, giving a vicious cycle of anxiety, tension and repressed aggression. This situation is typical of the older old person, particularly someone who has been institutionalised.

Neugarten *et al.* (1961) developed a specific attitude scale to assess the psychological well-being and morale of old people. Sidney & Shephard (1977a) used a form of scoring for this test that assessed five components of morale: self-concept, mood, zest for life, congruence of desired and achieved goals, and fortitude. Average scores were 14.5 + 2.9 in the men and 12.3 + 4.2 in the women. Other studies of elderly populations (D.L. Adams, 1969; Neugarten *et al.*, 1961; Wood *et al.*, 1969) have yielded very similar results. Edwards & Klemmack (1973) found that scores on this test were positively correlated with educational level, income and perceived health, and were negatively correlated with age.

Perceived Attitudes to Exercise

An attitude may be defined as a relatively stable behavioural trait, reflecting both the direction and intensity of feelings, belief and action. It is usually assessed by a questionnaire or scaling methods, although there may be discrepancies between the attitudes thus reported and the behaviour of the individual. Attitudes towards physical activity are generally more positive in those who take regular exercise than in those who do not (McPherson *et al.*, 1967; McPherson & Yuhasz, 1968; D.V. Harris, 1970). Kenyon's inventory (Kenyon, 1968) measures perceived attitudes towards activity as a social experience, a means for health and fitness, the pursuit of vertigo, an aesthetic experience, a cartharsis of tension, an ascetic experience and a game of chance (Table 4.8). Scores range from 8 to 56 points per item, a high score indicating a positive attitude. Relative to Canadian high-school students (Kenyon, 1968) and middle-aged volunteers (Massie & Shephard, 1971), the elderly subjects valued exercise more as an aesthetic experience and as a means for health and fitness. They also appreciated the social, cathartic and ascetic aspects of sports, but no more so than younger individuals. The sensation of vertigo was less attractive to the elderly women than to the younger age groups.

Table 4.8   Attitudes towards physical activity, as assessed by the Kenyon (1968) inventory. Data for high-school children (Kenyon, 1968), middle-aged men (Massie & Shephard, 1971) and elderly men and women (Sidney & Shephard, 1977a). Scores range from 8 to 56, a high score indicating a favourable attitude

| Concept of activity | MALE SUBJECTS | | | FEMALE SUBJECTS | |
	High school	Middle age	Elderly	High school	Elderly
Social experience	45.6 ± 6.7	45.9 ± 5.1	46.9 ± 7.7	46.3 ± 6.6	46.1 ± 7.4
Health & fitness	44.3 ± 6.8	45.7 ± 6.3	48.2 ± 6.3	43.9 ± 7.4	49.2 ± 5.6
Pursuit of vertigo	38.9 ± 8.5	33.7 ± 12.5	38.6 ± 8.7	35.5 ± 10.0	30.9 ± 11.5
Aesthetic experience	43.1 ± 9.5	47.7 ± 6.6	49.2 ± 6.1	48.7 ± 7.1	51.0 ± 4.3
Cartharsis of tension	45.2 ± 8.1	46.5 ± 6.7	45.9 ± 10.7	46.5 ± 2.5	48.0 ± 5.3
Ascetic experience	34.3 ± 8.9	32.2 ± 7.7	34.2 ± 6.3	32.9 ± 9.6	33.8 ± 9.9
Game of chance	32.4 ± 10.0	30.4 ± 10.1	29.7 ± 10.1	32.0 ± 10.0	29.7 ± 8.8

Motivation to Participate in an Exercise Programme

A number of authors have asked in an unstructured fashion why people choose to join an exercise programme. The President's Council on Fitness (1973) questioned a large sample of US citizens. Reasons cited by those who were exercising regularly included 'good health' (23 per cent), 'generally a good thing' (18 per cent), and 'to lose weight' (13 per cent). A relatively small percentage were doing so because they enjoyed it, and only 3 per cent had been advised to exercise by their physician. Excuses offered by those who were not exercising regularly included 'lack of time' (13 per cent), 'adequate exercise at work' (11 per cent), 'medical reasons' (8 per cent) and 'age' (5 per cent). The non-participants were generally the older, less well educated, and less affluent members of the sample, and they were less likely to have participated in exercise programmes at school. D.V. Harris (1970) questioned middle-aged men, and she also noted that those who were physically active had a history of previous participation, including attendance at summer athletic camps and membership of school and college sports teams; typically, their parents had encouraged participation in sports from an early age, and they enjoyed both competition and the feeling of fatigue that followed strenuous activity. Heinzelman & Bagley (1970) established an exercise programme for middle-aged workers at the US National Aeronautics and Space Administration headquarters. Volunteers joined this programme (1) to feel better or healthier, (2) to reduce the chance of a heart attack, and (3) to assist medical research. Other less frequently cited motives included a desire for health knowledge, recreation, fun and a variation in routine.

Motivation to exercise seems similar in other countries. Brunner (1969) questioned middle-aged Israeli men enrolled in a fitness programme. Their primary reasons for participation were a desire to keep physically fit and an associated feeling of well-being. The main reason cited by those who chose not to participate was a lack of time. Terraslinna *et al.* (1970) sent a questionnaire to 1,708 middle-aged managers and executives in Finland asking about willingness to participate in a programme of physical activity. Some 46 per cent of the sample were willing, 24 per cent were unwilling and 30 per cent did not reply. The most important reasons for participation were to improve health (63 per cent), to improve fitness (17 per cent) and to control body weight (7 per cent). Those who were interested in the programme in general lived close to the exercise facility, had an above average level of current activity, were aware that their current activity was insufficient for them, and (contrary to some other studies) were likely to be cigarette smokers.

The surveys mentioned to this point have involved the middle-aged rather than the elderly. Sidney & Shephard (1977a) analysed responses to 'open-ended' questions in their pre-retirement exercise class. The most frequently cited motive for joining the class was to improve health (Table 4.9). A second important motivator was the provision of a specific programme for the elderly, with appropriate physical facilities, instructions on how to exercise safely, and opportunities for regular supervised activity. Not one of the Canadian sample had received any suggestion of the merits of physical exercise from their personal

Table 4.9   Perceived motivation for joining a physical activity programme. Responses of elderly men and women (Sidney & Shephard, 1977a). An arbitrary score of 3 has been assigned for the first listed reason, 2 for the second reason and 1 for the third reason. Not all participants listed three reasons

Perceived motive	MEN		WOMEN	
	Cumulative score	Rank	Cumulative score	Rank
Physical health				
Improve fitness or health	18	1	37	1
Body appearance, weight control	5		8	
Medical advice	0		0	
Psychological well-being				
Increased vigour and alertness	0		13	3
Relief of tension, anxiety, aggression, relaxation	0		0	
Social				
To socialise, make friends	0		2	6
Pressure to join from others	0		3	
Recreational/hedonistic				
Fun, curiosity	7	4	7	5
Programme and facilities				
Exercise instruction	14	2	27	2
Exercise testing	5		12	
Altruism				
To assist science	9	3	12	4

physician. Other reasons cited by occasional class members were a desire to assist research, enjoyment of physical activity (particularly in the men), and anticipation of increased vigour and mental alertness (particularly in the women). Benefits anticipated from the programme were also commonly related to health and fitness. Some psychological gains were anticipated, but few subjects expected any social benefits, and no one thought there would be any improvement in the ability to perform physical work. Despite the multiplicity of gymnasia and other exercise facilities in Toronto, some of the group blamed their previous inactivity upon a lack of suitable programmes and physical facilities. This suggests that if the activity of the elderly is to be increased, it will be necessary not only to construct recreational facilities, but to establish special classes geared to the social needs and interests of the senior citizen.

Class leaders should finally be aware that the motives that initiate participation often differ from those that sustain interest (Stiles, 1967; Heinzelman, 1973). Stiles (1967) studied a 'representative' group of adults who had chosen to engage in sport, and he concluded that a fear of incapacitation and a desire for buoyant health were frequently responsible for the initiation of activity in this group. Other less common motives were a desire to compete and a history of family or personal involvement. However, continued involvement depended on the thrill or enjoyment of participation, the challenge and satisfaction of mastering different skills, the desire to better one's performance, a feeling of well-being engendered by the activity, maintenance of health and fitness and (although not often admitted) attainment of the desired self-image.

Retirement, Hospital Admission and Institutional Care

Retirement

It has often been assumed that retirement is a traumatic landmark in life, associated with a profound reduction of both mental and physical activity. Thus Sauvy (1970a) writes of the psychological effects that arise from stopping the rhythm of work — feelings of loneliness, uselessness, futility and aimlessness, with an unavoidable tendency to become obsessed by thoughts of old age and death. E. Cumming & Henry (1961) developed the theory that in an industrial nation men were integrated into society by their work. Disengagement thus developed on giving up work — 'many of the relationships between a person and other members of society are severed, and those remaining are altered in quality'. Ego energy declined, and the elderly person became increasingly self-preoccupied and unresponsive to normative controls.

More recent research has questioned this negative approach to the retirement years. Beverfelt (1971) found that while 26 per cent of Norwegian workers dreaded retirement, 51 per cent were actually looking forward to a cessation of employment. The advantages seen for retirement were greater opportunities for leisure activities (50 per cent) and a chance to rest (20 per cent). The main disadvantages were thought to be a reduction in income (32 per cent) and difficulty in passing the time (19 per cent). A positive attitude towards retirement was more frequent in women than in men, and those with poor health more commonly wished to cease work than those whose health was still excellent. Shanas (1971a) also commented that many people who had retired missed nothing about their work, except perhaps the money that they earned. Only a quarter to a tenth of the retired population would like to be employed, these being mostly recently retired individuals who were still in good health. Neugarten & Havighurst (1969) reanalysed the data of E. Cumming & Henry (1961), and questioned whether disengagement was either a natural consequence of aging or a contributor to well-being. In their view, old people were happiest when they remained well integrated into the remainder of society.

Sidney & Shephard (1977c) were able to compare daily activity diaries for two groups of elderly women, one seen immediately before, and the other soon after retirement (Table 4.10). The study confirmed that in the first few years after ceasing work, the new-found leisure was filled with various physically demanding projects. Thus, the retired group spent much less time sitting than those who were still employed, devoting their additional minutes to standing, walking and driving about the city. The total of light and moderate work was rather comparable for the two groups, but the period spent on heavy work jumped from 2 to 18 minutes per day in those who were retired. Little extra time was taken in bed after work had ceased, and indeed the retired were so busy that they actually allocated 17 minutes less per day to eating than was the case for those who were still working.

The picture of active retirement is perhaps less typical of the older senior citizen. Burch & Collot (1972) studied representative groups of men and women > 65 years of age who were living at home in three suburbs of Paris and in a small Californian town. Only 16 to 20 per cent of the Parisians belonged to organisations such as recreational

Table 4.10   A comparison of activity diaries for elderly employed women and those recently retired. Times per day, measured over a typical week (Sidney & Shephard, 1977c)

Activity	Employed (min)	Retired (min)	Difference (min)
Sitting	429	277	− 152
Standing	126	192	+ 66
Walking	123	173	+ 50
Driving and riding	42	63	+ 21
Personal hygiene	55	59	+ 4
Eating	102	85	− 17
Light work	55	78	+ 23
Moderate work	61	38	− 23
Heavy work	2.3	18.4	+ 16.1
Sleeping	444	455	+ 11

associations, clubs and trade unions, and many of this percentage attended meetings once a month or less. Reasons given for non-participation included lack of interest, not feeling the need, excessive age, bad health, difficulty in moving about and lack of time; a number of the women were occupied in minding grandchildren or ailing husbands. Work around the house was the most frequent source of activity (38 per cent) followed by parish or volunteer work (13 per cent), hobbies (9 per cent), participation in entertainment (7 per cent) and participation in social organisations (4 per cent). As many as 33 per cent of the French sample said that they had no activities. One popular pursuit was a stroll to the park, the main reason given for this being the exercise obtained from walking. Nevertheless, 50 to 60 per cent of the old people did not visit the public gardens. This was attributed to a lack of nearby gardens (20 per cent), lack of time (17 per cent), difficulty in moving (15 per cent), an adequate garden of their own (15 per cent), lack of interest (14 per cent), bad health (12 per cent), and tiredness (5 per cent). In California, club membership was much more popular, 54 per cent of the sample belonging to some type of social group. However, this was often informal in nature, and only 16 per cent participated in any kind of organised recreation. The perceived reason was 'lack of transport', although in fact about a third of the clubs and organisations in the area were willing to provide cars to and from their meetings. Other pursuits were minimal. Some 5 per cent enjoyed an afternoon walk in the park, 5 per cent had a hobby, and 4 per cent engaged in volunteer work for a church or community organisation.

Hospital Admission and Illness

Illness and hospital admission are frequent accompaniments of old age. Kaiser (1970) asked subjects which aspect of aging affected them to the greatest extent. Conditions affecting the locomotor system were cited by 17.7 per cent of his sample, central nervous system problems (including loss of memory and insomnia) by 15.7 per cent, deterioration in the special senses by 14.6 per cent, skin conditions by 14.4 per cent, general tiredness by 10.5 per cent, waning function of the sexual organs by 9.2 per cent and specific conditions of the heart and blood vessels by 7.1 per cent.

Hospital admissions are not only more common in the elderly, but they also tend to be for longer periods. Unfortunately, the decline of function that accompanies immobilisation of a young person (Taylor *et al.*, 1949; Saltin *et al.*, 1968; Fried & Shephard, 1969, 1970; Bassey & Fentem, 1974; Carswell, 1975) proceeds more rapidly in the aged. Phillipen (cited by Kaiser, 1970) reported that old people suffered an 18 per cent loss of muscle strength with as little as a week in bed. Complications such as thrombosis of varicose veins, embolism, pneumonia, renal stones and pressure sores are frequent consequences of hospital admission in this age group.

Institutionalisation

Casual inspection of most geriatric institutions suggests that there is almost no physical activity on the part of the residents. The majority of those who are not bed-ridden spend their days sitting in somnolent fashion in the lounge. One may suspect that over-liberal administration of sedatives contributes to this sad spectacle.

Formal scientific data on activity levels after institutionalisation seems limited to assessments of daily energy consumption (Table 4.2). The figures confirm the impression of extreme inactivity.

Implications for Nutrition

Many dietary studies such as the detailed survey conducted by Nutrition Canada (1976) unfortunately give no consideration to the activity patterns of those examined.* However, it is a necessary requirement of homeostasis that the usage of nutrients by physical

---

* Activity measurements were considered but rejected because of the practical difficulties involved.

activity be made good in the diet. In this section we shall note current recommendations concerning the food intake of the elderly, consider theoretical problems of nutrition in older people, examine present standards of nutrition and make some suggestions regarding the diet of the senior citizen.

Recommended Intake of Nutrients

Since activity decreases progressively with aging, there must be a parallel decrease of overall food intake if gross obesity is to be avoided. It is difficult to assess individual patterns of physical activity accurately, and practical checks are most conveniently based upon regular weighing and measurements of skinfold thicknesses. Because lean tissue is generally decreasing, the target weight should be somewhat below the 'ideal' value of the Society of Actuaries (1959).

Recent recommendations concerning the intake of individual nutrients are summarised in Table 4.11. These figures, proposed by British and Canadian authorities, are generally duplicated in reports from other nations. Note that smaller caloric allowances are made for elderly women in Canada than in the UK. The demand for most minerals and vitamins (except thiamine) is independent of the overall energy expenditure so that it becomes progressively more difficult to ensure adequate nutrition as a person becomes older.

Theoretical Problems in the Aged

There are many theoretical reasons why old people can become malnourished. Poverty may restrict the types of food that can be bought, and perhaps more importantly it may deny the use of an efficient stove, refrigerator and utensils for preparing nutritious and appetising meals. Poor eyesight, gross tremor or crippling arthritis of the hands may hamper both the purchase of food and its subsequent cooking. Appetite may be limited by loss of the senses of taste and smell, by a lack of teeth, by poorly fitting or uncomfortable dentures, and by difficulty in swallowing (dysphagia). A reduced secretion of hydrochloric acid and enzymes by the stomach may restrict the absorption of iron and the digestion of proteins, while malfunction of the gall bladder can cause flatulence and a dislike of fatty foods. Often there may be psychological reasons for a restriction of eating. Refusal to take adequate meals may become a means of protest against grievances, real or imaginary. Loneliness and isolation do not encourage the preparation of elaborate meals, and there may be a loss of morale, with little desire to stay alive. Many old people have never been taught

Table 4.11 Recommended intake of nutrients for sedentary subjects (data of Department of Health and Social Security, UK, 1969; and Nutrition Canada, 1976)

Sex & age	Body weight kg	Energy intake MJ	Energy intake kcal	Protein g	Thiamine mg	Riboflavin mg	Nicotinic acid mg equiv	Ascorbic acid mg	Vitamin A µg	Vitamin D µg	Ca mg	Fe mg
MEN												
35 – 65 yr	65	10.9	2,600	65	1.0	1.7	18	30	750	2.5	500	10
65 – 75	63	9.8	2,350	59	0.9	1.7	18	30	750	2.5	500	10
over 75	63	8.8	2,100	55	0.8	1.7	18	30	750	2.5	500	10
> 66 yr (Canada)	70	8.4	2,000	56	1.4	1.7	18	30	1,000	2.5	800	10
WOMEN												
18 – 55 yr	55	9.2	2,200	55	0.9	1.3	15	30	750	2.5	500	12
55 – 75	53	8.6	2,050	51	0.8	1.3	15	30	750	2.5	500	10
over 75	53	8.0	1,900	48	0.7	1.3	15	30	750	2.5	500	10
> 66 yr (Canada)	56	6.3	1,500	41	1.0	1.2	13	30	800	2.5	700	9

the principles of good nutrition. Milk, fresh fruit and vegetables were much less readily available seventy years ago. Present habits show much faddism, with a choice of diet on the basis of self-indulgence, prejudice, apathy and fears of 'the wrong food', 'indigestion' and 'constipation'. Lastly, a proportion of the elderly are mentally disturbed, and thus incapable of attending adequately to their nutritional requirements.

Some authors have suggested that these various problems are compounded by a poor absorption of food and an increased protein requirement. Southgate and Durnin (1970) made a careful study of differences between intake and excretion of total calories, protein, fat and pentosan in small groups of young adults (mean age 21 years) and elderly subjects (mean age 74 years). They found no evidence for a reduction in the efficiency of digestion and absorption of foodstuffs with aging. Occasional investigators (Swendseid & Tuttle, 1961; Tuttle *et al.*, 1965) have claimed that people over the age of 50 years need larger amounts of nitrogen, particularly the amino acids methionine and lysine. However, other authors (Horwitt, 1953; Schulze, 1954; Watkin, 1964) have sustained a nitrogen balance on protein intakes as low as 0.35 g/kg, with no difference of requirements between the young and the elderly (Roberts *et al.*, 1948; Albanese *et al.*, 1957; Watts *et al.*, 1964). Widdowson & Kennedy (1962) have further noted that a negative nitrogen balance is likely to develop in the elderly rat, irrespective of the quality of the diet that is provided.

Current Nutritional Status

There have been reports of widespread malnutrition in the elderly (for example, G.F. Taylor, 1968, in the UK, and the Citizens' Board of Enquiry into Hunger and Malnutrition in the US, 1968). Berry (1968) suggested that 4 per cent of 1,200 elderly patients admitted to British hospitals were suffering from sufficient protein lack to cause oedema; unfortunately, no biochemical or dietetic studies were advanced to support this view.

The bulk of present evidence (Table 4.12) suggests that at or immediately following retirement, the average person in an affluent Western nation is more likely to show signs of overnutrition than undernutrition. Further, even in the oldest age groups the average intake of nutrients is not greatly reduced if data are expressed per kilogram of body weight (Gillum & Morgan, 1955; Gillum *et al.*, 1955a-c). Nevertheless, the intake of some items is only a little in excess of recommended levels. Shortages can thus arise if food intake

Table 4.12   Observed intake of nutrients in elderly subjects

Sex and age		Energy intake		Protein	Thiamine	Riboflavin	Nicotinic acid	Ascorbic acid	Vitamin A	Vitamin D	Ca	Fe
		MJ	kcal	g	mg	mg	mg equiv	mg	μg	μg	mg	mg
MEN												
55 – 64	(1)	10.8	2,570	92				115	2,009			16
65 – 74	(1)	9.5	2,260	78				92	1,081			14
65 – 74	(2)	9.8	2,340	75	1.1	1.6	16.8	43	1,131	3.3	910	12
75 +	(1)	9.2	2,190	76				97	1,639			14
75 +	(2)	8.8	2,100	68	0.9	1.4	13.6	38	1,089	2.6	880	11
65 +	(6)	8.6	2,056	72	1.1	1.8	28	85	1,113		709	13
WOMEN												
55 – 64	(1)	7.4	1,760	62				90	1,358			11
65 – 74	(1)	7.4	1,760	64				88	1,057			11
65 – 74	(2)	7.5	1,790	59	0.8	1.3	11.5	40	1,021	2.3	795	9
60 – 69	(3)[a]	8.3	1,990	62	0.9	1.1	9.2	31	1,063	1.8	845	11
60 – 69	(4)[b]	8.9	2,130	62							758	11
75 +	(1)	6.2	1,485	51				76	582			9
75 +	(2)	6.8	1,630	54	0.7	1.1	10.2	34	883	2.1	725	9
70 – 80	(5)	7.9	1,900	57					860			10
65 +	(6)	6.4	1,530	54	0.9	1.5	21	87	1,008		619	10

References

(1) Gillum *et al.* (1955a, b, c).
(3) Durnin *et al.* (1961a) — elderly women living alone
(5) Exton-Smith *et al.* (1965)
(6) Nutrition Canada (1976)

(2) Dept. of Health & Social Security (UK) (1972).
(4) Durnin *et al.* (1961b) — elderly women living with their families

is further restricted by bed rest or alcoholism.

One source of detailed information is a survey conducted by the UK Department of Health and Social Security (1972). This report covered 879 people over the age of 65 years living in six different areas of Britain. Participation rates ranged from 51 per cent to 79 per cent. Some 1.5 per cent of the sample were judged to be helpless, 3 per cent were mentally confused and 22 per cent had significant physical limitations; 13 per cent of the men and 40 per cent of the women were living alone. Twenty-seven of the group were regarded as malnourished, mainly on the basis of excessive thinness. Although only 3 per cent of the sample, Davidson *et al.* (1972) pointed out that on a national basis this amounted to some 150,000 people. Twelve had major medical disorders, in seven there were socio-economic problems, and in eight there was no obvious reason for the limitation of food intake. Twelve of the twenty-seven, all from one area, were said to have protein/calorie malnutrition, but Durnin (1973) stressed that this is a difficult diagnosis to reach; it was supported by biochemical analyses in only one or two cases. Medical examinations were carried out on 789 of the group. Fifty-seven had disorders of the lips (angular stomatitis or cheilosis), but in only four subjects was this related to a deficiency of riboflavine. Frank scurvy was diagnosed in two subjects, and the condition was suspected in three others. There also appeared to be some relationship between low back pain and a deficient intake of vitamin D. It was concluded that income had surprisingly little direct effect on diet; the only observable factors contributing to malnutrition were biologically advanced age, limited mobility and specific pathologies.

A particularly detailed examination was made on 88 subjects with a daily food intake of less than 6.3 MJ (1,500 kcal). Only eight of this group revealed one well-established index of protein deficiency (Hutchinson *et al.*, 1951) — a low pseudo-cholinesterase level. Reasons for the limited food intake included dieting (fourteen subjects, all women), reduced activity due to strokes, crippling arthritis or mental depression, gastro-intestinal disorders, difficulty in preparing food and senile degenerative states. Twenty-two of the group were regarded as having a 'better than average' general health, despite their apparently low level of food intake. This suggests that the recommended intakes of Table 4.11 may be generous, particularly for women.

Biochemical tests were carried out on many of the sample. Table 4.13 summarises the proportion of subjects failing to meet arbitrary minimum levels of normality. A substantial proportion were deficient

Table 4.13   Percentage of elderly subjects failing to meet arbitrary blood concentrations for selected nutrients. Based on data of UK Department of Health and Social Security, 1972, and Nutrition Canada (1976)

| Variable | Lower limit | Percentage failing to meet standards | | | | CANADA | |
		MEN 65–74 %	MEN 75+ %	WOMEN 65–74 %	WOMEN 75+ %	MEN >65 %	WOMEN >65 %
Serum albumin	3.5 g/100 ml	10.7	15.3	10.2	13.6	0.3	0.1
Serum vit. B_{12}	100 pg/ml	0.5	2.6	1.2	0.7	–	–
Serum folate	3 ng/ml	14.8	14.5	10.6	18.0	~ 25	~ 23
Leucocyte ascorbic acid	7 μg/10^8 cells	6.3	15.9	2.6	5.7	–	–
Serum iron	60 μg/100 ml	15.9	16.9	20.5	24.6	11.2	4.9
Haemoglobin	13 g/100 ml	5.5	9.6		5.7	5.7	
	12 g/100 ml			8.1	5.3		4.0

in serum albumin, serum iron, serum folate and leucocyte ascorbic acid.
This does not necessarily imply overt malnutrition, but it does indicate
a reduced margin against a further deterioration in the dietary intake of
essential foods.

Specific Nutrients

1. Protein   The recommended intake is met by the average old person
(Table 4.12). At 1 g/kg, the daily ingestion of protein substantially
exceeds the minimum needed for nitrogen balance (0.35 g/kg). Thus,
even if the total intake is restricted by bed rest or hospitalisation, it
is unlikely that a deficiency will develop. Should the diet appear
marginal, a daily half pint of milk will provide an additional 8 g of
protein.

2. B Vitamins   The normal intake of thiamine and riboflavin is at or
slightly below the recommended level (Brin, 1968). There have also
been suggestions that the diet of the elderly is deficient in folic acid
(Batata *et al.*, 1967; Girdwood *et al.*, 1967). Reduction of activity
could thus cause a shortage of the B vitamins, although in practice it is
quite rare for clinical deficiency symptoms to develop.

3. Ascorbic acid   Ascorbic acid intake is much more marginal in
Britain than in California (Table 4.12). Brin (1968) found deficiencies
relative to recommended levels, but there was no evidence that these
were sufficient to cause scurvy. One biochemical measure of the
adequacy of ascorbic acid intake is the content of this compound in
the leucocytes. In a survey of Edinburgh citizens aged 62 to 94 years,
Milne *et al.* (1971a) found values of 23.9 $\mu g/10^8$ cells in men,
compared with recommended minima of 7 $\mu g/10^8$ cells. While levels
were lower in hospitals and old people's homes (Kataria *et al.*, 1965;
Andrews *et al.*, 1966), again no clinical scurvy was seen.

4. Fat soluble vitamins   There may be some deficit of fat soluble
vitamins in patients with biliary disease due to their voluntary
avoidance of fat. In the average old person (Table 4.12), the intake
of vitamin A appears to be more adequate than that of vitamin D.
Exton-Smith *et al.* (1965) found that the diet of elderly Londoners
provided only 2.3 μg of vitamin D per day. However, evidence linking
this somewhat limited intake with the development of osteomalacia
was not very convincing (Exton-Smith, 1968). In many elderly subjects,
problems are compounded by an indoor life with lack of sunlight and

deficient synthesis of vitamin D in the skin.

5. Calcium   Many old people seem prejudiced against drinking an
adequate amount of milk. There have also been suggestions that calcium
absorption decreases with aging (Bogert *et al.*, 1966). Some reports
have linked a low serum calcium with a diminution of bone thickness
(UK Dept. of Health & Social Security, 1972). However, D.A. Smith
et al. (1968) compared 152 normal women with 97 subjects giving a
history of severe back pain or recent fracture. They were unable to
find any difference between the two groups with respect to calcium
intake, absorption or excretion; further, the intakes of protein,
phosphates and vitamin D were similar for the two groups. The
problem of osteomalacia (Chapter 3) is probably complex, with
contributions from skeletal disuse, diminished androgen secretion and
reduced cutaneous synthesis of vitamin D.

6. Iron   We have noted previously (Table 3.10) that healthy old people
do not often suffer from low haemoglobin levels. However, marrow
stores of iron are relatively small, and severe anaemia can develop as a
sequel to gastro-intestinal bleeding (Will & Groden, 1965). Lesser
degrees of haemoglobin deficiency are sometimes seen in association
with an overall limitation of food intake.

General Dietary Recommendations

Existing food patterns for Canadian subjects are summarised in Table
4.14. When recommending diet for the elderly, any changes must be
introduced gradually, to encourage compliance. It is a formidable
undertaking to attempt to modify the eating habits of seventy or eighty
years! Since the total calorie intake is likely to be small, it is advisable
to avoid 'empty' calories such as pastry, confectionery and alcohol.
Emphasis should be placed on such items as green vegetables, milk,
eggs, meat and moderate amounts of whole wheat bread. If there are
biliary problems, fried food should be avoided, and the overall intake
of fat should be reduced to perhaps 25 per cent of energy requirements. Rich and highly spiced foods are also badly tolerated. Hot
meals are more easily digested than cold, and where the appetite is
flagging it is helpful to resort to smaller but more frequent meals.
    If an old person is incapacitated, he should be encouraged to avail
himself of special facilities such as 'meals on wheels'. Salt intake may
be restricted for medical reasons; care must then be taken to avoid
salt depletion, particularly during warm weather, when exercising hard

Table 4.14   Principal sources of various nutrients for Canadians aged 65 years and over. Based on data of Nutrition Canada (1976)

Nutrient	Source												
	Dairy products		Meat, poultry, fish, eggs		Cereal products		Fruit		Vege-tables		Fats, oils		Other	
	M %	F %	M %	F %	M %	F %	M %	F %	M %	F %	M %	F %	M %	F %
Calories	12	15	22	18	29	31	5	8	7	7	8	7	16	13
Protein	18	22	47	40	20	22	1	2	6	6			6	6
Fat	15	20	38	32	16	18		1	3	3	21	20	5	5
Carbohy-drate	7	9			44	44	11	17	12	11			24	19
Fibre					28	26	19	26	42	39			10	9
Calcium	56	58	6	4	18	18	4	5	7	7			8	8
Iron	2	2	32	27	34	34	7	9	12	12			14	14
Vitamin A	16	16	29	34	3	3	3	4	22	22	20	14	6	5
Thiamine	8	10	24	19	40	39	6	10	17	16			5	5
Riboflavin	30	33	24	21	27	26	3	4	7	6			9	9
Nicotinic acid	11	13	47	43	21	24	2	3	9	8			9	8
Vitamin C	6	4		1	1		47	62	45	31			1	1
Free folate	16	15	14	13	22	18	16	25	28	25			4	3

and when sweating from inter-current infections. Fluid intake should be sufficient to sustain a urine flow of 1.5 litres per day. Under conditions of rest, this implies a daily intake of 2 litres of fluid, and if there is increased sweating several additional litres of water or dilute saline may be needed (Kavanagh & Shephard, 1975a). Coffee or tea gives a useful stimulation of gastro-intestinal motility, which in the old person is often decreased to the point of constipation. However, coffee should be avoided late at night, particularly if there are complaints of insomnia. Finally, if there are dental problems or difficulty in swallowing, it may be necessary to mince foods prior to serving.

5 TRAINING FOR THE SENIOR CITIZEN

Since working capacity is substantially curtailed by aging, training programmes have practical importance even if they bring about relatively small physiological gains. In this chapter, we will consider the responses of the average senior citizen to a programme of progressive endurance training. The following chapter will examine specific characteristics of the elderly athlete.

Optimum Training Regimen

The optimum training regimen for an elderly person is marked by safety, effectiveness, a strong motivational appeal, and low unit cost.

Safety

The risks that exercise will provoke a musculo-skeletal injury or provoke a cardiac dysrhythmia inevitably increase as a person becomes older. We have noted in Chapter 3 that some exercise programmes for middle-aged and older citizens have had a more than 50 per cent toll of sprains, strains and bone injuries within the first few weeks of conditioning. Such statistics inevitably have a strong negative impact upon the motivation of both the injured individual and other members of his exercise class. Factors contributing to a high injury rate include: (1) clumsiness associated with lack of recent practice of a skill and deterioration of balance, (2) obesity, increasing the strain per unit section of tendon, (3) shortening of tendons associated with many years of inactivity, (4) failure to take an adequate 'warm-up', (5) violent calisthenics, especially rapid twisting movements and excessive stretching, (6) too rapid a progression of training, with exercise continuing when the subject is more than pleasantly fatigued, (7) exercise on a hard, uneven or icy surface, and (8) the use of shoes with inadequate heels and poor ankle support. If a subject is obese, or gives a history of back, leg, or foot problems, particular care is needed. Walking rather than jogging and calisthenics should be suggested for such individuals, at least initially. Tired and aching muscles are also a warning sign; if symptoms are more than slight at the beginning of the next class, the rate of progression is too fast, and the exercise prescription should be moderated for a few days until recovery has occurred.

176

There is a small risk that injudicious exercise may precipitate cardiac arrest or ventricular fibrillation (Shephard, 1974a; 1977a). Haskell (1976) collected a total of 949,568 man-hours of experience from 86 exercise clubs. Considering all available information, the risk of cardiac arrest was 1 in 29,674 man-hours; in recent years, a more cautious approach to operation of the clubs has apparently reduced the risk to 1 in 268,922 man-hours. The population of most exercise classes is male, and the average age is about 45 years. It is likely that the risks of gymnasium attendance increase at least in proportion to the rise in overall likelihood of a heart attack. Risks for a class of 65- to 70-year-old men would thus be at least ten times those for 45-year-olds (that is, 1 in 27,000 man-hours), while risks for elderly women would be about a third of the male figure. The main hazard is probably an intrusion of the 'type A' personality upon performance in the gymnasium. Individuals with this characteristic assume that they can accomplish their intended fitness goal in a third of the time if they exceed prescribed exercise by a factor of three! Games such as squash and tennis arouse an insatiable desire to trounce their opponent, irrespective of his proficiency. In class gymnastics, the 'type A' man is unwilling to admit that he is tired. Social and business problems are brought into the gymnasium, and items such as the warm-up, warm down and showering are rushed because other commitments prevent a leisurely enjoyment of the exercise hour. Shephard & Kavanagh (1978a) attempted to identify other characteristics of the person who succumbs to a heart attack during exercise, but with little success. Possible warning signs include a high cigarette consumption, a high resting blood pressure and abnormalities of the exercise electrocardiogram (ST segmental depression and dysrhythmias). Catastrophe is less likely if a safe level of exercise has been defined by a careful stress test and if the subject has been taught to hold his training intensity below this safe level, as monitored by palpation of his carotid pulse rate. It also seems important to avoid sustained isometric exercise and straining against a closed glottis (Valsalva manoeuvre).

Effectiveness

There is some danger that caution in the exercise prescription may preclude the development of an effective training programme; a nice judgement must be made between necessary prudence and timid incompetence. If the objective of training is to improve cardio-respiratory endurance, then the main determinants of effectiveness are the intensity of training and the initial fitness of the subject (Shephard,

1968a). There is general agreement that in a young person training does
not occur at efforts of less than 50 per cent of maximum oxygen
intake (Shephard, 1968a; 1975; 1977d; Davies & Knibbs, 1971; Pollock,
1973); unless the exercise is prolonged (Durnin *et al.*, 1960) or the
subject is unfit, the threshold heart rate may be 140-150 per minute
(Karvonen *et al.*, 1957). The necessary heart rate is lower in an old
person, partly because the maximum heart rate decreases with age,
and partly because initial fitness levels are low. Initial prescriptions
should be individually tailored so that heart rates are no higher than
120-130/min, to avoid musculo-skeletal and cardiac problems; however,
there should be progression to training rates of 140-150/min as soon as
observation in the gymnasium and formal exercise tests show such
advancement to be safe. The aim should be to attain 30 minutes of
vigorous activity three or four times per week, although in the first
few weeks it may be necessary to split individual bouts of training into
two fifteen minute stints.

If body weight is to be reduced, it is important that individual
exercise sessions are of sufficient duration to build up a substantial
energy usage. In this respect, an hour of brisk walking is more effective
than five minutes of jogging. The average 65-year-old may commence
with an added expenditure of 150 kcal (0.6 MJ) per session, and
progress to 300 kcal (1.2 MJ) per class. If there is substantial obesity,
correction of the problem can be speeded by an equal (150-300 kcal,
0.6-1.2 MJ) restriction of food intake.

If it is hoped to restore lean mass, some work with weights may be
permitted, providing there is no history of hypertension or cardiac
problems. However, it is important that individual efforts be kept
short enough to avoid a substantial rise of blood pressure, and that
intervals between repetitions be long enough to allow the oxidation
of accumulated metabolites. Muscle hypertrophy demands an
adequate quantity and quality of dietary protein, although as we have
seen, protein deficiency is not a common problem in Western society.
Some lean tissue is restored by measures to develop cardio-respiratory
fitness, and such muscle-building is probably adequate for most elderly
people. Certainly, care must be taken not to develop a heavily muscled
body while leaving the heart in poor condition.

If there is concern about bone weakness (osteomalacia and osteoporosis), the emphasis must be upon weight-bearing activities. Studies
on astronauts under 'zero-gravity' conditions have shown that exercise
in the absence of gravitational stress does little to prevent decalcification
of the bones. Again, activity should move in tandem with dietary

checks on such items as calcium intake, calcium/phosphorus ratio and vitamin D intake. Added exposure to sunlight will help by increasing synthesis of vitamin D in the skin.

Motivation

Certain expectations of the elderly with regard to exercise programmes were noted in the previous chapter. It seems important that they appreciate the existence of a class tailored to the specific needs of the senior citizen, and view this as a place where they can obtain instruction on a safe and effective regimen. There is a strong desire for well qualified leadership, and it is critical to find an instructor with a warm, out-going personality — a person who appreciates not only the strengths, but also the weaknesses of the elderly. An over-zealous instructor can have a markedly negative effect on both enthusiasm and body image if he makes unrealistic demands upon the class members. The main objectives of class participants seem an improvement in health and fitness and the 'feedback' of results should thus concentrate on presenting any gains in these variables.

The individual exercise prescription should build upon local facilities and available equipment, since the old person may have neither the funds nor the inclination to make a major investment in travel, specialised clothing or gear. Note should be taken of the skills and interests of the participant, and any previous training or special aptitudes should be exploited. Personality should also be considered; extroverts react best in a group situation, but introverts find more satisfaction if a major part of their prescription is filled alone or with a single close friend.

Possible lack of transport should be remembered, and where feasible the formal part of any programme should be taken to where the old people are located. Poor memory should be helped by diary records of requirements and accomplishments, and if attendance flags conscience should be stimulated by use of the telephone. Finally, reliance should not be placed on the supposed endless free time of the elderly. In fact, many old people remain very busy after retirement, and where possible the exercise counsellor should recommend building at least a part of the required activity into the normal duties of the week, such as walking the dog and mowing the lawn with a hand mower.

Cost

Group activity is usually more successful than an individual programme, both in arousing interest and in sustaining motivation. The main practical objection to the group approach is its cost. A class leader can hardly provide effective supervision for more than thirty people at one time. In Canada, a recently qualified physical education graduate might lead such classes for $15 per hour, or 50 cents per participant. Stated in such terms, the expense does not seem prohibitive, but if there are four sessions per week the cost becomes at least $100 per year. To this must be added an allowance for the rental of locker and shower facilities, and (in winter at least) the rental of a gymnasium. Other necessary expenses include a medically supervised exercise test perhaps once per year ($50 to $100), and a simpler test by paramedical personnel at three month intervals ($5 to $10 per test). From such statistics, it becomes apparent that commercial gymnasia with membership fees of $300 to $600 per year are not making an exorbitant profit.

Many old people do not have $300 per year to invest in exercise. A municipality may consider an exercise class as a worthwhile charge upon its budget if it reduces the number of senior citizens who require very expensive institutional care. Once an appropriate pattern of exercise has been taught and monitored for a few months, it may also be possible to cut back the number of supervised exercise classes to one per week, or even one every eight weeks (Kavanagh & Shephard, 1978), giving class members a home prescription that specifies a walking or jogging distance and time, with a pulse rate ceiling and a note of any warning symptoms. The periodic return to a formal class provides continuing motivation for the subject, opportunity for discussion of both exercise and other aspects of life-style, and a check on the suitability of the current activity prescription.

Typical Programme

It may finally be useful to describe a typical programme as followed by one group of sedentary 65-year-old subjects in Toronto (Sidney & Shephard, 1977a-c; 1978a,b). Since they were participating in a training experiment, they met four times per week. However, a similar format could have been adopted with one class per week or one class in eight weeks, instruction for the intervening periods being given as a home prescription, and compliance with the prescription being monitored by a daily activity diary (Figure 5.1).

Each class was of approximately 60 minutes duration. The first 15 minutes were devoted to calisthenics and stretching exercises. Most subjects expect such exercises as part of a fitness programme, and they

DAY	Main Activities	Time Actually Active (min)	Points
Sunday	1. Jogging 1 mile	12 min	2
	2. Skiing	30 min	3
	3. —	—	—
Monday	1. Jogging 1 mile	12 min	2
	2. Walking 1½ miles	30 min	0
	3. —	—	—
Tuesday	1. Jogging 1 mile	12 min	2
	2. Squash	10 min	1½
	3. Walking 3 miles	60 min	1½
Wednesday	1. Squash	10 min	1½
	2. Walking 1 mile	20 min	0
	3. —	—	—
Thursday	1. Jogging 1 2/20 miles	12 min	3
	2. Skating	30 min	2
	3. Walking 3 miles	60 min	1½
Friday	1. Jogging 1 1/20 miles	12 min	3
	2. Squash	10 min	1½
	3. —	—	—
Saturday	1. Golf	9 holes	1½
	2. Walking 1 mile	20 min	0
	3. —	—	—
		Total Points for Week	26

Figure 5.1   Example of an activity diary used to monitor personal exercise. Subjects are required to give details of the three most significant voluntary physical activities they have undertaken each day. Sheets are returned to the exercise counsellor on a weekly basis. (From the author's text *Alive, Man! The Physiology of Physical Activity*.)

provide both a 'warm-up' and an increase of flexibility. During the next 30 minutes, subjects followed an individually prescribed sequence of brisk walking interspersed with slower-paced recovery periods. In the early weeks of training, approximately equal distances (400 m) were covered by fast (6-8 km/h) and slow (4 km/h) walking. The aim was to reach a heart rate of 120-130/min during the fast walking. To check upon the intensity of effort, subjects were taught the technique of pulse counting by light carotid palpation, and the accuracy of their counting was verified by an observer and by the use of a portable tape recorder. As training continued and the condition of the individual permitted, the distances covered in the fast activity phase were increased and the recovery distances were decreased; in this way, the more co-operative subjects progressed to training heart rates of 140-150/min within 6 to 7 weeks. Prescriptions were further augmented to sustain these heart rates for the remainder of the year of training. The final fifteen-minute period of each class was occupied by a slow walking warm-down. Subjects were also encouraged to find new sources of activity in their leisure time, walking instead of using their cars and dispensing with unnecessary power equipment around their homes.

Cardio-Respiratory Changes

Opinions regarding the effectiveness of cardio-respiratory training in the elderly vary widely. At one extreme, Hollmann (1964) claimed that persons over 60 years of age made little adaptation to effort unless they had undergone conditioning at some earlier point in life. Benestad (1965) also found no gains of maximum oxygen intake when men aged 70 to 80 years underwent six weeks of training. Roskamm (1967) and Wilmore *et al.* (1970) agreed that men aged 50 years and over failed to improve as much as younger groups, while Kilböm (1971) stated that training benefits were less pronounced in women once they reached the age of 50 years. At the opposite extreme, there have been reports of anticipated or even of unusually large gains of maximum oxygen intake in old people with a history of many years of physical inactivity (Barry *et al.*, 1966a; de Vries, 1970, 1971; Tzankoff *et al.*, 1972; Stamford, 1973; Adams & de Vries, 1973; Sidney & Shephard, 1978a). The prime objective of this section will be to consider the extent of cardio-respiratory gains in the elderly in relation to the frequency and the intensity of training. However, it will be necessary to make some preliminary examination of training indices.

Indices of Training Response

It might seem a simple matter to compare the gains of maximum oxygen intake when young and older subjects undertake a specified period of endurance training. However, in practice the analysis is beset by several pitfalls, including problems in the matching of training and trainability, differences in methods of measuring and expressing changes of maximum oxygen intake, and a possible specificity of training at certain intensities of effort.

1. Matching of training and trainability   Young subjects are more easily persuaded to undertake vigorous training than are an older population. It is thus vital to ensure that comparisons are made between groups that have received an equal training stimulus. Matching should probably be on the basis of relative rather than absolute stress; for example, both young and elderly groups should be required to exercise for a fixed period of weeks at 60 per cent of aerobic power.

The training response is inversely related to the initial fitness of the subjects (Shephard, 1968a). Groups must thus be equated in terms of their trainability. Several Scandinavian reports (Kilböm *et al.*, 1969; Saltin *et al.*, 1969; Kilböm, 1971) have prejudiced their analysis by matching young and older subjects in terms of absolute aerobic power; the elderly were thus more fit than the younger subjects, and started the experiment with a handicap of lesser trainability. The ideal comparison seems between groups that are initially at the same percentage of age-related normal standards of maximum oxygen intake.

2. *Measurement and expression of data*   The optimum basis for the measurement of training response is probably to demonstrate an increase in the directly measured maximum oxygen intake. However, there may be hesitancy to ask older subjects to undertake a test of this severity, and even if it is attempted, a plateau of oxygen consumption may not be realised. If the symptom-limited maximum oxygen intake is substituted, there is a danger that the fears of the subject or the observer may bias the results of the first examination in a downward direction. At a second test, confidence will be greater, and a higher 'maximum' may be recorded in the absence of any conditioning; this could account in part for the very large (38 per cent) gains that Barry *et al.* (1966a) found over three months of conditioning.

We have seen (Chapter 3) that in elderly subjects predictions of maximum oxygen intake have a substantial systematic error (24.7 per cent, M; 15.4 per cent F) and a large coefficient of variation (14.5 per cent, M; 16.0 per cent, F). Saltin *et al.* (1969) cautioned that predictions could be further distorted by a decrease of maximum heart rate as conditioning developed. However, in accord with several other authors (Benestad, 1965; Hanson *et al.*, 1968b; Pollock *et al.*, 1971; Hollmann & Liesen, 1972; Tzankoff *et al.*, 1972), we have not observed a significant decrease. In the experiment of Sidney & Shephard (1978a), the average maximum heart rate of thirteen elderly men went from 169 ± 15 to 165 ± 15/min with conditioning; corresponding data for sixteen elderly women were 162 ± 13 and 157 ± 10/min. Subjects must also be habituated to the laboratory and the test procedure before the first definitive test is undertaken, but if this precaution is observed, sub-maximum tests can yield a reliable index of change in an individual (Wright *et al.*, 1978).

3. *Specificity of training response*   Some years ago, Roskamm (1967)

commented on a specificity of training, high intensity interval work improving all-out performance, while more moderate continuous training improved the physical working capacity at a heart rate of 130/min. Benestad (1965) trained his elderly subjects by interval running; he found that while there was an improved performance during sub-maximal work, there was no change of maximum oxygen intake. Sidney & Shephard (1978d) had rather similar findings. During the early weeks of training, when the exercise intensity was light (heart rates of 120-130/min), the largest gains were seen in the PWC_{130} rather than the PWC_{150}, but this trend was reversed as the group progressed to more intensive effort. In the second seven weeks of training, the directly measured maximum oxygen intake increased by a further 4 per cent, whereas the predicted maximum oxygen intake (based on the heart rate during sub-maximum work) showed continuing gains of only 1 to 2 per cent.

Responses to Maximum Effort

1. Maximum oxygen intake   Benestad (1965) found no gains of directly measured maximum oxygen intake when thirteen men aged 70-81 years carried out 5-6 weeks of interval training. However, a fairly high level of initial fitness (maximum oxygen intake 27 ml/kg min, 1.21 mM/kg min) and the brevity of conditioning may explain the absence of response. In contrast, Barry *et al.* (1966a) reported a remarkable 38 per cent increase of 'maximum oxygen intake' in five men and three women who followed a three month programme of interval training. At the initial test, the work tolerance in four of the eight subjects was limited by local muscle weakness, fatigue or motivational factors, and in the remaining four subjects the test was halted because of electrocardiographic changes; both 'maximum' heart rate (126 beats/min) and 'maximum' lactate concentration (40 mg/ 100 ml, 5.4 mM/l) were low, and suggestive of sub-maximal rather than maximal effort. After training, the subjects either chose to push themselves harder, or were allowed to do so, so that the apparent gains of maximum oxygen intake were accompanied by large increases in maximum heart rate, systolic blood pressure, lactic acid concentrations and respiratory minute volume. Although increases were in symptom-limited performance rather than true plateau values of oxygen intake, their practical importance should not be minimised; subjects were able to accomplish 38 per cent harder physical effort before the work-load became intolerable for them.

For reasons of safety, Sidney & Shephard (1978a) deferred direct measurements of maximum oxygen intake until their elderly subjects had participated in a preliminary conditioning programme for seven weeks. Unfortunately, much of the 'regulatory' component of training had already been completed at this stage. Nevertheless, subsequent gains of maximum oxygen intake totalled 4 per cent from week 7 to week 14, and 5 per cent from week 7 to week 21. The total response to week 21 was largest in subjects who elected a high intensity and a high frequency of training (19.5 per cent, 5.8 ml/kg min, 0.26 mM/kg min). No further gains were registered in the five women and four men who continued to train hard for the remainder of the year. Nevertheless, there is now unequivocal evidence that old people who train hard can induce a substantial increase in their directly measured maximum oxygen intake over the first few months of conditioning.

2. Sub-maximal predictions Predictions of maximum oxygen intake confirm that training can be induced in the elderly, given a suitable regimen of endurance exercise. Several authors (Stamford, 1972, 1973; Adams & de Vries, 1973) have reported a reduction in heart rate at a fixed sub-maximum work-load; assuming their subjects were habituated to the test procedure, this would imply an improvement of predicted aerobic power. De Vries (1970) exercised 68 men aged 51 to 87 years for a total of six weeks; perhaps because the training period was short, the predicted maximum oxygen intake of the test group increased by only 5 per cent, and there was an almost equal gain in control subjects. Eight of the test group continued their training for 42 weeks, and at this stage showed an 8 per cent increase over their initial predicted aerobic power. Sidney & Shephard (1978a) found a larger response when 42 men and women entered a one year training study; in the first seven weeks, gains of predicted aerobic power averaged 15 per cent, with a further (insignificant) 1-2 per cent improvement over the next seven weeks. Twenty-two subjects (10 men and 12 women) completed the one year programme; the final gain (24 per cent) was at least as large as would have been anticipated in younger subjects. As in some other comparisons (Roskamm, 1967; Kilböm, 1971; Getchell & Moore, 1975), increases of predicted aerobic power were shown equally by men and women. However, the response varied with the self-selected regimen of training (Figure 5.2). Sidney & Shephard (1978a) classified their subjects on the basis of attendance and intensity of effort. Their high frequency group averaged 3.3 sessions per week, while the low frequency group 1.5 sessions per week during the first seven weeks, and 1.0 sessions per week thereafter.

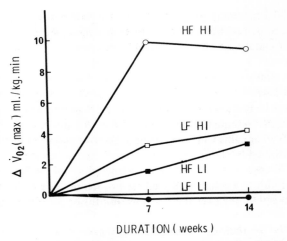

Figure 5.2   Changes in predicted maximum oxygen intake of four groups of elderly subjects electing respectively a high frequency/high intensity (HF, HI), low frequency/high intensity (LF, HI), high frequency/low intensity (HF, LI) and low frequency/low intensity (LF, LI) training regimen. Data of Sidney & Shephard (1978a).

Effort was classified as high or low intensity on the basis of observation and pulse counts. The largest response (32.9 per cent gain in seven weeks) was seen in the high frequency/high intensity group. The next greatest response (10.0 per cent in seven weeks) was in the high intensity/low frequency group. The low intensity/high frequency group showed a relatively small change in the first seven weeks, but by the fourteenth week had almost equalled the gains in the high intensity/low frequency group (total change of 10.0 per cent).

The rapid nature of the gains in maximum oxygen intake is in keeping with previous studies of young (Cunningham & Hill, 1975; Saltin *et al.*, 1968) and middle-aged (Saltin *et al.*, 1969; Massie & Shephard, 1971) subjects, but contrasts with our experience in post-coronary patients (Kavanagh *et al.*, 1973), where the maximum oxygen intake continued to increase well into the second year of conditioning. The attendance of the high frequency/high intensity group did not falter as the programme continued, and their intensity of effort increased from 60 per cent of their initial maximum oxygen intake to 70 to 80 per cent of their final aerobic power. The plateauing of the training response thus seems to reflect the attainment of physiological potential rather than any inadequacy of the conditioning programme. Early changes are presumably regulatory in type (Holmgren, 1967b; Saltin *et al.*, 1969); smaller structural changes, including a loss of body fat and an increase of lean mass continued throughout the year of observation.

While the largest response was obtained from high intensity/high frequency exercise, it is important to stress that a more moderate intensity of effort (a heart rate of 120-130/min, equivalent to about 60 per cent of aerobic power at the age of 65 years) also produced some response over a longer period. Where the subject is unable or unwilling to withstand a very vigorous programme, there thus remains virtue in encouraging him to pursue more moderate effort.

3. Cardiac responses We have already noted the small and statistically insignificant decrease of maximum heart rate in response to training. Some authors have found small associated increases of stroke volume (L.H. Hartley *et al.*, 1969; de Vries, 1970; Kilböm & Åstrand, 1971; Rousseau *et al.*, 1973), but the majority of the subjects studied have been middle-aged rather than elderly. Niinimaa & Shephard (1978) found no changes in 65-year-old men and women over 11 weeks of conditioning. In younger subjects, training can also lead to a widening of the maximum arterio-venous oxygen difference (Ekblöm, 1969; Ekblöm *et al.*, 1968; Kilböm, 1971; Rousseau *et al.*, 1973), but existing studies do not show such a response in the elderly (L.H. Hartley *et al.*, 1969; Kilböm & Åstrand, 1971; Niinimaa & Shephard, 1978). It is unlikely that training can increase the density of muscle capillaries in the elderly. Peripheral oxygen extraction may be helped by increases in the activity of cytochrome oxidase (Kiessling *et al.*, 1974) and aerobic enzymes (Clausen, 1969; Gollnick & Hermansen, 1973), but this is often offset by greater perfusion of inactive muscle (Clausen *et al.*, 1973) and the viscera (Clausen, 1969).

Responses to Sub-Maximum Effort

Increased economy of effort after conditioning is suggested by smaller increments of most cardio-respiratory variables during sub-maximum effort. Barry *et al.* (1966a), Benestad (1965), Shneidman (1972); Stamford (1972, 1973) and Sidney & Shephard (1978a) all observed a lower heart rate at a given work-load, while several authors have commented on parallel increases in the oxygen pulse (the volume of oxygen transported per heart beat, Barry *et al.*, 1966a; de Vries, 1970; Adams & de Vries, 1973). In the experiments of Niinimaa & Shephard (1978) training-related change in this last index was small and statistically insignificant. De Vries (1970) found no change of cardiac output, stroke volume, total peripheral resistance or mean tension time index (a measure of cardiac work-load) when the trained subjects were retested at a fixed work-load of 75 watts. Niinimaa & Shephard (1978) also saw no change of stroke volume with conditioning, but because the heart rate was slower, they noted a small (5-7 per cent) decrease in cardiac output at a given work-load. De Vries (1970) and Stamford (1972, 1973) both found a decrease of systolic blood pressure, with no change of diastolic pressure.

Some authors have found no alteration in the ventilatory cost of sub-maximum effort after training (Benestad, 1965; Barry *et al.*, 1966a; Adams & de Vries, 1973). De Vries (1970) noted that while ventilation remained constant at a given external work-load, it was increased at a given heart rate. There was an associated increase of vital capacity, so that the proportion of the vital capacity used with each breath remained constant. Barry *et al.* (1966a) tested subjects at what had initially been their limiting exercise, and at this load they saw a decreased accumulation of lactic acid after conditioning.

Recovery Curves

One well-recognised sign of conditioning is a faster recovery of the heart rate following both sub-maximum and maximum effort. Sidney & Shephard (1978a) found that after seven weeks of training, the heart rate during the first six minutes of recovery from a sub-maximal bicycle ergometer test was 6-10 beats/min slower than at the beginning of the experiment; after fourteen weeks of training, the decrement was 9-17 beats/min, with significant additional slowing of the heart rate during the first two minutes post-exercise (Figure 5.3). While all groups showed some change, as with the data taken during exercise the largest response was in the high frequency/high intensity exercise group, and the smallest response in the low frequency/low intensity group.

Resting Cardio-Respiratory Data

1. Respiratory system   There are reports that training can augment the vital capacity of young subjects, particularly where the exercise involves the chest musculature (Delhez *et al.*, 1967-8); however, it is difficult to exclude the possibility that a part of the reported gain has been due to a learning of technique (Mills, 1949). Some experiments on elderly subjects have shown quite a large response. Thus de Vries (1970) found a 5 per cent gain, after 6 weeks and a 20 per cent gain after 42 weeks of endurance training; further,

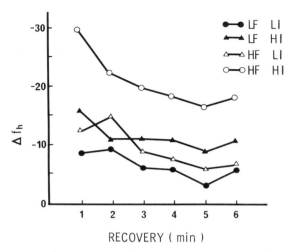

Figure 5.3   Influence of fourteen weeks endurance training on the recovery heart rate following sub-maximal effort on the bicycle ergometer. Data of Sidney & Shephard (1978a) for four groups of elderly subjects who elected respectively low frequency/low intensity (LF LI), low frequency/high intensity (LF HI), high frequency/low intensity (HF LI) and high frequency/high intensity (HF HI) training. Difference of heart rate (Δf_h) between initial and fourteen week tests.

learning of technique did not occur in this experiment, since the control subjects showed no change of vital capacity. Other observations on elderly men and women (Barry *et al.*, 1966a; Adams & de Vries, 1973; Sidney & Shephard, 1978a; Niinimaa & Shephard, 1978) have found no training effect. Niinimaa & Shephard (1978) concluded that a response was more likely if the initial vital capacity was low; in their series, initial readings were already well up to previously published normal standards. An increase of vital capacity depends partly on a strengthening of the thoracic muscles, partly on changes in the elasticity of the chondral cartilages, and partly on ability to alter the shape of the chest wall. While muscle hypertrophy is still possible in an older person, it presumably becomes progressively more difficult to induce alterations of chest mobility with aging.

There is no evidence that training can restore the closing volume of the lung (Chapter 3) towards more youthful values (Niinimaa & Shephard, 1978). This is not surprising, since the increase of closing volume reflects a loss of elasticity in the finer structure of the lungs (Anthonisen *et al.*, 1969-70), and this is an irreversible process.

Cross-sectional studies (Bates *et al* , 1955; F. Newman *et al.*, 1962; Holmgren, 1965) have shown a higher resting pulmonary diffusing capacity in the well-trained individual. Longitudinal studies on young and initially sedentary subjects show small effects on both resting and exercise diffusing capacity (Rosenberg, 1967; Anderson & Shephard, 1968). Short-term training (six weeks) leaves the diffusing capacity unchanged at a given sub-maximal oxygen intake, but maximum diffusing capacity is increased by some 5 per cent, due to a larger maximum cardiac output (Anderson & Shephard, 1968a). Longer training (three months) yields an increase of diffusing capacity in sub-maximum effort (Rosenberg, 1967). On the other hand, Niinimaa & Shephard (1978) found that in elderly subjects conditioning brought about a decrease of diffusing capacity at a given sub-maximal work-load, a change that might have been predicted from the parallel decrease of cardiac output.

2. Cardio-vascular system   A slow resting heart rate is a well-recognised feature of the well-trained young person. One report (Adams & de Vries, 1973) found a 3 beat/min decrease in elderly participants in an exercise class compared with a 4 beat/min increase in controls. However, a slowing of the resting pulse is not a common finding when older people undergo conditioning (Boucher, 1959; Stamford, 1972, 1973; Sidney & Shephard, 1978a; Niinimaa & Shephard, 1978), even though other variables indicate an improvement of cardio-respiratory performance. One reason may be that training has a limited effect upon the cardiac stroke volume of an older person.

In the healthy young adult, it is doubtful whether exercise can influence systemic blood pressure. Reductions are more likely in subjects with hypertension, and most studies of middle-aged and older subjects have shown some response (Barry *et al.*, 1966a; de Vries, 1970; Jokl *et al.*, 1970; Stamford, 1972, 1973; Sidney & Shephard, 1977). The mean change of systolic pressure in one series was as much as 20 mm Hg (2.67 kPa). Several authors (de Vries, 1970; Jokl *et al.*, 1970; Sidney & Shephard, 1978a) have also observed small (3-8 mm Hg, 0.4-1.1 kPa) decreases of diastolic pressure. Sidney & Shephard (1978a) found that over a year of progressive endurance training, the systolic pressure decreased from 132 to 115 mm Hg (17.6 to 15.3 kPa), while the diastolic reading dropped from 87 to 81 mm Hg (11.6 to 10.8 kPa). However, it is difficult to rule out all possibility of habituation in these experiments. Even where control groups have been established, the experimental subjects have necessarily had more contact with the laboratory and the investigator.

Early Scandinavian workers attached great importance to the total blood volume and the total haemoglobin level as indices of endurance fitness (Holmgren, 1967a). On current evidence, these variables are probably more important to sustained than to brief (1-5 minute) bursts of maximum work. Benestad (1965) noted significant increases of both total blood volume and total haemoglobin when his elderly subjects underwent five weeks of intensive training. However, there was no change in the haemoglobin content of unit volume of blood.

Electrocardiographic Findings

A reversal of abnormal electrocardiographic findings would be a particularly potent argument in favour of participation in an exercise programme, in view of the association between an abnormal exercise electrocardiogram and sudden death. Several authors have made cross-sectional comparisons of e.c.g. abnormalities between athletes and the general population (Chapter 6). There have also been some occupational comparisons — for example Blackburn (1969a) commented that the incidence of post-exercise ST segmental depression was less in farmers than in relatively sedentary railway clerks.

More weight must be given to the results of longitudinal studies. Salzmann *et al.* (1969) found that 79 per cent of subjects who showed an improvement of physical fitness also showed decreases in ST abnormalities, improvements in the e.c.g. record being directly related to exercise adherence and the resultant reduction in heart rate at a given work-load. After training, Bruce *et al.* (1969) found a 10 per cent decrease of heart rate during sub-maximal work, with a 40 per cent lessening of ST segmental depression; on the other hand, ST depression was unchanged if subjects were pushed to what was generally an increased symptom-limited maximum effort. Several other authors (Mazzarella *et al.*, 1966; Kilböm *et al.*, 1969; Detry & Bruce, 1971; Costill *et al.*, 1974) have observed lesser ST abnormalities at a given work-load, but no change in responses at a fixed heart rate after training. This would imply that the beneficial effect of conditioning was attributable simply to a reduction of heart rate and thus cardiac work-load at a given external effort. Kilböm (1969) commented that training led to an increase of ST segment elevation during both rest and work; however, the two women in their series who had a significant initial ST depression showed no improvement after training.

Kavanagh *et al.* (1973) carried out experiments with a group of middle-aged post-coronary patients. Their data is interesting, since some reversal of ST depression was seen, not only at a given work-load, but also at a given heart rate. Because of the nature of the disease, some of their subjects initially had quite marked ST depression. Demonstration of a positive response was favoured by the intensity of training, some of the subjects being conditioned to the point where they could complete a marathon race in as little as 210 minutes!

Sidney & Shephard (1977d) examined the effects of fourteen weeks vigorous training on the electrocardiograms of 42 elderly subjects. Under resting conditions, there was a very slight slowing of the heart rate, insignificant at seven weeks, and just significant at fourteen weeks (average change 5.4 beats/min). There was also some elevation of the ST segmental voltage at rest, the average change amounting to 0.03 mV at seven weeks, and 0.04 mV at fourteen weeks. The extent of this positive deviation varied with the pattern of training; the high frequency/high intensity group showed an elevation of 0.06 mV, and the high frequency/low intensity group also had an increase of 0.05 mV, but there were no changes in the low frequency/high intensity and the low frequency/low intensity groups. The significance of the ST elevation is not yet fully understood. Sjöstrand (1950) has related the phenomenon to a slow heart rate, and Saltin & Grimby (1968) have commented that many endurance athletes show quite marked ST elevation. Kilböm (1971) previously described a similar change when she trained middle-aged women. However, the displacement is sufficiently large that an argument can be made for considering it when calculating the ST depression induced by exercise.

In order to evaluate changes in the exercise ST response, Sidney & Shephard (1977d) calculated linear regression equations relating ST segmental voltage to heart rate before and after training; in this way, it was possible to calculate the ST voltage corresponding to a fixed heart rate (120/min) before and after fourteen weeks of training. The average results were −0.03 mV before and + 0.03 mV after conditioning, with rather similar responses in men and women. Eleven of 39 subjects initially showed a clinically significant ST depression (> 0.1 mV at 85 per cent of maximum oxygen intake), but after the fourteen weeks of training five of these eleven had improved to the point where the depression was less than 0.1 mV at the selected 'target' heart rate; a further two men who had not resolved their abnormality at fourteen weeks did so over an additional 35 to 40 weeks of progressive endurance training.

Although ST depression during exercise is associated with an adverse prognosis, it has yet to be shown that reversal of the ST change improves prognosis. Certainly, interpretation is complex. It is tempting to attribute the lessening of ST depression to an improvement of collateral blood supply to an ischaemic area of myocardium, but angiocardiographic studies do not support the view that exercise increases collateral flow in the middle-aged and elderly subject. A second and more plausible hypothesis is that a strengthening of the cardiac muscle and a reduction of mean ventricular radius decrease the work-load sustained by unit volume of cardiac tissue at any given external effort. This would imply a relief of myocardial oxygen lack without the resolution of cardiac atheroma or the development of new vascular channels. A further possibility is that the well-trained subject releases less intramuscular potassium at a given intensity of effort (Blomqvist, 1969); this would also reduce the magnitude of ST segmental changes. Lastly, it should be stressed that in keeping with the tradition of cardiology, Sidney & Shephard (1977d) referred all measurements to the 'iso-electric' potential; however, if they had taken account of the resting ST elevation induced by training, then they would have found no reduction in the downward displacement of the record induced by exercise.

Body Composition and Muscle Strength

A number of authors have found rather small changes of body composition when elderly subjects have followed programmes of endurance training. Barry *et al.* (1966a) found no change of body weight after three months of bicycle ergometer training. Pařízková & Eiselt (1968) compared body fat and lean mass in four groups of subjects. One had participated in intensive physical training throughout life, a second had trained recreationally, a third was sedentary and the fourth was initially sedentary, but had trained for three years immediately prior to observation. No significant differences in the percentages of body fat and lean mass were found between the four groups. De Vries (1970) found an 0.9 kg diminution of body weight and a 0.9 per cent decrease of fat after six weeks of interval training, but changes were no larger after 42 weeks of conditioning. A second study on elderly women (Adams & de Vries, 1973) showed no change of subcutaneous fat after three months of conditioning, although the exercise group lost 0.5 kg in weight, compared with a gain of 1.4 kg in control subjects.

In contrast with these rather negative findings, Sidney *et al.* (1977) found a substantial loss of body fat when elderly men and women participated in regular endurance exercise involving an additional daily

Table 5.1   Mean changes in skinfold thickness (mm and % loss) after seven and fourteen weeks of training. Data of Sidney *et al.* (1977) for thirteen elderly men and twenty-five elderly women

Site of skinfold measurement	Duration of training					
	7 weeks			14 weeks		
	mm	%	P	mm	%	P
Subscapular*	− 1.2	− 7.0	<.025	− 2.9	− 16.9	<.001
Triceps*	− 0.9	− 5.5	NS	− 2.3	− 14.1	<.001
Biceps	− 1.1	− 11.1	<.05	− 1.7	− 17.2	<.005
Suprailiac*	− 0.7	− 4.3	NS	− 2.1	− 12.9	<.005
Chin*	− 0.4	− 3.5	NS	− 1.1	− 9.7	<.001
Waist*	− 0.9	− 4.3	NS	− 2.3	− 10.9	<.01
Mid-axillary	− 0.1	− 0.6	NS	+ 1.1	+ 7.0	NS
Juxta-nipple*	− 4.0	− 19.4	<.005	− 3.9	− 18.9	<.001
Thigh	− 1.4	− 5.4	<.05	− 2.8	− 10.9	<.001
Calf	− 1.9	− 11.9	<.01	− 2.8	− 17.6	<.001
Knee*	− 2.5	− 9.8	<.005	− 2.6	− 10.2	<.01
Suprapubic*	+ 0.1	+ 0.3	NS	− 1.0	− 3.4	NS
Average of 8 skinfolds (mm)	− 1.6	− 8.0	<.005	− 2.4	− 12.1	<.001
Predicted body fat (%)	− 1.1	− 4.1	<.025	− 2.2	− 8.3	<.001

*

Table 5.2   Average percentage loss of fat according to self-selected pattern of training. Data of Sidney *et al.* (1977)

Variable	Group[a]	Duration of training			
		7 weeks	p[b]	14 weeks	p[b]
Average	LF LI	− 0.8	NS	− 1.4	NS
skinfold	LF HI	− 1.4	NS	− 1.9	NS
thickness	HF LI	− 1.5	NS	− 2.9	< .005
(mm)	HF HI	− 2.4	< .05	− 3.1	< .01
Predicted	LF LI	− 0.8	NS	− 1.9	< .05
body	LF HI	− 1.1	NS	− 2.4	< .05
fat	HF LI	− 0.9	NS	− 2.0	< .025
(%)	HF HI	− 1.6	NS	− 2.7	< .05

[a]   LF = low frequency training; HF = high frequency training; LI = low intensity training; HI = high intensity training

[b]   Statistical significance of change relative to initial value

energy expenditure of 150-300 kcal (6.3-12.6 MJ). Within seven weeks, there was an average decrease in skinfold thickness of 1.6 mm, and by fourteen weeks the decrease was 2.4 mm, with significant losses at ten of the twelve measurement sites (Table 5.1). Corresponding estimates of fat loss were 1.1 and 2.2 per cent respectively. Ten men and twelve women continued to train for up to one year, with an ultimate 3.3 mm decrement in skinfold thickness, corresponding to about three quarters of the fat burden normally accumulated over adult life (Shephard, 1977d). Nevertheless, total body weight remained unchanged, suggesting that there was an associated increase in lean muscle mass. Fat loss did not differ significantly between men and women, but was proportional to the frequency and the intensity of effort selected by the subject (Table 5.2). Persons training at a low frequency and intensity of effort lost fat at only one of twelve sites, after seven weeks of training, and three of twelve sites after fourteen weeks. In contrast, persons training frequently and at a high intensity lost fat at five and six sites after seven and fourteen weeks of training respectively, the overall fat loss for this group amounting to 2.7 per cent in fourteen weeks.

Further evidence of an increase in lean mass was obtained from measurements of ^{40}K (Sidney *et al.*, 1977); the data indicated a 4 per cent increase of total body potassium over the year of training, some 70 per cent of this gain developing between the 14th and the 52nd weeks of conditioning. Differences of response with pattern of training were small, although the largest gain (5 per cent) was seen in the high frequency/high intensity exercise group.

Many authors have found little change of muscular strength when elderly subjects have participated in brief periods of cardio-respiratory training. Thus Barry *et al.* (1966b) observed no change of either elbow or leg strength in response to a programme that stressed bicycle ergometer training. De Vries (1970) noted a small improvement in strength of the elbow flexors, 6 per cent after six weeks and 12 per cent after 42 weeks of conditioning. It may be significant that the latter subjects spent longer per session (20-25 minutes rather than 10-15 minutes) in performing calisthenic exercises. Sidney *et al.* (1977) found a small (5 per cent) increase in right (but not left) handgrip after fourteen weeks of conditioning. In their programme, also, the main emphasis was on cardio-respiratory conditioning, and perhaps for this reason a larger gain of knee extension force was observed (11 per cent at seven weeks of training, 13 per cent after one year of training). Chapman *et al.* (1972) adopted a specific programme of weight lifting, and with this type of regimen they were able to induce significant increments in the strength of the index finger, with associated improvements in the mobility of the metacarpophalangeal joint; responses of the elderly subjects were judged to be as large as would have been found in young men undertaking an identical training programme.

E.L. Smith & Babcock (1973) reported small but statistically significant increases in the bone mineral content of elderly men and women following eight months of either light calisthenics (2.6 per cent gain) or physical therapy (7.8 per cent). However, the technique used (E.L. Smith, 1971) measures the mineral content on only one segment of the body (the radius), and there is no guarantee that the changes observed in this one area are typical of the body as a whole. Sidney *et al.* (1977) used the neutron activation technique to obtain similar information. In their subjects, there was no gain of bone calcium over the year of training, final values being 99.7 ± 7.0 per cent of the initial readings. However, it may be significant that the small group of four subjects who persisted with a low frequency/low intensity programme showed an appreciable loss of calcium (9 per cent) over the same period.

Hormone Secretion

There is limited information concerning training induced alterations in the blood levels of several hormones, including growth hormone, cortisol and insulin.

Growth Hormone

In young subjects, both cross-sectional and longitudinal comparisons suggest that exercise more readily induces an increase of growth hormone concentration in untrained than in trained individuals (Sutton *et al.*, 1969; L.H. Hartley *et al.*, 1972a). Elderly subjects, in contrast (Figure 5.4) show an augmented response to sub-maximum effort after 9-10 weeks of endurance training (Sidney & Shephard, 1978b). In support of this observation, there is evidence that even in young subjects training abolishes the secondary drop of growth hormone levels at exhaustion, with a parallel improvement of endurance as depot fat is used in place of muscle glycogen (L.H. Hartley *et al.*, 1972b). It is conceivable that in the untrained elderly person, a combination of low muscle glycogen levels and a limited responsiveness of the hypothalamus and pituitary glands lead to a sub-optimal release of growth hormone in sub-maximum exercise; conditioning might thus restore hypothalamic sensitivity and augment the release of growth hormone. As we have noted above, Sidney *et al.* (1977) found good evidence that their programme of progressive endurance exercise caused a substantial mobilisation of subcutaneous fat.

A heightened growth hormone response may also help to conserve body proteins, always a problem in a person who is attempting to rid himself of excess fat. Growth hormone normally acts as a 'biochemical amplifier', enhancing the work-induced synthesis of muscle protein (Goldberg, 1967; Goldberg & Goodman, 1967). Greater quantities of growth hormone may be needed for this purpose in the elderly subject. Not only is there a lesser production of androgens, but small glycogen reserves and a poor peripheral circulation sometimes force the body to use protein as a fuel during sustained exercise. Furthermore, there are indications that aging reduces the sensitivity of the target cells to a given level of growth hormone (Szanto, 1975). Even if the growth hormone does not increase the rate of protein synthesis directly, mobilisation of depot fat will conserve glycogen and thus reduce protein breakdown during exercise. However, the experiments of Sidney *et al.* (1977) suggest that there is some increase of protein formation; as we have seen, there was an appreciable increase of lean mass when elderly subjects completed a year of endurance training.

A recent experiment of Szanto (1975) supports the concept that secretion of growth hormone is enhanced by training. He compared active and sedentary elderly men. Both showed an equal decrease of growth hormone concentrations in response to glucose administration, but the recovery of normal levels occurred much faster in the active

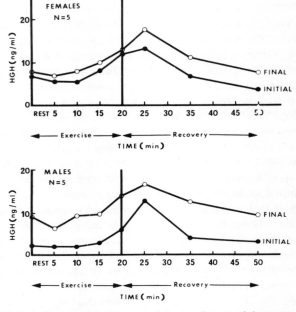

Figure 5.4   Influence of endurance training on the growth hormone response to a progressive exercise test in elderly men and women. Data of Sidney & Shephard (1978b); subjects exercised on the treadmill to 85 per cent of maximum oxygen intake before and after ten weeks of conditioning.

than in the sedentary group.

Cortisol

Cortisol levels do not seem to be increased by physical activity unless the effort is pursued to a stressful level. Viru & Akke (1969) found that in animals, training reduced the exercise-induced rise of cortisol concentrations. Cross-sectional comparisons of fit and unfit human subjects have yielded conflicting information, with reports of larger (Frenkl *et al.*, 1969) and smaller (Sutton *et al.*, 1969) exercise responses in poorly trained individuals. Longitudinal studies (Hartley *et al.*, 1972a,b; Amundsen & Balke, 1974; Sidney & Shephard, 1978b) are unanimous in showing no change of response after training in either young or elderly subjects.

Insulin

Diabetes is a common concomitant of loss of physical condition in the elderly, particularly if there is an accumulation of body fat. There is evidence that a regular programme of endurance training can do much to correct maturity onset diabetes, reducing or eliminating the need for insulin treatment. However, it has yet to be clarified whether this reflects usage of excess glucose by the exercise, an encouragement of muscle glycogen storage, or an enhanced secretion of insulin.

Psychological Gains from Training

As with physiological studies, many of the analyses relating psychological gains to chronic activity are cross-sectional in type. Any observed differences between active and inactive groups, although suggestive, are susceptible to at least two alternative explanations: (1) psychological problems may keep the inactive person from participation in an exercise programme, and (2) physical disability may be responsible for both the psychological problems and the restriction of physical activity. Longitudinal studies are generally more satisfactory, although also open to error. Benefit may be derived from group support or the encouragement of the class leader rather than from exercise *per se*. Furthermore, subjects may think it discourteous to suggest that they have not benefited from training, while the drop-out process necessarily gives a selective elimination of those with adverse reactions to exercise.

General Reactions

Many authors have commented on an increased sense of well-being that is associated with regular physical activity (Scott, 1960; Benestad, 1965; Cooper, 1968; W.P. Morgan, 1968; D.V. Harris, 1970; Morgan *et al.*, 1970; Reville, 1970; Massie & Shephard, 1971). However, there is relatively little objective data to support such claims, at least in healthy individuals (Hammett, 1967; Morgan *et al.*, 1970).

Barry *et al.* (1966b) found no changes of personality, cognition or motivation with training, despite remarkable increases of physical performance. R.R. Powell (1974) noted gains of cognition but no changes of behaviour when institutionalised geriatric mental patients were exercised. Stamford *et al.* (1974), also working with geriatric mental patients, observed that significant improvements in tests of general knowledge accompanied a physiological training effect; their control subjects showed neither physiological nor psychological gains.

Perceived Health

Cheraskin & Ringsdorf (1973) reported that Cornell Medical Index scores were significantly lower in old people who were taking regular daily exercise than in subjects who were inactive. Furthermore, scores on that part of the questionnaire dealing with psychological health (sections M to R) were lower for the daily exercisers (Table 4.6, p. 156). Palmore (1970) noted a correlation between perceived health and good health practices, particularly exercise participation. Poor health was defined as (1) more than two weeks of bed rest, (2) more than three visits to the doctor, or (3) hospitalisation within the past year. Complaints in these three categories were four times more frequent in elderly subjects who took little regular exercise. Further, twice as many of the inactive group said that their health had deteriorated over the preceding year. Unfortunately, it is hard to distinguish cause and effect in such relationships. Sidney & Shephard (1977b) conducted a longitudinal experiment on elderly men and women, and found little change of Cornell Medical Index scores with training. However, there was a significant decline in positive responses to section K (miscellaneous diseases), while subjects taking high frequency/high intensity exercise also showed a decrease of complaints relating to anxiety (section O of the Index).

Manifest Anxiety

The subjects of Sidney & Shephard (1977a) showed a modest overall decline of manifest anxiety scores in response to training. Reductions were unrelated to gains of aerobic power, and were largest in the group pursuing high frequency but low intensity training; this suggests that the observed change was related to group support rather than to physical activity itself. In keeping with this suggestion, Massie & Shephard (1971) could not demonstrate any change in manifest anxiety when middle-aged men improved their aerobic power by endurance training. Similarly, Polkins *et al.* (1973) in young women and Popejoy (1967) in middle-aged women observed training responses only in those subjects with high initial anxiety scores. McPherson *et al.* (1967) reported significant decreases of manifest anxiety following 24 weeks of training, but changes were much less marked in normal subjects than in patients who had recently sustained a myocardial infarction; among the latter group, participation in light recreational activity also reduced anxiety scores.

Life Satisfaction Index

Scores for the Neugarten Life Satisfaction Index were unchanged when elderly subjects participated in a programme of endurance training (Sidney & Shephard, 1977a).

Self-Concept

Some authors have described an improvement of self-image with training. Thus Heinzelmann & Bagley (1970) randomly assigned 381 middle-aged coronary prone men to exercise and control groups. After eighteen months of conditioning, the exercise participants manifested a more positive self-image, with associated increases in stamina and energy, more positive feelings of health and a greater ability to deal with stress. Likewise, McPherson *et al.* (1967) observed positive changes in self-image after 24 weeks of conditioning, gains being larger in cardiac 'post-coronary' patients than in normal subjects. In contrast, Massie & Shephard (1971) observed no change of either perceived or ideal body image when a group of middle-aged men underwent 28 weeks of vigorous training, this despite substantial improvements in aerobic power, muscle strength and percentages of body fat.

Presumably, much depends upon the initial body image; if this is good and in reasonable accord with the perceived ideal image, there is much less scope for improvement with training. Sidney & Shephard (1977a) found little change in average scores on the Kenyon test instrument when elderly subjects had completed three months of endurance exercise. However, those who trained the hardest showed a significant improvement in their actual body image, bringing it closer to the desired image; those who exercised less had small and statistically insignificant improvements; while those who exercised the least showed an insignificant widening of the discrepancy between actual and ideal images. Similarly, on McPherson's 'The Real Me' test, subjects who achieved little or no gain of aerobic power had a decline of mood score, whereas subjects with moderate or large gains of maximum oxygen intake improved their mood.

These findings have important implications for programming. Improvements of body image undoubtedly encourage a subject to persist with an exercise programme. On the other hand, it would appear that over-zealous encouragement of a low frequency/low intensity exerciser can have the negative effect of weakening body image. A nice judgement is thus needed to provide effective conditioning without excessive persuasion. Individual exercise prescriptions must be reviewed by a class leader who is not only enthusiastic, but is sensitive to the physical limitations of an aging population.

Attitudes

Sidney & Shephard (1977a) repeated the Kenyon attitude tests after their elderly subjects had completed fourteen weeks of conditioning. The group as a whole showed an increase on only one scale (physical activity as the relief of tension). However, those subjects who attained a high frequency and a high intensity of exercise also showed larger scores on the scales rating activity as a social experience, as health and fitness, as beauty of movement, and as an ascetic experience. In contrast, subjects who trained infrequently at a low intensity of effort showed a significant decline of scores for the scale rating activity as a means to health and fitness.

General Implications

Many exercise programmes are plagued by high drop-out rates, 50 per cent or more of recruits being lost within the space of six months. A successful programme will thus exploit favourable changes of attitude, and sustain the interest of participants by the demonstration not only of physiological gains but favourable changes in health, mood and manifest anxiety. There is scope for a feedback of information through the periodic repetition of both simple fitness tests and self-evaluations of psychological state. Furthermore, caution is necessary to avoid the negative impact of loss of health (through excessive fatigue and minor injuries) or a deterioration of body image (through a discrepancy between the expectations of the class leader and the actual achievements of the subject).

Activity Patterns

Participation in an exercise class necessarily gives a fairly high level of energy expenditure for a part of the day. However, much of the potential for training and the usage of excess calories could be dissipated if subjects reduced their activity for the remainder of the day as a consequence of participation in the conditioning programme.

Sidney & Shephard (1977c) compared diary sheets for eleven elderly subjects before and after completing twelve months of endurance training (Table 5.3). After training, less time was spent driving cars (particularly by the men) and performing ablutions (particularly by the women), with corresponding increments in the time allocated to active pursuits. The final daily energy consumption (2,500 kcal/day, 10.5 MJ/day in the men; 2,264 kcal/day, 9.5 MJ/day in the employed women; 2,212 kcal/day, 9.3 MJ/day in recently retired women) was greater than in many previous surveys of the elderly.

Table 6.3 Body composition of older participants in track competitions

Age	Height (cm)				Weight (kg)		Excess weight (kg)		Body fat (%)		Lean body mass (kg/cm)		Mileage per week	
	(1)	(2)	(3)	(C)	(1)	(C)	(1)	(C)	(1)	(2)	(1)	(2)	(1)	(2)
MEN														
< 40	175.2	—	—	176.7	69.9	80.0	−0.3	+ 9.4	13.9	—	0.339	—	27.6	—
40 – 50	174.7	180.7	162.6	176.2	69.4	81.7	+ 0.7	+ 11.6	14.5	11.2	0.339	0.352	42.0	40.4
50 – 60	172.6	174.7	163.9	173.1	66.0	77.1	−1.3	+ 9.2	14.4	10.9	0.327	0.343	38.4	42.0
60 – 70	172.3	175.7	162.9	171.5	68.7	77.4	+ 1.3	+ 10.8	14.4	11.3	0.339	0.339	26.6	29.7
> 70	165.3	175.6	156.6	—	61.0	—	−5.7	—	11.1	13.6	0.325	0.329	—	20.0
WOMEN	164.9	—	—	161.8	57.1	62.0	−1.3	+ 5.1	22.8	—	0.268	—	23.3	—

References

(1) Kavanagh & Shephard (1977b)
(2) Pollock (1974)
(3) Asano *et al.* (1976)
(C) Bailey *et al.* (1974) – control subjects, Saskatoon

The implication is that they had accumulated at least 12 kg of fat relative to their more active contemporaries.

Montoye *et al.* (1957) documented a similar rapid weight gain in former US university class athletes. Up to the age of 45 years, weight gain was less than in their sedentary classmates (Figure 6.1), but thereafter they put on more weight than those who did not win 'letters' for a specific sport at university.

Lean Tissue

We have noted that in the series of Saltin & Grimby (1968), the older orienteers were 6-7 kg lighter than younger age groups, suggesting that there was a substantial loss of lean tissue with aging. In contrast, the track competitors studied by Pollock (1974) and Kavanagh & Shephard (1977b) showed almost no decrease of lean tissue in older age categories (Table 6.3); both of these latter populations were still running 30-40 miles (48-64 km) per week.

Some authors (such as C.T.M. Davies, 1972) have argued that athletes maintain a large heart and other 'dimensional' effects of endurance training as they become older. The subjects examined by C.T.M. Davies (1972) showed a rise of cardiac volume from the 20 to 60-year-old age group. This may be partly an artefact of sampling, with the inclusion of more active subjects in the older age categories. However, Kavanagh & Shephard (1977b) had similar findings in their sample of Masters' Athletes. The heart volume, expressed per kg of body weight, increased from 12.0 ± 2.3 in those under the age of 40 to 12.5 ± 1.7 at ages 40 to 50, 12.4 ± 1.7 at ages 50 to 60, 13.9 ± 2.8 at ages 60 to 70, and 13.2 ± 3.0 at ages 70 to 90 years. A study of female swimmers suggested that the cardiac volume was well maintained for a few years, even if training was relaxed (Eriksson *et al.*, 1971). On the other hand, Saltin & Grimby (1968) reported that the heart volume of inactive orienteers had already dropped to 11.1 ml/kg at the age of 45 years (compared with 15.0 ml/kg in those who remained active). Over the next two decades, heart volumes diminished even in orienteers who claimed to be persisting with their sport, a figure of 13.2 ml/kg being observed at the age of 65 years.

It seems likely that the Masters' Athletes are an unusual group, in that their enthusiasm for hard endurance training is often initiated in middle age; cardiac volumes thus tend to increase in this group as they become older. However, most other types of athlete show a steady decline in the rigour of their training, and this is ultimately associated with some loss of lean tissue.

Blood Chemistry

Irrespective of activity patterns, serum cholesterol levels were relatively high in the elderly orienteers examined by Saltin & Grimby (1968); average values were 286 mg/100 ml, 7.4 mM/l, and 266 mg/100 ml, 6.9 mM/l for the active and inactive groups. However, serum lipids were higher for inactive (1.85 mM/l) than for active subjects (1.10 mM/l).

Muscular Strength

The only published information on the muscular strength of continuing athletes is a 25-year longitudinal study of physical education teachers (Asmussen & Mathiasen, 1962). This group was presumably more active than the general population, but nevertheless the loss of handgrip force was at least as great as in sedentary subjects:

	Left hand		Right hand	
	Age 23/24	Age 50/51	Age 23/24	Age 50/51
Men (N)	473	382	533	434
Women (N)	321	226	360	261

Cardio-Respiratory Function

Maximum Oxygen Intake

Some authors (Hollmann, 1965; Dehn & Bruce, 1972) have suggested that maximum oxygen intake deteriorates more slowly in the continuing athlete than in the sedentary subject. However, the rates of functional loss cited for the continuing athletes (0.70 and 0.56 ml/kg min per year, 31.3 and 25.0 μM/kg min per year) are much as in cross-sectional studies of the general population, raising the suspicion that the apparent rate of aging of their control groups was exaggerated by an increase of body weight and a decline of habitual activity.

Dill *et al.* (1967) reported a loss of 0.67 ml/kg min per year (29.9 μM/kg min per year) in champion runners who were still active. Cross-sectional data for track competitors is summarised in Table 6.4. The loss of maximum oxygen intake from age 45 to 65 (6.1-8.3 ml/kg min, 0.27-0.37 mM/kg min) seems appreciably less than the 4-5 ml/kg min (0.18-0.22 mM/kg min) per decade encountered in sedentary subjects. However, this is probably an expression of habitual activity patterns for the two populations rather than any more general effect of endurance training upon the aging of aerobic power. While the

Table 6.4 Cross-sectional studies on the aging of maximum oxygen intake in track and field athletes and orienteers; data expressed in ml/kg min STPD (ml) and mM/kg min (mM)

| Age (yrs) | Track and field competitors | | | | | | Orienteers | |
| | Ref (1) | | Ref (2) | | Ref (3) | | Ref (4) | |
	(ml)	(mM)	(ml)	(mM)	(ml)	(mM)	(ml)	(mM)
< 40	49.6	2.21	—	—	—	—	—	—
40 − 50	49.9	2.23	57.5	2.57	49.7	2.22	57	2.54
50 − 60	46.0	2.05	54.4	2.43	45.1	2.01	53	2.37
60 − 70	41.6	1.86	51.4	2.29	42.2	1.88	43	1.92
> 70	29.0	1.29	40.0	1.79	38.9	1.74	—	—

References

(1) Kavanagh & Shephard (1977d) − predicted maximum oxygen intake
(2) Pollock (1974) − direct maximum oxygen intake
(3) Asano *et al.* (1976) − direct maximum oxygen intake
(4) Saltin & Grimby (1968) − direct maximum oxygen intake

general population shows a substantial decline of voluntary activity between 25 and 65 years of age (Chapter 4), many Masters' competitors first become interested in serious competition around 35 or 40 years of age. In the youngest age group, we are thus comparing a Masters' athlete who has recently initiated training with a member of the general population who is still taking some voluntary recreational activity, while in subsequent decades the comparison is between an increasingly well-trained veteran runner and an average citizen who has become almost completely inactive. Irrespective of mechanisms, the Masters' candidate has a substantial advantage in terms of his capacity to perform endurance work; at the age of 65 years, his maximum oxygen intake is close to that anticipated in a sedentary 25-year-old adult.

Saltin & Grimby (1968) have provided cross-sectional data for orienteers. Their findings are similar to those for the track competitors, with an annual loss of aerobic power amounting to 0.34 ml/kg min (15.2 μM/kg min) in those who remained physically active, and 0.40 ml/kg min (17.9 μM/kg min) in those who have taken up the sport.

We may conclude that both longitudinal and cross-sectional data offer a tantalising suggestion that the rate of loss of maximum oxygen intake develops less rapidly in the continuing endurance athlete than in the general population. However, much further work will be needed to distinguish the possible contributions of differences in activity

Table 6.5 Resting systemic blood pressures for elderly athletes, compared with the values of Masters *et al.* (1964) for the general population

Age (years)	Kavanagh & Shephard (1977b)		Pollock (1974)	
	mm Hg	kPa	mm Hg	kPa
< 40	124/79	16.5/10.5	—	—
40 − 50	120/77	16.0/10.3	117/76	15.6/10.1
50 − 60	127/77	16.9/10.3	129/81	17.2/10.8
60 − 70	128/77	17.1/10.3	122/78	16.3/10.4
> 70	140/86	18.7/11.1	141/83	18.8/11.1

Age (years)	Asano *et al.* (1976)		Master *et al.* (1964)	
	mm Hg	kPa	mm Hg	kPa
< 40	—	—	127/80	16.9/10.7
40 − 50	117/70	15.6/9.3	130/82	17.3/10.9
50 − 60	132/79	17.6/10.5	137/84	18.3/11.2
60 − 70	135/82	18.0/10.9	143/84	19.1/11.2
> 70	157/78	20.9/10.4	146/82	19.5/10.9

patterns and selective sample attenuation to the apparent advantage of the athlete.

Systemic Blood Pressures

Cross-sectional data are available for three groups of elderly track competitors (Table 6.5). All values are marginally lower than published norms obtained on sedentary subjects. This supports the finding of a small reduction of systemic pressures with endurance training (Chapter 5).

Vital Capacity

There have been two longitudinal studies of vital capacity, both in physical education teachers. Asmussen & Mathiasen (1962) found quite a small change over 25 years (0.2 litres in men, 0.25 litres in women), while I. Åstrand *et al.* (1973) could not detect any loss of vital capacity over 21 years. These observations may indicate some protective effect of sustained physical activity upon pulmonary function, but two possible sources of bias relative to cross-sectional studies of the sedentary population are that few physical education students smoke, and spirometer designs were improved substantially between the initial and final dates of these experiments.

Electrocardiographic Findings

Some authors have expressed a fear that the large heart of the athlete could predispose to myocardial ischaemia. Opinions differ with respect to the incidence of electrocardiographic abnormalities. Holmgren & Strandell (1959) reported a high frequency of ST segmental abnormalities in former competitors, but other investigators (Pyorala *et al.*, 1967; Saltin & Grimby, 1968) have found a normal or even a low incidence of pathological records. Discrepancies in such reports may relate to differences in the training intensities sustained as the athletes became older.

Kavanagh & Shephard (1977b) obtained both resting and exercise electrocardiograms on 135 participants in the World Masters Track competition. Subjects in their sample were still running 30-40 miles (48-64 km) per week. Seventeen of the group showed occasional ventricular premature systoles at rest, but in all except two of these subjects the record became normal during exercise. Four athletes showed other abnormalities of the resting electrocardiogram, including a previously unrecognised old myocardial infarction, a right branch bundle block, and two cases with minor changes in the T wave. None of these findings was considered a contraindication to participation in an endurance training programme.

The principal abnormality encountered during exercise was a substantial (> 0.1 mV) depression of the ST segment. Fifteen of 135 tracings showed such an abnormality (Kavanagh & Shephard, 1977b), a somewhat smaller proportion than would have been anticipated in a random sample of the general population of comparable age (35 to 91 years), despite the fact that the athletes were exercised to a much higher absolute work-load than that tolerated by sedentary subjects. This seems in line with the lessening of ST depression observed when sedentary older subjects undertook a programme of vigorous endurance training (Chapter 5). Possible explanations include not only development of the coronary collateral circulation, but also a lessening of the rise in serum potassium with effort, and a reduction in the work-load per unit mass of heart muscle secondary to either cardiac hypertrophy or a change in the average dimensions of the heart.

Injury Experience

We have noted previously that some training programmes for the elderly have been marred by a very high toll of musculo-skeletal problems. It is disturbing to find that injuries are at least equally frequent in the Masters' competitors, despite twenty years experience of techniques, presumably with an associated conditioning of the muscles and tendons used in running. Kavanagh & Shephard (1977b) reported that among those attending the World Masters' competitions in Toronto, 57.2 per cent had suffered an injury of sufficient severity to interrupt training during the previous year. Of those injured, 39.6 per cent had experienced at least one week of disability, a further 26.7 per cent had been incapacitated for one to four weeks, and 33.7 per cent had been affected for more than four weeks. All three categories of track competitor were implicated (sprinters 58 per cent, middle-distance runners 68 per cent, and long distance runners 54 per cent).

There have been occasional suggestions that a lack of essential nutrients contributes to a high injury rate. Many of the Masters' athletes were taking dietary supplements, but this group (63 per cent injured) fared somewhat worse than those who did not supplement their normal diet (49 per cent injuries). In particular, large doses of vitamin C (> 500 mg/day) were apparently of no benefit (64 per cent injuries in subjects taking mega-doses of this vitamin). It may be unavoidable that an older person will push himself to the point of occasional injury if he wishes to excel in international competition. However, injuries can be avoided in sedentary old people if their rate of training is suitably graded (Chapter 5), and until the contrary has been proven, it would seem wrong to regard the current injury rates for Masters' athletes as inevitable.

Dietary Foibles

Older athletes are generally a health-conscious population, as can be gauged from their interest in dietary supplements. In the series of Kavanagh & Shephard (1977b), 62 per cent were taking one or more regular dietary supplements, the practice being more common in middle-distance (67 per cent) and long-distance (73 per cent) than in sprint runners (29 per cent). The catalogue of items taken included vitamin C, vitamin B mixtures, wheat germ oil, yoghurt, vitamin E and yeast extract. A number, particularly among the English contestants, were also keeping to a vegetarian diet.

Longevity

The longevity of the athlete provides a convenient overall assessment of the effects of vigorous physical activity on the aging process. Interest in this question was stimulated about a century ago by the belief that participation in vigorous sport would greatly curtail the human life-span. The Rev. Charles Wordsworth, originator of the Oxford and Cambridge boat race, noted 'we used to be told that no man in a racing boat could expect to live to the age of 30' (P. Hartley & Llewellyn, 1939). In 1869, Mr Frederick Skey (then consultant surgeon to St Bartholomew's Hospital in London) wrote: 'The University Boat Race as at present established was a national folly' (ibid., 1939). This point of view was almost immediately disproven by J.E. Morgan (1873) in England and Meylan (1904) in the United States, with subsequent reiteration of the safety of rowing by Knoll (1938) in Germany. Nevertheless, as recently as 1968 a rumour was circulated that all members of the Harvard 1948 rowing crew had died of various forms of cardiac disease, and it was necessary for Quigley (1968) to stress that the 36 individuals most intimately affected by such a rumour were still very much alive.

Problems of Analysis

Before looking in detail at the evidence, it is necessary to stress certain problems that arise when comparing the longevity of an athlete with that of a less active person.

The age of death of the athlete has commonly been obtained from the obituary column of an alumnal magazine (for example, W.E. Anderson, 1916; Rook, 1954), from a sporting almanac (for example, Hill, 1927), or in the case of high-school athletes, from the death records of state and county (for example, Wakefield, 1944). While some of the authors concerned went to great trouble to verify their facts, there is an inevitable risk with such an approach that a proportion of deaths will be overlooked, thus overestimating the longevity of the average athlete.

Early comparisons were with the general population or with life expectancy tables prepared by the assurance companies. This is not altogether fair, since the university graduate and even the senior high-school student of the mid-nineteenth century enjoyed substantial socio-economic advantages relative to the average citizen (P. Hartley & Llewellyn, 1939; Dublin, 1932; Rook, 1954; Prout, 1972). Other students attending the same university provide a better control group (Dublin, 1932; Rook, 1954; Montoye *et al.*, 1956, 1957), although there remains a danger that the death of an indifferent graduate will be less widely reported than that of a star athlete or a renowned scholar. Further, there is no guarantee that a person who fails to win a place on a university sports team is inactive — indeed, some of the 'control' series have been men renting locker space in university gymnasia (Polednak, 1972a,b).

Often the sample size has been inadequate, particularly when attempts have been made to stratify data in terms of type of sport and cause of death. In the attempt to obtain a sufficient sample of athletes, and to ensure that the majority were dead at the time of analysis, studies have been extended far back into the nineteenth century. This has exposed the control population, and to a lesser extent the privileged university graduates, to a period of rapidly changing medical and social care. Furthermore, many of the early fatalities are from conditions such as tuberculosis which are no longer prevalent. The dates of death are usually recorded precisely, but many of the early records have vague descriptions of the terminal illness that are hard to reconcile with modern classifications of disease.

The majority of studies give little information on life-style subsequent to graduation. If physical activity is to modify longevity, it seems likely that the activity must continue into middle and old age. However, as we have noted earlier in this chapter, many ex-athletes ultimately pursue a less healthy pattern of life than their contemporaries. Montoye *et al.* (1957) found that at the age of 35, the non-athletic graduates of Michigan State University had gained over 8 kg of weight, while the ex-athletes had gained only half as much. However, in subsequent years the weight of the non-athletes stabilised, while that of the ex-athletes continued to increase. Thus, after the age of 45, the ex-athletes showed the larger weight gain (Figure 6.1). Up to 45 years, a large percentage of the ex-athletes continued to participate regularly in some sports activity, but in older subjects this comparison also favoured the non-athlete. In contrast to the American experience, Karvonen *et al.* (1974) noted that Finnish cross-country skiing champions pursued their sport for at least twenty years, and a large proportion of contestants retained skiing as a hobby in later life (Karvonen, 1959).

Life-Span of Rowers

Much of the available information refers to rowing. This is undoubtedly one of the more strenuous forms of physical activity, and in the team events the pace of effort is largely outside the control of the individual sportsman. Data is summarised in Table 6.6. Morgan (1873) followed up 294 oarsmen who had participated in the Oxford versus Cambridge

Table 6.6   Mean life-span of oarsmen and control groups with lower levels of activity. Based on data collected by Yamaji & Shephard, 1978

Authors	Subjects	N	Year of birth[a]	Life-span	Control group
Morgan (1873)	Oxford & Cambridge	294	1808 – 1848	+ 2 years	Average Englishman
Meylan (1904)	Harvard	152	1831 – 1871	+ 2.88 years	Mortality tables
Dublin (1928)	Ten US universities	576	1859 – 1884	94.1%[b]	American Men Table of Mortality
L. Cooper *et al.* (1937)	Ormend Coll., Australia	100	1864 – 1884	75.5%[b]	Mortality tables
P. Hartley *et al.* (1939)	Oxford & Cambridge	513	1808 – 1841	87.8%[b]	Mortality tables
			1842 – 1872	76.7%[b]	
			1872 – 1902	85.1%[b]	
			1903 – 1907	93.5%[b]	
Rook (1954)	Cambridge	167	1850 – 1900	67.08 years	67.43 years (325 random students) 69.41 years (362 intellectual students)
Polednak (1972)	Harvard	133	1860 – 1889	66.8 years	67.1 years (3,287 classmates)
Prout (1972)	Harvard	90	1861 – 1881	67.79 years	61.54 years (90 classmates) $p < 0.05$
	Yale	82		67.91 years	61.56 years (82 classmates) $p < 0.05$
	Combined	172		67.85 years	61.55 years (172 classmates) $p < 0.01$

a   Where date of race stated, assumed that students 21 years old at time of competition
b   Actual deaths expressed as percentage of expected value for control series

boat race between 1829 and 1869. The group lived some two years longer than the 'average Englishman' of insurance tables. Meylan (1904) carried out a parallel study on 152 men who rowed in the Harvard University crews from 1852 to 1892; again, the crew members lived 2.88 years longer than indicated by an insurance table ('American Experience Table of Mortality'). Dublin (1928) obtained a larger sample by collecting information from ten US universities; actual deaths were only 94.1 per cent of the figure predicted from the 'American Men Table of Mortality'. L. Cooper *et al.* (1937), in a small study from Ormend College, Australia, and P. Hartley & Llewellyn (1939) had essentially similar findings.

Greenway & Hiscock (1926) were probably the first to point out that not only athletes but also non-athletic graduates had a favourable life-expectancy. In their sample, the ratio of actual to expected deaths for non-athletes was only 83 per cent when measured against the 'American Men Ultimate Table'. In 1932, Dublin corrected the deficiency in his earlier study, comparing the experience of 4,976 athletes with 38,269 general college graduates and 6,500 men earning scholastic honours. The athletes (who included the 576 oarsmen) lived approximately as long as the general graduates, but some two years less than those winning scholastic honours. A comparable study of 834 Cambridge athletes (including 167 oarsmen) was carried out by Rook (1954). The mean age at death for all athletes was 67.97 years. The oarsmen lived for 67.08 years, compared with 67.43 years for 379 randomly selected students and 69.41 years in 382 'intellectuals' selected from the same university; in making his comparison, Rook excluded deaths due to war and accidents, an important distinction, since the personality that leads athletes to excel in competition also contributes to their involvement in dangerous ventures (Greenway & Hiscock, 1926). By way of example, eight of the 152 oarsmen studied by Meylan (1904) were killed accidentally; excluding these subjects, the advantage over the general insurance tables would have been 5.09 rather than 2.88 years. Polednak (1972b) also restricted his comparison to those dying of natural causes; the average age of death was 66.8 years for 133 Harvard oarsmen, compared with 67.1 years for 3,287 classmates who rented gymnasium lockers but did not represent their university at any sport.

The most recent examination of the fate of the oarsmen is that of Prout (1972). He compared 172 graduates of Harvard and Yale who had rowed at least once in the four mile intervarsity race with an equal number of classmates; unlike the earlier studies, he found the oarsmen to have a six year advantage over their classmates (P < 0.01). Although superficially a convincing statistic, the difference rests mainly on the premature demise of subjects selected as controls for his investigation.

Other Classes of Athlete

Although the main focus of research interest has been the competitive rower, there are some reports describing longevity for other classes of sportsman (Table 6.7). Inter-sport comparisons are of interest because of (1) differences of personality and body build between the various classes of sportsmen, (2) differences in the intensity and duration of activity required for the various sports and (3) differences in the likelihood that the sport will continue to be pursued in middle and old age.

Track and field sports have traditionally attracted the less privileged socio-economic groups, particularly in the United States. However, with the exception of the early study of Anderson (1916) they fare quite well in comparison with the crew members. Running has the advantage that it can be continued into later life without assembling a team, and the track competitor may also have advantageous features of body build.

A second favoured group are the cricketers. Hill (1927) concluded that they lived substantially longer than the general English population. Among those born 1800-49, deaths were only 67 per cent of expected at age 65 years. Amateurs fared slightly better than professionals. Both groups had substantially fewer deaths than the oarsmen of 1808-41, whose mortality was 87.8 per cent of expected (P. Hartley & Llewellyn, 1939). In a more recent study (Rook, 1954), the cricketers continued to enjoy a small advantage of about one year relative to crew members. This has been attributed (without great evidence) to the contemplative aspects of cricket.

Assessments of Rugby and American football have varied. In the series of Dublin (1928) and Rook (1954), the football players lived longer than crew members. Reed & Love (1931) found that West Point graduates who earned letters in football lived 0.25 to 1.25 years longer than the average military graduate, but 0.5 years less than other classes of athlete. More recently, Polednak (1972) found no advantage of life expectancy in amateur football players, and in the mainly professional series of Largey (1972) there was a substantial disadvantage. This may reflect the ever increasing emphasis upon weight rather than skill in American football.

Table 6.7 Mean life-span[b] for various classes of sportsman. Based on data collected by Yamaji & Shephard (1978)

Sport	Anderson (1916)[a]		Dublin (1928)[a]		Rook (1954)[a]	Polednak (1972)		Largey (1972)[c]	
Track and field	62%	(276)	91.8%	(1,076)	67.41 years (203)	66.9 years	(186)	71.3 years	(23)
Cricket					68.13 years (116)				
Crew	45%	(171)	94.1%	(576)	67.08 years (167)	66.8 years	(133)		
Rugby football					68.84 years (218)				
American football	58%	(213)	88.3%	(1,233)		66.6 years	(135)	57.4 years	(120)
Baseball	47%	(148)	98.0%	(1,111)		65.2 years	(107)	64.1 years	(630)
Boxing								61.6 years	(107)
Two or more sports						67.2 years	(85)		

a Actual deaths expressed as percentage of expected values for control series
b With the exception of the data of Anderson (1916), deaths from war and accident have been excluded
c Mainly professionals, drawn from *Who was who in American Sports*

Data on cross-country skiing champions comes from Scandinavia, where life-expectancy is typically greater than in North America. Schnohr (1971) compared the mortality of 297 Danish skiers born between 1880 and 1910 with that of the general male population. Over the age range 25 to 50 years, mortality was only 61 per cent of the expected figure (p < 0.05); on the other hand skiers > 50 years had the same mortality experience as the general population. Karvonen *et al.* (1974) carried out a somewhat similar study of 396 Finnish champion skiers; this group was born between 1845 and 1910, and was followed until 1967. Life expectancy was 3 to 4 years greater than for the general male population. The authors noted that the athletes had a low blood pressure, seldom smoked and continued physical activity into their later years.

Wakefield (1944) has contributed the only specific study of basketball. He followed 2,919 boys who had played in the finals of the Indiana State tournaments from 1911 to 1935. The observed deaths were only 67.9 per cent of the figure anticipated for the general population. Again, a tall ectomorphic body build may confer some advantage on this group; it is also possible that not all deaths were traced in the Wakefield series.

Kitamura (1966) studied a mixed group of 1,655 university athletes; at all ages from 48 to 72 years, the percentage of survivors was substantially greater than for 3,069 medical graduates of Tokyo University.

It seems fair to conclude that while the life-expectancy of rowers does not differ from that of appropriate controls, there are some classes of athlete who lived longer than might be anticipated (for example skiers, basketball players, track and field participants and cricketers). It remains to be determined whether this is a consequence of physical activity, or whether the advantage is dependent on some initial factor of selection for these sports.

Degree of Achievement

Athletic competition is associated with an adverse mortality to the extent that it attracts the achievement-oriented individual. Polednak & Damon (1970) noted that participants in the 'major' sports of US universities (baseball, football, crew, track, ice hockey and tennis) tended to live less long than those electing the 'minor' sports (basketball, cricket, fencing, golf, lacrosse, polo, swimming and wrestling). In a further analysis, Polednak (1972b) found that life-expectancy diminished in proportion to the number of sports 'letters' that were won – 67.1 years for one, 66.4 years for two and 65.5 years for three or more 'letters'.

Body Build

It is widely recognised that if a person allows his body weight to rise by more than a small amount, his life-expectancy diminishes (Sinclair, 1953; Society of Actuaries, 1959). There is also evidence that specific body 'types' have a characteristic life-span. In particular, the plump, endomorphic body build is destined for a short life, at least in our present culture (Spain *et al.*, 1963; Damon *et al.*, 1969; Biorck, 1972; Sheehan, 1973). It is thus possible that part of any difference in the life-expectancy of a given class of athlete is related to the innate physical characteristics of the person who performs well in that discipline. One expert on somatotyping (Carter, 1970) con- cluded that distance runners were typically ectomesomorphs and mesoectomorphs, American football and baseball players were endo- mesomorphs, basketball players were low ectomesomorphs and rowers were mesomorphs.

Rook (1954) arbitrarily classified his athletic population into heavy (N = 251) and lightweight (N = 315) groups. The heavyweights comprised those rowing at a weight of over 76 kg, rugby backs, hammer and weight men. The lightweights were rowers < 76 kg, runners and rugby forwards. Despite the simplicity of this scheme of classification, Rook found that the lightweight athletes lived an average of 1.73 years longer than the heavyweights. Among the track and field group, 57 per cent of the short-distance and 56 per cent of the long-distance runners, but only 34 per cent of the hammer and weight men lived to the age of 70.

Polednak & Damon (1970) were able to make a more precise analysis, since all of their sample were photographed and given an anthropometric rating while attending Harvard. The athletes as a class were shown to be fatter, more muscular and stockier than the non-athletes. Further, differences were more marked for 'major' than for 'minor' athletes.

Cause of Death

The propensity of the athlete to meet a violent death has already been noted. Other causes of death are examined in Table 6.8. There is substantial evidence that in an older, coronary-prone man, vigorous and unaccustomed exercise can precipitate both myocardial infarction and sudden death (Shephard, 1974a). To the extent that

Table 6.8 Causes of death among athletes (per cent of known causes). Based on data collected by Yamaji & Shephard (1978)

Cause of death	Meylan (1904)	Anderson (1916)	Greenway & Hiscock (1926)	Bickert (1929)	Knoll (1938)	Van Mervenne (1941)	Wakefield (1944) Ath	Wakefield (1944) Cont	Rook (1954) Ath	Rook (1954) Cont	Pomeroy & White (1958) Ath	Pomeroy & White (1958) Cont	Montoye et al. (1957) Ath	Montoye et al. (1957) Cont
Influenza, pneumonia, bronchitis	13.6	11.3	25.0	10.0		8.0	10.5	11.4	8.9	10.5	10.3	4.8	2.0	5.0
Heart, vascular disease	18.2	7.5	3.1	40.2		25.0	16.3	13.3	36.4	41.5	37.9	49.0	66.0	56.0
Genito-urinary disease									5.2	7.1	4.6	3.7		
Cancer & tumours	4.5			10.1		9.0			13.9	12.8	12.6	13.6	12.0	14.0
Tuberculosis	4.5	22.6	6.2	9.1	3.2	10.0	13.8	20.9						
Accidents, war, homicide	36.4	17.0	43.8	10.4	36.8	21.0	34.0	17.3	11.1	7.0	19.5	5.7	10.0	13.0
Suicide									1.1	0.0	4.6	1.8	4.0	3.0
Total cases	32	58	36	264	155	100	123		541	198	126	24,026	114	86
Total cases, cause known	22	53	32	231	155	100	123		439	142	87	24,026	114	86

ex-athletes are more likely to engage in strenuous exercise, they have an increased risk of such episodes.

Glendy *et al.* (1937) reported that former athletes who had partici-pated extensively in their sport had an increased risk of becoming coronary patients. Unfortunately, in many early studies the cause of death is uncertain, and comparisons between athletes and control groups yield conflicting information. Greenway & Hiscock (1926) found fewer deaths from heart disease in Yale athletes than in control subjects; however, 43.8 per cent of their sample died from other than natural causes, and in a further 11.1 per cent the reason for death was ill-defined or unknown. Dublin (1928) reported that the death rate from heart disease was 12 per cent greater than expected in athletes over the age of 45. In several subsequent comparisons, differences between athletes and control populations have been quite small and within the bounds of statistical error (Rook, 1954; Pomeroy & White, 1958; Schohr, 1971). Montoye *et al.* (1957) concluded that not only were there no differences in the causes of death for athletes, but that there was no difference in the relative proportions of sudden and of lingering deaths between the two groups.

More recently, Polednak (1972a,b) reported some statistically significant findings. Coronary disease was more common in 'major' than in 'minor' and non-athletes, with the greatest risk for those who completed in three or more sports. This could reflect not only the influence of physical activity itself, but also the effects of personality, physique and habits in later life. As we have noted above, although the Scandinavian skier continues to pursue his sport to an advanced age, Montoye *et al.* (1957) found that the North American ex-athlete was heavier, less active and more likely to smoke and to drink than the person who was not a formal athlete while at university. It might be hypothesised that vigorous activity would increase the systemic blood pressure and thus increase the risk of cerebral vascular accidents. However, a recent study by Paffenbarger & Wing (1967) showed that only 7 per cent of 'stroke' victims had participated in athletics at college, compared with 16 per cent of controls.

Conclusion

It seems almost impossible to determine from the present data whether athletic activity influences longevity in general or the risk of cardio-vascular disease in particular. In some North American studies, there is a suggestion that sport participation has an adverse effect, but this could be no more than a response to initial body build and personality, or an adverse life-style after completion of an athletic career. Equally, some studies of continuing athletes such as the Scandinavian skiers suggest a favourable effect of the sport, but it is difficult to dissociate this from the associated lean body build and life-long abstinence from cigarettes that are the mark of an endurance competitor.

The incidence of some diseases shows little relati
the subject. However, the occurrence of other cor
influenced by senescence. This can be illustrated b
mortality figures for various diseases against age (Fi   ~ome
instances, the mortality for a specific pathology incr ~~s much more
steeply than the death rate for all causes. Atherosclerosis, myocardial
degeneration, hypertension and cancer all show such a characteristic,
arousing the suspicion that aging predisposes to development of the
condition. On the other hand, the frequency of deaths from liver
cirrhosis actually diminishes in those over the age of 60 years, making
it unlikely that aging is implicated in this process. With some conditions
such as respiratory infections, the incidence is not increased in the
elderly, but the likelihood of a fatal outcome to an attack is greater
than in a young person.

The common causes of death are illustrated in Figure 7.2 and
Table 7.1. In a child or young adult, the main hazard is some form of
accident, but in the elderly the main problems are coronary heart
disease, cerebro-vascular accidents, respiratory disease, other forms of
arterio-sclerotic disease and neoplasms. The proportion of deaths
attributable to the various conditions varies somewhat between a total
national population (Figure 7.2), general hospital and geriatric wards
(Table 7.1), but nevertheless all statistics emphasise the dominance of
cardio-vascular, respiratory and neoplastic disease.

The present chapter will not attempt a detailed consideration of
every possible geriatric pathology. Rather, it will examine possible
interactions between physical activity and some of the more common
conditions that afflict the elderly.

Cardio-Vascular Disease

Arterio-Sclerosis and Athero-Sclerosis

Arterio-sclerosis is a generic term applied to any form of vascular
degeneration associated with thickening and loss of resilience in the
arterial wall. Athero-sclerosis is one specific variety of degeneration
associated with an accumulation of fat in the intimal lining of the
vessels and an increase of connective tissue in the underlying sub-

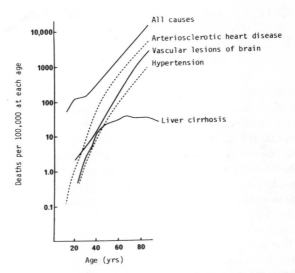

Figure 7.1   Mortality from all causes and from specific diseases. Note that deaths from some conditions increase more rapidly than would be predicted from age alone, while deaths from other conditions actually diminish in the older age groups. Based on data of Kohn (1963).

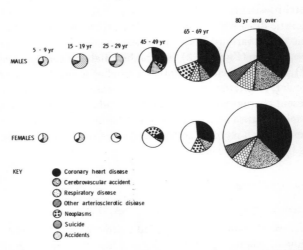

Figure 7.2   Principal causes of death for each sex at different ages. Based on Canadian vital statistics for 1971 (Lalonde, 1974). The area of each circle is proportional to total deaths in a given age group.

Table 7.1   Common causes of death in the elderly, as seen in the experience of a General Hospital and a Geriatric Unit (based on the data of Timiras, 1972)

Cause of death	General hospital				Geriatric unit	
	65-69 yrs	70-74 yrs	75-79 yrs	Over 80 yrs	80-89 yrs	Over 90 yrs
	%	%	%	%	%	%
Cancer	29	27	27	24	10	7
Cardio-vascular	25	25	32	36	40[a]	40[a]
Respiratory system	14	12	13	10	24[b]	25[b]
Digestive system	12	9	13	16	—	—
Nervous system	11	9	8	6	9[c]	—
Renal tract	4	7	5	3	—	—
Other	5	1	2	5	16	28

[a]   Athero-sclerosis and myocardial degeneration
[b]   Broncho-pneumonia and chronic bronchitis
[c]   Cerebral thrombosis

intima. The pathological consequences depend on the site. In the aorta, a bulging weakness of the vessel (aneurysm) may form. In the coronary arteries, the various types of ischaemic heart disease are seen, and in the cerebral vessels cerebro-vascular conditions such as strokes may appear.

Almost all animal species show some degree of athero-sclerosis, and it has for this reason been considered as an inevitable accompaniment of aging. Lindsay & Chaikoff (1963) noted lesions in both domestic and wild species, although both the incidence and the severity of the condition was greater in captive animals. This may reflect not only differences in habitual physical activity with domestication (Wissler *et al.*, 1969) but also changes in the type and amount of food, coupled with altered social and emotional pressures. Rabbits develop athero-sclerosis quite rapidly if fed a diet rich in cholesterol; nevertheless, the animals remain free of the secondary responses to lipid infiltration that cause disability and death in man unless local injury of the vessel wall is caused by drugs, cauterisation or a surgical operation. In other species, it is much harder to induce any athero-sclerotic change. The rat, for example, requires not only a diet rich in cholesterol and triglycerides but also thiouracil treatment (to decrease cholesterol metabolism) and cholic acid administration (to increase the digestion and absorption of cholesterol).

Table 7.2   Types of lipid found in normal and diseased aortae. Based on data of E.B. Smith (1965)

Type of specimen	Cholesterol ester %	Free cholesterol %	Triglyceride %	Phospholipid %
Normal intima, age 15 years	12.5	20.8	24.8	41.9
Normal intima, age 65 years	47.0	12.2	16.6	24.2
Fatty streak	59.7	12.7	10.0	17.6
Fatty nodule	64.8	13.9	8.7	13.6
Fibrous plaque	54.1	18.4	11.1	16.6
Calcified plaque	56.3	22.4	6.5	14.8

Man apparently shows a clear-cut sequence of vascular degeneration (Timiras, 1972), with fatty streaks appearing in the aorta during the first year of life, in the coronary arteries during the second decade, and the cerebral arteries during the third decade. Fibrous plaques are found from the second decade onwards, and clinical consequences such as heart attacks, strokes, gangrene of the limbs and aneurysm of the large vessels, from the fourth decade. There are related changes in the composition of the accumulated fat (Table 7.2). Aging leads to an increase in the percentage of cholesterol esters and a decrease of phospholipids. However, this change is not identical with that found in atheromatous deposits.

Ischaemic Heart Disease

Athero-sclerosis of the coronary arteries can cause a reversible oxygen lack in cardiac muscle when the activity of the heart is increased by effort or emotion (anginal pain). If the oxygen lack is of sudden origin (for example, haemorrhage into an atheromatous plaque, thrombosis over a plaque or lodgement of a plaque embolus), it can cause irreversible damage to a segment of heart muscle (myocardial infarction). Repeated minor episodes of irreversible myocardial oxygen lack can also lead to progressive myocardial degeneration.

1. Anginal pain   We have noted already that as many as 30 per cent of old people show an acute depression of the ST segment of the electrocardiogram during vigorous effort (Table 3.20), and that this is usually interpreted as evidence of a disparity between the oxygen demands of cardiac work and the oxygen supplied by the coronary vessels. Some individuals show marked ST depression without developing characteristic anginal pain; nevertheless, there is a general correlation between the occurrence of ST depression and the onset of anginal symptoms.

Oxygen extraction from the capillary vessels of the heart is relatively complete even under resting conditions. If the work-load of the heart is increased by exercise or emotional excitement, the necessary additional oxygen can be supplied only by dilatation of the coronary vessels. A young person may show a five- or six-fold increase of coronary blood flow, but this is impracticable in rigid, athero-sclerotic vessels. Partly because vascular resistance is a power function of vessel radius, and partly because the main impedance to blood flow is in the small arterioles, the occurrence of angina is almost always a portent of gross obstruction of the major coronary vessels (Ellerstad, 1975).

Typically, there is a history of pain brought on by vigorous exercise, such as hurrying uphill in cold weather. Cold precipitates symptoms by causing cutaneous vaso-constriction, and thus a greater rise of systemic blood pressure for a given physical effort. There may also be a reflex spasm of the coronary vessels, initiated by the impingement of cold air on receptors in the airways. Symptoms are usually relieved by 1 to 2 minutes of rest or slow walking. Nitro-glycerine is also an effective remedy, apparently because it reduces the systemic blood pressure. The pain may abate if the exercise is continued. This characteristic reflects either an increase of coronary blood flow, as diastolic pressure rises, or an opening up of alternative vascular pathways to the heart muscle in response to increasing oxygen lack. However, most clinicians do not recommend attempting to walk through an attack, as this can occasionally provoke a left-sided heart failure (Parker *et al.*, 1966).

Anginal pain can be extremely debilitating. All forms of physical activity, including sexual intercourse, are severely limited (Kavanagh & Shephard, 1977a), and the patient becomes very depressed. Most medical treatments are only palliative. The rise of blood pressure associated with isometric work can be avoided through appropriate regulation of occupational and leisure activities. Exposure to cold air can be tempered by use of a 'jogging mask' (Kavanagh, 1970). Bouts of hard physical work may be prefaced by one or two trinitrin tablets. Often, misery is such that the patient is glad to accept surgery to by-

Table 7.3   A comparison of responses to continuous and interval training in post-coronary rehabilitation (Kavanagh & Shephard, 1975b). All patients had undergone an initial period of continuous training. At the beginning of the experimental year, 6 patients with angina and 20 of the remaining 35 patients were transferred to an interval training programme

| Patient group | Predicted aerobic power | | | | | |
| | ml/kg min STPD | | | mM/kg min | | |
	Initial	Final	Δ	Initial	Final	Δ
Continuous	25.2	35.9	10.7	1.13	1.60	0.48
training	± 5.8	± 9.8	± 7.8	±0.26	±0.44	±0.35
Interval training						
with frequent	19.9	28.9	9.0	0.89	1.29	0.40
angina	± 7.4	± 7.4	± 8.1	±0.33	±0.33	±0.36
without frequent	23.6	30.0	6.4	1.05	1.34	0.29
angina	± 7.0	± 4.9	± 7.3	±0.31	±0.22	±0.33

pass the atheromatous obstruction. Angiograms frequently show that the graft remains patent for six months or less, and controlled trials show little improvement of prognosis relative to conservatively treated individuals (Ellerstad, 1977). Nevertheless, the power of faith is such that many patients seem to obtain several years of relief from their angina following surgery.

The wisdom and merit of progressive exercise therapy for the anginal patient is still hotly disputed. Some authors have argued that vigorous effort may encourage the opening up of alternative vascular pathways to areas of ischaemic heart muscle, with permanent relief of the angina. However, attempts to demonstrate formation of a 'collateral' blood supply in man have been at best equivocal (Kattus & Grollman, 1972). Progress with a standard programme of endurance training is disappointing, but dramatic gains of maximum oxygen intake can be achieved through an interval training plan (Table 7.3), intervals being of sufficient length to allow recovery from anginal sensations (Kavanagh & Shephard, 1975b). The gain of maximum oxygen intake implies that more work can be accomplished for a given heart rate, and many of the ordinary daily tasks are brought below the angina threshold by persistent conditioning. Strengthening of the skeletal muscles can also reduce the rise of blood pressure, and thus the likelihood of angina at a given external work-load. If a subject gives a history of angina when using his arms, the alternatives are to avoid the activity concerned (occasionally difficult if the individual is still employed), or to strengthen the relevant muscles. We have not seen reversal of ST segmental changes at a given heart rate in anginal patients. Improvement of the blood supply to the myocardium is indeed unlikely, but the load on individual heart muscle fibres could theoretically be reduced through hypertrophy of the heart wall.

2. *Myocardial infarction* A number of recent books have discussed interactions between physical activity and myocardial infarction (Naughton *et al.*, 1973; Semple, 1973; Zohman & Phillips, 1973; Kavanagh, 1976). Their general focus has been on male patients in early middle age, although it is plain from Figure 7.2 that the problem of myocardial infarction becomes progressively more frequent in older age groups. In part, this reflects the increased prevalence of two major risk factors, diabetes and hypertension (Hammond & Garfinkel, 1969).

Some of the postulated mechanisms for the causation of infarction (haemorrhage into an athero-sclerotic plaque, impaction of an embolus from a fragmented plaque and development of a severe relative oxygen insufficiency) could well be induced by vigorous physical activity. However, other pathologies such as the formation of a thrombus on the surface of an ulcerated plaque seem more likely to occur when an individual is asleep. A review of data for patients attending the Toronto Rehabilitation Centre suggested that about a quarter of the non-fatal episodes were precipitated by physical activity (Shephard, 1974a). It was estimated that activity had increased the hazard by a factor of 6-12 (Shephard, 1977a), leading to a corresponding deficit of episodes during normal sedentary pursuits and bed rest. Peculiar characteristics of the activity implicated were: (1) effort of unusual intensity, for which the subject was ill-prepared; (2) effort of unusual duration; and (3) effort accompanied by emotional stress. Specific examples from our laboratory files include: a lengthy canoe portage, made twice a year on opening and closing a summer cottage; a day spent by a sedentary executive in fixing two-inch screws into a concrete basement wall; a day spent by a geologist in sorting 50-pound crates of rock collected during a sabbatical year; three hours of highly competitive tennis after many years of absence from the courts; defence of a curling championship; a janitor's sprint up a long apartment staircase to attend to a broken water main.

To the extent that an elderly person has become reconciled to a waning of physical prowess, such feats of imprudent activity are less

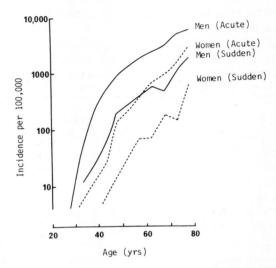

Figure 7.3 The influence of age on total 'acute' deaths from ischaemic heart disease and sudden deaths. Data of Romo, 1972. 'Acute' deaths include all cases dying within one month of the onset of symptoms. Sudden deaths are cases dying within the first hour of the onset of symptoms.

likely to occur than in a younger adult. This view is borne out by the statistics. In older age groups, a smaller proportion of ischaemic heart disease deaths occur suddenly (Figure 7.3), and if all ages are considered the association between strenuous activity and death is rare (Wikland, 1971; Romo, 1972).

There is continuing controversy regarding the merits of exercise in the prevention and treatment of coronary attacks. Again, much of the available evidence refers to early middle age rather than old age. Epidemiological studies suggest some protection from both occupational and leisure activity (Kannel, 1967; Brunner, 1968; J.N. Morris *et al.*, 1973; Paffenbarger & Hale, 1975), although in most instances it is difficult to rule out a bias due to the subject's self-selection of an active or an inactive life-style (J.N. Morris *et al.*, 1956). In older age groups, relative weight has progressively less influence on the chances of developing a fatal heart attack (Table 7.4); this presumably reflects the confounding influence of an increasing loss of lean tissue. On the other hand, lack of regular exercise becomes progressively more important as a risk factor. Presumably, those who

Table 7.4 Influence of relative weight and exercise habits on relative mortality from coronary heart disease at selected ages (based on data of Hammond & Garfinkel, 1969)

Sex and age	Relative weight		Relative mortality Habitual exercise			
	<90%	>120%	Heavy	Moderate	Slight	None
MEN						
40 − 49	1.00	2.25	1.00	1.23	1.36	1.80
50 − 59	1.00	1.55	1.00	1.11	1.26	1.31
60 − 69	1.00	1.27	1.00	1.26	1.73	2.18
70 − 79	1.00	1.19	1.00	1.55	2.13	2.85
WOMEN						
40 − 49	1.00	2.18	1.00	1.11	1.33	—
50 − 59	1.00	1.79	1.00	1.23	1.52	1.00[a]
60 − 69	1.00	1.58	1.00	1.05	1.80	1.92
70 − 79	1.00	1.14	1.00	1.53	2.50	3.53

[a] Limited sample

report that they are still taking 'heavy' exercise at the age of 70 to 79 years are a health conscious segment of the total population. It is also arguable that continued good health is the reason such subjects are able to sustain heavy exercise.

There can be little dispute concerning the practical benefits of exercise-centred rehabilitation following myocardial infarction. Patients who have been virtually bed-ridden can be restored to normal life, and some have progressed to the point of running a 42 km marathon event in as little as three and a quarter hours (Kavanagh *et al.*, 1977a). There are corresponding gains of maximum oxygen intake, mood and morale. However, the effects of conditioning upon mortality are less clearly established. The experience of uncontrolled exercise programmes is uniformly good. For example, Kavanagh & Shephard (1977c) followed 610 well-documented cases of myocardial infarction for an average of 36.5 months. During this period, they saw only 35 deaths, no more than 24 of which were attributable to a recurrence of the myocardial infarction. Their annual rate of fatal re-infarctions was thus 1.29 per cent, compared with 4 to 5 per cent in most conservatively treated series (Weinblatt *et al.*, 1973). In contrast, preliminary reports from trials where patients have been allocated in random fashion to heavy and light exercise programmes have indicated little difference of mortality experience between the two groups (Rechnitzer *et al.*, unpublished data). The simplest explanation of this paradox would be that patients recruited to uncontrolled exercise programmes are a selected population with an inherently favourable prognosis. Comparing the Toronto series (Kavanagh & Shephard, 1977c) with the patients enrolled in the Health Insurance Plan of New York (Weinblatt *et al.*, 1973), the exercised group had some advantage in terms of age (49 rather than 54 years) the frequency of hypertension (23.1 per cent, rather than 33.4 per cent) and elevated serum cholesterol (7.5 per cent rather than 24.7 per cent). On the other hand, 97.2 per cent of the Toronto sample showed residual abnormalities of the resting electrocardiogram, as against 77.6 per cent in the New York series. Allowing for these differences in the two samples, we should have seen 49 deaths (2.6 per cent per annum) rather than 35 deaths (1.89 per cent per annum). It seems difficult to explain this advantage other than in terms of a protective effect of the exercise programme. There are two possible explanations why this has not been demonstrated in controlled experiments. Possibly patients in the latter type of trial have not undertaken sufficiently severe training, and possibly much of the benefit arises as a by-product of exercise, through cessation of smoking, control of diet, weight reduction and so on. Such benefits might be gained almost equally by a 'control' group, obscuring the real benefits of the total programme offered to the patient. In support of this view, current data for the Southern Ontario multicentre trial (Rechnitzer *et al.*, unpublished) show a low rate of mortality not only in the high intensity exercise group (1 per cent per annum) but also in the 'controls' who are receiving only light recreational activity (1.3 per cent per annum).

There is a particular need for further study of responses of the older post-coronary patient to an exercise training programme. Kavanagh *et al.* (1973b) found that after the first year of rehabilitation, patients tended to sort themselves into two groups. The first group continued to increase their weekly training mileage and developed large gains of maximum oxygen intake. The second group apparently were unable to progress beyond an exercise prescription of ten miles per week and had disappointingly small improvements in aerobic power; this latter type of patient seemed physiologically older, and was more likely to show angina and/or hypertension. It was thus suggested that the older myocardium was less capable of responding to vigorous training following infarction. However, the authors could not rule out the possibility that motivation was poorer in the older subjects; once their children had been educated and the house mortgage repaid, there was probably less incentive to devote long hours to conditioning.

3. Myocardial degeneration   The general decline of cardiac performance with age is well recognised (Chapter 3). There is a decrease of both resting and maximum cardiac output that parallels corresponding changes in oxygen consumption, a decrease of right ventricular work, and a variable change of left ventricular work, depending on the relative magnitudes of the reduction in cardiac output and the increase of systemic blood pressure (Harrison & Reeves, 1968; Toscani, 1971). Furthermore, while a young person readily accepts a sustained increase of cardiac work-load, in old age an equivalent stress frequently gives rise to cardiac failure. Thus a young subject notices the palpitations of a fast heart rate if he is suffering from thyrotoxicosis, but the older patient complains of the shortness of breath associated with a failing heart. Advancing years increase the probability of cardiac failure as a complication of many other circulatory problems, including a high systemic blood pressure, a minor disorder of the heart valves, or an excessive infusion of intravenous fluids.

The cause of reduced myocardial function remains controversial. Some authors have regarded it as a normal manifestation of aging (Dock, 1966; Toscani, 1971), attributable to such factors as a wasting of heart muscle, a loss of elasticity with prolongation of the relaxation phase of the cardiac cycle (T.R. Harrison *et al.*, 1964), fibrotic changes in the valves of the heart, and a modification of catecholamine production or sensitivity (Toscani, 1971). Others have blamed infiltrative disease. Pomerance (1965) found amyloid material in the hearts of 12 per cent of men who died after the age of eighty years; while minor lesions probably have little functional significance, extensive anyloidosis could well be one cause of senile cardiac failure. It is quite likely that the majority of cases are due to chronic myocardial oxygen lack and fibrosis secondary to diffuse coronary vascular disease, but this hypothesis is difficult to prove or disprove, since almost all older adults show both athermomatous plaques and small myocardial scars at autopsy.

In our present context, it is worth noting that one commonly cited pathology in the 76 exercise death reports collected by Jokl (1958) was chronic myocardial degeneration (eight cases). The frequency of this condition may have been somewhat over-stated, since a number

236 Activity and the Pathology of Aging

of the reports were from before World War II. Nevertheless, it seems reasonable to postulate that repeated small myocardial infarctions can produce a situation where the resting cardiac output is well tolerated, but sustained and strenuous activity pushes the subject into cardiac failure. According to Bruce (1957), patients with a seriously reduced cardiac reserve report a marked need for rest even after mild physical activity. In addition to persistent and undue fatigue, an inadequate cardiac response to exercise usually causes an acute shortness of breath (dyspnoea), while a restriction of blood flow to the heart itself may produce anginal pain. Inadequate blood flow to the peripheral tissues may give the skin a bluish hue (peripheral cyanosis). The pulse count typically rises over the day, with a slow and incomplete recovery during rest pauses. In some instances, the tasks of a normal day are completed without obvious difficulty, yet the heart is brought sufficiently close to acute failure that there is a paroxysm of dyspnoea on lying down and attempting to sleep.

Simple indications of an adverse response to exercise testing include an absence of the anticipated rise of systemic blood pressure, accumulation of a substantial oxygen debt and a slow recovery of heart rate and ventilation after cessation of effort. Measurements of cardiac stroke volume show a decrease rather than an increase as the intensity of work is augmented. Myocardial contractility is also impaired. Approximate values for this variable can be derived from the simultaneous recording of the carotid pulse wave, the electrocardiogram and the apical heart sounds. In some instances more accurate assessment by echocardiography or cardiac catheterisation may be justified.

While there is probably merit in persuading subjects with diffuse myocardial disease to preserve their existing function through cautiously prescribed effort, the intensity of such activity must be held below the level at which left ventricular failure begins to occur. Once failure has developed, there is little alternative to a combination of traditional medical therapy and rest until the heart is again operating on the favourable (compensated) portion of its pressure/volume curve (Figure 7.4).

Peripheral Vascular Disease

Athero-sclerosis and other forms of peripheral vascular disease can lead to partial or complete obstruction of the main arterial supply to the limbs. The practical consequences include intermittent claudication and amputation subsequent to the development of gangrene.

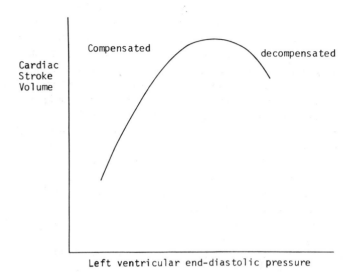

Figure 7.4   To illustrate the concept of decompensated heart failure. An increase of left ventricular end-diastolic pressure in a failing heart leads to a vicious cycle of decreasing stroke volume and further increase of left ventricular end-diastolic pressures.

1. Intermittent claudication   Intermittent claudication is a severe muscular pain, typically occurring in the calf (Gillespie, 1960). It is brought on by modest exercise (such as walking 200 metres), and is relieved by rest. Like the analagous anginal pain of the heart, it reflects an acute oxygen lack in the affected muscle. The condition is not particularly common, since it is essentially a problem of males with a high cigarette consumption. Many of this group die of lung cancer or are incapacitated by chronic bronchitis or angina before there is sufficient impairment of calf blood flow to cause claudication. Isacsson (1972) found a prevalence of 2.8 per cent in a random sample of 55-year-old men living in Malmo, Sweden. However, the condition is seen most often in the elderly; 38 per cent of the 171 cases collected by Singer & Rob (1960) were aged 60-69 years. While the main risk factor is undoubtedly a high cigarette consumption, venous occlusion plethysmography shows a significant relationship between calf blood flow and leisure activity (Isacsson, 1972).

    Many patients are rather vague about the amount of activity needed to induce pain, and in order to evaluate therapy it is necessary to make objective measurements either of calf blood flow or of the time to claudication; exercise may be a standard treadmill walk, or a rhythmic lifting of the body weight by the calf muscles once every second (Stein, 1956; Christie *et al.*, 1968). The traditional treatment has been surgical (excision of the thrombus, vascular graft or lumbar sympathectomy). However, Singer & Rob (1960) noted that the condition of 20 out of 22 patients receiving conservative treatment was either unchanged or improved, and a recent review (*British Medical Journal*, 1976) suggested that only 20 per cent of patients required surgical intervention. The prognosis of the local vascular lesion seems to depend greatly on the properties of the blood — initial viscosity, plasma fibrinogen level and susceptibility of the red cells to auto-oxidation (Dormandy *et al.*, 1973).

There have been reports that the walking distance to the onset of claudication can be extended by a programme of regular exercise over a period of some months (Hedlund & Porjé, 1964; Larsen & Lassen, 1966). The suggested mechanism is the development of a collateral blood supply to that part of the limb beyond the site of obstruction. Larsen & Lassen (1966) could not demonstrate that training produced an increase of maximal blood flow as measured by the Xenon-133 method. However, Sanne & Sivertsson (1968) found a 30 per cent decrease in the resistance of collateral blood vessels when cats were given five weeks of treadmill exercise following deliberate occlusion of the femoral artery.

Other practical suggestions for the patient with intermittent claudication include (1) the taking of a peripheral vaso-dilator drug prior to vigorous exercise, (2) the wearing of adequate and well-insulated shoes, especially in cold weather, and (3) correction of any anaemia. Clinicians have traditionally recommended Buerger's exercises. These require holding the legs elevated at 45 to 90 degrees for three minutes, three or four times per day, followed by three minute periods with the legs dependent. The rationale of such exercises is to improve collateral flow through a reactive vaso-dilatation, but it is conceivable that any benefit from the exercises is attributable to a strengthening of the affected muscles (Clausen & Lassen, 1971; Hirai, 1974).

Irrespective of treatment, the subsequent mortality of the claudicant patient is high; deaths are attributable largely to coronary thrombosis and cerebral thrombosis or haemorrhage (Singer & Rob, 1960; Gillespie, 1960).

Table 7.5 Successful use of a prosthesis by elderly subjects.
Based on data of Clarke-Williams (1973). Success is defined as daily
walking on the prosthesis for at least six months

Age at amputation (years)	Single amputation			Double amputation		
	Success %	Failure %	Death %	Success %	Failure %	Death %
60 – 69	56	44	–	67	34	–
70 – 79	55	27	18	40	40	20
Over 80	48	31	21	46	31	23

2. Amputations   In some 10 per cent of patients with peripheral
vascular disease, mainly those who are also suffering from diabetes
(Aitken, 1961; Bloor, 1961), the onset of gangrene in the affected
limb makes an amputation necessary. Young adults who have had an
amputation following a traffic accident often make a very complete
adaptation to their disability, but in elderly subjects problems are
frequent due to both a limited physical capacity and associated
disabilities. Less than a half of those who receive an amputation for
ischaemia learn to walk on their prostheses (Warren & Kihn, 1968;
Table 7.5), and some authors have alleged that many patients wear the
devices only to visit the orthopaedic clinic (Charlesworth & Baker,
1973).

Kavanagh *et al.* (1973a) used an arm ergometer test to predict the
maximum oxygen intake of a group of 27 older subjects who had
undergone amputation for peripheral vascular disease. Seventeen of
eighteen men and two of nine women were able to reach the minimum
heart rate (122 beats/min) required for application of the Åstrand
prediction procedure. All figures for maximum oxygen intake were
extremely low (Table 7.6). It is well recognised that in healthy young
subjects the maximum oxygen intake is some 28 per cent smaller for
arm than for leg work, with a corresponding displacement of the heart
rate/oxygen consumption relationship during sub-maximal work
(Simmons & Shephard, 1971a), but even if allowance is made for
this factor, the maximum oxygen intake is still only 50 to 60 per cent
of normal for healthy old people (Table 3.18). Because of tissue loss
in the amputated limb, it is difficult to express results per kilogram
of body weight. If the 67-year-old men seen by Kavanagh *et al.* had
weighed 77.4 kg (as in our normal sample from Saskatoon, Table 6.3),
their aerobic power would have been only 10.6 ml/kg min, 0.47 μM/

Table 7.6   Predicted aerobic power of elderly amputees (based on data of Kavanagh *et al.*, 1973a)

Sex and age	Predicted aerobic power	
	l/min STPD	mM/min
MEN		
50.2 ± 8.2 yrs	1.29 ± 0.37	57.6 ± 16.5
67.0 ± 1.9	0.82 ± 0.18	36.6 ± 8.0
74.7 ± 3.4	0.78 ± 0.25	34.8 ± 11.2
WOMEN		
66.0[a]	0.81	36.2

[a] Only two subjects

kg min. In fact, many seem to have been somewhat lighter than the general population. Assuming that 10 per cent of body weight was removed by an above-knee amputation, and 4 per cent by a below-knee operation, the excess weight relative to the 'ideal' value of the Society of Actuaries (1959) would have been − 1.7 ± 8.2 kg in the men, and 1.6 ± 1.4 kg in the women. It could be that some patients lost more tissue than our arbitrary 10 per cent allowance for surgery, but it is also likely that there was substantial muscular wasting secondary to inactivity after operation.

The actual working capacity is in many instances even poorer than suggested by predictions of maximum oxygen intake, since tests have to be halted for marked ST segmental depression and/or anginal pain before the theoretical maximum heart rate has been reached. Eighteen of the 27 patients exercised by Kavanagh *et al.* (1973a) developed a horizontal or downward sloping ST segmental depression greater than 0.1 mV. Nine of these eighteen had a history of previous myocardial infarction. The other nine had previously been accepted as free of cardiac involvement on the basis of a normal resting electrocardiogram; nevertheless, they developed a highly significant ST depression (average 0.29 ± 0.16 mV, range 0.11 to 0.60 mV) at an average load of only 40.7 Watts (range 25-50 Watts).

The frequency of complications was further brought out (Kavanagh *et al.*, 1973a) in a larger series of 62 amputees (44 men aged 65.4 ± 11.5 years, and 18 women aged 67.2 ± 11.9 years, all with a history of peripheral vascular disease). Thirty of this sample gave a history of previous heart trouble, including myocardial infarction (22 cases),

Table 7.7   Energy cost of ambulation with prostheses. Based on data
of O'Hara, as reported by Durnin & Passmore (1967)

Speed of walking (km/h)	Predicted normal cost KJ/min/65 kg	Cost after amputation			
		Above knee KJ/min/65 kg	%	Below knee KJ/min/65 kg	%
3.6	13.8	19.1	138	–	–
4.0	15.1	21.0	139	16.3	108
4.8	17.2	25.6	149	19.1	111

digoxin therapy (18 cases), cardiac failure (3 cases) and angina (3 cases).
Twenty-eight of the sample also showed abnormalities of the resting
electrocardiogram (evidence of past myocardial infarction, T-wave
abnormalities, dysrhythmias and varying degrees of heart block).
Twenty-three patients (including thirteen of those with a history of
cardiac complications) had a diastolic pressure of more than 100 mm Hg
(13.3 kPa). Other complications included diabetes (10 cases),
vascular emboli (3 cases), osteomyelitis (1 case), gangrene (1 case) and
poplitteal aneurysm (1 case). It was further considered that rehabilitation was adversely affected by cerebral muscular involvement (4 cases),
chronic alcoholism (4 cases), blindness (1 case), deafness (1 case) and
gross obesity (1 case).

Having regard to these various problems, it is scarcely surprising
that less than 50 per cent of elderly subjects succeed in using their
prostheses. The cost of movement is related to the total weight of the
limb, but is increased three-fold if the movement is initiated with a
stiff knee. Many amputees have a very inefficient action in the early
phases of ambulation, and the energy cost of using an above-knee
prosthesis can be three or four times as great as normal walking. This is
plainly incompatible with the impaired cardiac performance of many
elderly subjects, and attempts to use the prosthesis may precipitate
heart failure. Once learning of the new skill has been accomplished,
the handicap is much smaller. Table 7.7 shows some British data
from the Roehampton clinic. Others have had a similar experience.
Molen (1972) found a 20 per cent increase in the energy cost/speed
relationship for below-knee amputees, while Corcoran (1971) set the
added cost of walking with an above-knee prosthesis at 10 to 15 per
cent in a young person, and 25 to 100 per cent in an older individual.
Ralston (1961) and James (1973) pointed out that this load is

mitigated, since those who succeed in walking usually slow their speed to the point where the energy expended per minute remains much as before amputation.

The likelihood that the prosthesis will be accepted can be increased by a suitable programme of rehabilitation, aimed at improving cardio-respiratory performance and strengthening the muscles in the trunk and the remaining limbs (Vitali & Redhead, 1967). Where possible, this should begin before amputation, and if walking is impracticable because of intermittent claudication, ulceration or gangrene, the possibility of conditioning by arm work (Simmons & Shephard, 1971a) should be explored. It is vital to avoid a further deterioration of physical condition during the post-operative period, and early ambulation should thus be encouraged. A pylon can be used except where eyesight is poor or balance is impaired. Where there has been a double amputation, it is sometimes helpful to commence ambulation on short rocker pylons, thus lowering the centre of gravity of the body (Clarke Williams, 1973). The arms should be supported by a light walking frame rather than crutches, since the confidence of the patient is readily destroyed by even a single fall.

A proportion of elderly patients have such severe cardiac impairment that they cannot be trained to the point of handling a prosthesis. With such individuals, false hopes are created by the fitting of an artificial limb, and it is preferable to commence training in the use of a wheelchair. Voigt (1968) maintained that the energy needed to propel a wheelchair on level ground was as little as 10 Watts, so that the energy cost of such transportation was less than that of walking at a comparable speed. However, heart rates as high as 150/min are sometimes encountered when a wheelchair is operated by an elderly amputee. One explanation of this paradox is that much of the effort is sustained by the small muscles of the forearm (Barr & Glaser, 1977), which may be operating with a relatively low mechanical efficiency (4 to 7 per cent according to estimates by Glaser *et al.*, 1977). A second possibility is that the early estimates of work-load were wrong; more recent figures from Stoboy *et al.* (1971) have indicated an average energy expenditure of 43 Watts (3.15 kcal/min, 13.2 kJ/min) during free movement at a speed of 3.0 km/h. Although such costs are substantially higher than the figures reported by Voigt (1968), they are still not much larger than the normal cost of walking (Table 7.7).

Stroke

A 'stroke' is a sudden and persistent loss of neural function having a focal distribution consistent with a vascular cause. The many possible pathologies include haemorrhage (both sub-arachnoid and intra-cerebral) and cerebral oxygen lack secondary to thrombosis, embolism, atheroma or arteritis; however, in old people athero-sclerosis is the commonest responsible factor. More than three-quarters of all strokes are seen in those over the age of 65 years, the incidence rising steeply with age; statistics for the United Kingdom and the United States show approximately 3 cases per 1,000 between the ages of 55 and 64 years, 8 per 1,000 between 65 and 74, and 25 per 1,000 in those older than 75 (Whisnant *et al.*, 1971). The incidence of stroke and of cerebral athero-sclerosis is especially high in Japan (Nakamura *et al.*, 1971), and this has been linked to the prevalence of hypertension in the orient. Hypertension is the most clearly identified risk factor (WHO, 1971). Attempts to demonstrate an effect of sedentary living have as yet been inconclusive (Kannel, 1971). If habitual activity does influence the risk of subsequent cerebro-vascular disease, it may prove to be a rather indirect effect, through control of other risk factors such as obesity and cigarette smoking.

A half of all stroke victims die within the first four weeks of the acute episode. About a half of the survivors have a recurrence, usually in the first three years after the primary attack (Acheson & Hutchinson, 1971). There is also a heavy mortality from various complications (as much as 17 per cent per year, Marquardsen, 1969).

Conventional muscle strengthening exercises may merely reinforce abnormal movement patterns, and an important part of rehabilitation is to teach the patient to discard unwanted movements (Bobath, 1970). The sensations of movement must also be relearnt through the careful use of tactile and proprioceptive (position-sensing) stimulation. Some of the mass flexion and extension movements which appear in the early phases of recovery can be exploited and modified to form skilled movements (Brunnstrom, 1971). However, a stable gait can be attained even when there is only minimal recovery of skilled leg movements (Perry, 1969).

A successful return to normal home life depends on a careful assess-ment of function, using either simple scales of locomotion and self-care attainment (Gordon & Kohn, 1966) or more formal measure-ments of muscular strength. The ergonomics of the home may need considerable thought (Shephard, 1974b). Doors may need modifica-tion to allow easier entry to rooms, hand supports and a lower tub side may be required in the bathroom, and floor coverings may need to be replaced to minimise the risk of slipping. Even the design of beds and chairs may have to be altered (Isaacs, 1973). The patient must also undergo a psycho-social transition (Parkes, 1971), establishing a balance between the hope needed to maximise his performance and the realities of the physiologically possible (New *et al.*, 1969).

Even when recovery is relatively complete, selective weakness of muscles can lead to much asymmetry of movement. This increases both the displacement of the centre of gravity during motion and also the cost of postural support. Spasticity, joint stiffness and the resort to trick actions all foster awkward and jerky patterns of movement, with particularly high energy demands for acceleration of the body parts (Ralston, 1964). Tremor adds further to the toll of unnecessary energy expenditure. At the same time, muscle wasting, an increase of body fat and a progressive deterioration of cardio-respiratory fitness restrict the ability to deal with these various handicaps. A large part of the available aerobic power may be used in a simple task such as level walking. The relative heavy demand soon creates a vicious cycle of fatigue, increasing inactivity, worsening efficiency and further fatigue.

Although there are many theoretical reasons why the hemiplegic patient should have a low mechanical efficiency, this expectation is not always borne out by the experimental data. Bard (1963) found an energy expenditure of 2.8 kcal/min, 11.7 kJ/min (116 per cent of predicted) when hemiplegic subjects were moving at a comfortable speed of 2.4 km/h, and 3.1 kcal/min, 13.0 kJ/min (94 per cent of predicted) when they were moving at their maximum speed of 3.5 km/h. Dr Terence Kavanagh and I have also observed lower than predicted energy expenditures in hemiplegic patients (unpublished experiments). Several factors are involved. It is always a difficult feat to collect expired gas after a stroke, because paralysis of the mouth leads to leakage of gas around the mouthpiece (Corcoran & Brengelman, 1970). Further, when the walking speed is close to a subject's tolerated limit, oxygen debts may be larger than when a healthy person is moving at the same velocity. Lastly, energy consumption is probably low in the flaccid muscles on the paralysed side of the body.

Gordon (1956) quoted some figures for the paraplegic. The inefficiency of walking was plainly worse when both of the lower limbs were paralysed. Values of 6.0 kcal/min, 25.1 kJ/min (233 per cent of predicted) and 6.3 kcal/min, 26.4 kJ/min (230 per cent of predicted) were seen in two subjects walking at respective speeds of 2.6 and 2.8 km/h. Such rates of energy expenditure obviously approach maximum performance for an old person with associated cardio-vascular disease. One of Gordon's two subjects accumulated an oxygen debt of 1.7 litres over 4 minutes, despite his slow rate of walking. He probably would have required a wheelchair for a longer journey. The other individual accumulated little oxygen debt, and could apparently have sustained the slow rate of walking for an extended period.

Following partial paralysis of a limb, the efficiency of poorly controlled movements can be improved by the use of a knee or ankle brace (Simonson & Keys, 1947; Gordon, 1956; Bard, 1963; Dasco *et al.*, 1963; Corcoran *et al.*, 1970). On the other hand, a spinal brace may increase energy expenditures, since the normal counterbalancing actions of the back, pelvis and shoulder girdle are all restricted.

Hypertension

While other diagnoses must be ruled out, the main cause of a high blood pressure in old age is 'benign essential hypertension'. The term 'essential' implies that the underlying pathology is unknown, and since there is no clear point of separation between normal and abnormal populations (Stamler *et al.*, 1967), it has been argued that the condition may be no more than an extreme form of the normal aging of the cardio-vascular system. We have noted earlier that the systemic blood pressure shows a steady rise from early adulthood to age 65, but that there is little increment of pressures thereafter (Chapter 3). The range of normality is wide (Master *et al.*, 1958), and symptoms of hypertension are not normally encountered unless pressures exceed the eightieth percentile of the population average. In elderly men, this threshold corresponds to readings of 191/103 mm Hg, 25.5/13.8 kPa, while in elderly women the upper limit of normality is somewhat higher (203/109 mm Hg, 27.1/14.5 kPa).

It is generally agreed that in young adults prognosis is improved if hypertensive individuals are treated with drugs that reduce their systemic blood pressure. However, in hypertensive patients over the age of 65 years, there is no good evidence that such therapy prolongs life or reduces the chance of a stroke. Indeed, if there are symptoms of mental deterioration, the condition of the patient may be worsened by the use of hypotensive drugs.

Most (Kilböm *et al.*, 1969; L.H. Hartley *et al.*, 1969; de Vries, 1970; Hanson & Nedde, 1970; Chrastek & Adimirova, 1970; Choquette & Ferguson, 1973; Jokl *et al.*, 1970) but not all (Frick *et al.*, 1963; Tabakin *et al.*, 1965; Ekblöm *et al.*, 1968) authors have

Table 7.8   Changes in systemic blood pressure with three years of
vigorous endurance training. Data of Kavanagh & Shephard
(unpublished) for normotensive and hypertensive 'post-coronary'
patients

	All subjects (n = 553)			Hypertensives (n = 141)		
	Initial	Final	Δ	Initial	Final	Δ
(mm Hg)						
REST						
Systolic	133 ± 17	127 ± 15	− 6 ± 17	161 ± 19	154 ± 12	− 7 ± 19
Diastolic	85 ± 9	87 ± 11	+ 2 ± 13	104 ± 9	103 ± 13	− 1 ± 12
EXERCISE[a]						
Systolic	169 ± 25	183 ± 29	+15 ± 25	172 ± 31	188 ± 30	+15 ± 27
Diastolic	96 ± 13	96 ± 12	− 0 ± 14	100 ± 12	99 ± 16	− 1 ± 18
(kPa)						
REST						
Systolic	17.7 ± 2.3	16.9 ± 2.1	−0.8 ± 2.2	21.5 ± 2.5	20.6 ± 1.5	−0.9 ± 2.5
Diastolic	11.4 ± 1.2	11.6 ± 1.4	0.2 ± 1.7	13.8 ± 1.2	13.7 ± 1.5	−0.1 ± 1.5
EXERCISE[a]						
Systolic	22.5 ± 3.3	24.5 ± 3.8	+2.0 ± 3.4	22.9 ± 4.1	25.0 ± 4.0	+2.0 ± 3.6
Diastolic	12.8 ± 1.7	12.8 ± 1.6	0 ± 1.9	13.3 ± 1.6	13.2 ± 2.1	−0.1 ± 2.5

[a]   Final loading, about 75 per cent of aerobic power

reported that regular physical exercise lowers the systemic blood
pressure, both in hypertensive and in normotensive individuals. Two
possible artefacts in such studies are (1) the improved fit of the blood
pressure cuff as subcutaneous fat is lost, and (2) a progressive
habituation of the subjects to the observer and test laboratory. We have
now followed a total of 553 middle-aged and older post-coronary
patients over three years of progressive and vigorous endurance training
(Kavanagh & Shephard, unpublished). During this time, we have seen a
small but highly significant decrease in the resting systolic pressure
(Table 7.8), accompanied by a small but significant increase in the
diastolic reading. At the maximum tolerated exercise loading, the
systolic pressure has shown a small increase, while the diastolic reading
has remained relatively unchanged. A total of 141 of our post-coronary
group had hypertension, with a resting systemic pressure of over
150/100 mm Hg (20.0/13.3 kPa). Changes in this sub-group were much

as observed in the total population. All of these subjects were well habituated to the test laboratory, and many showed relatively little fat loss; we can thus accept that the decrease in resting systolic pressure was not an experimental artefact. On the other hand, the extent of the change is too small to have great therapeutic significance.

Blood Lipids

We have discussed previously age-related changes in the body lipids (Table 7.2). A high blood cholesterol is well-recognised as one of the principal risk factors associated with the development of ischaemic heart disease and other manifestations of athero-sclerosis (Stamler *et al.*, 1972). A large proportion of the blood cholesterol is synthesised in the liver, and for this reason it seems inherently probable that exercise could help to control high blood lipid levels. There is some suggestive evidence to support this idea. The example of the Masai warriors is frequently cited (Mann *et al.*, 1955, 1964); this group supposedly eats large quantities of cholesterol rich foods, such as milk, meat and blood, yet maintains a low blood cholesterol by virtue of a high daily energy expenditure, presumably burning excess calories that would otherwise be converted to lipids. The same is true of Eskimos that have preserved their traditional life-style — they are reputed to eat much polyunsaturated fat, yet have low levels of serum cholesterol, β lipoproteins and triglycerides (Bang *et al.*, 1971; Draper, 1976; Sayed *et al.*, 1976). Nichols *et al.* (1976) found positive correlations between obesity and serum lipids in the coronary-prone 'white' man, weak in the case of cholesterol and moderate for non-fasting triglycerides. Ashley & Kannel (1974) also found that the weight gain of North American men over a sixteen-year period was matched by a parallel gain of serum cholesterol. Others have gone even further, concluding that much of the apparent influence of obesity upon the risk of a heart attack is due to the correlation between obesity and other danger signs such as a high serum cholesterol and a high systemic blood pressure (Keys *et al.*, 1959).

Because large amounts of cholesterol are synthesised in the body, individual differences of diet explain little of the normal variation in blood cholesterol levels (Medalie, 1970). Adherence to a cholesterol-free diet can give a substantial immediate lowering of blood cholesterol, but over the course of several weeks, values tend to move back towards their original level, presumably because of increased synthesis. Vigorous exercise does not do a great deal to lower the blood cholesterol unless it is associated with a negative caloric balance (Montoye *et al.*, 1959; Holloszy *et al.*, 1964; Goode *et al.*, 1966).

It is probable that the prevalence of athero-sclerotic heart disease could be reduced by a combination of prudent diet and adequate exercise from an early age. However, it is much less certain how far it is possible to correct advanced vascular changes through manipulation of blood lipid levels. Dietary modification studies involving a mental institution in Finland (Turpeinen *et al.*, 1968), a Veterans' Affairs hospital in Los Angeles (Dayton *et al.*, 1969) and a cancer detection clinic in New York (Rinzler, 1968) have all shown only marginal advantages of prognosis in the subjects allocated to a low fat regimen.

Chronic Chest Disease

Chronic obstructive lung disease (Shephard, 1976) is another important reason for a pathological response to exercise in the senior citizen. The two underlying processes of chronic bronchitis and emphysema are theoretically distinct, but in practice they are often co-existent and difficult to distinguish from one another.

Chronic bronchitis is diagnosed if the subject has a chronic or recurrent productive cough on most days for a minimum of three months per year in not less than two successive years (American Thoracic Society, 1962). There is an increase in the secretion and expectoration of sputum (Reid, 1960), with frequent episodes of superimposed infection (Birath *et al.*, 1964). Cigarette smoking, exposure to air pollution and a cold damp climate are all predisposing factors. The condition seems particularly common in England, where by the age of 65 some 50 per cent of unskilled labourers and 20 per cent of professional men are affected (Fletcher *et al.*, 1964; Holland *et al.*, 1965).

Emphysema is characterised by an abnormal enlargement of the terminal air spaces. In part, the condition is an expression of normal senescence, a loss of elastic tissue from the lungs leading to expiratory collapse of the larger air passages, difficulty in expiration and dilatation of the terminal airways. However, in the centrilobular form, where the lesion is localised to the end of the respiratory bronchioles, a vicious cycle of infection, destruction of the small airways and increased vulnerability to further infection may be suspected (G. Cumming & Semple, 1973).

Both forms of chronic obstructive lung disease have an insidious onset. At first, there may be no more than a slight breathlessness on hurrying, and the subject is inclined to dismiss this as an inevitable expression of aging. As the obstruction becomes more severe, there is a progressive increase in the work of breathing. Expiratory pressures often reach the limiting value where further effort leads to a decrease of flow (Grimby & Stiksa, 1970; Potter *et al.*, 1971). Eventually, a large part of the maximum oxygen intake is consumed by the respiratory muscles whenever exercise is attempted; nevertheless, it may not be easy to demonstrate an increase in the oxygen cost of physical activity (Filley, 1958; Levison & Cherniack, 1968; Shuey *et al.*, 1969), because a larger part of the total work-load is performed anaerobically (Eldridge, 1966; Shuey *et al.*, 1969; Marcus *et al.*, 1971). The respired gas is poorly distributed. and particularly in emphysema the gas exchange is restricted by a destruction of pulmonary capillary vessels (Bedell & Adams, 1962; Gabriel, 1972).

In the early stages of disease, the patient may compensate for these handicaps by increasing his exercise ventilation (Colin *et al.*, 1972; Spiro *et al.*, 1975). Such cases, the 'fighters' or 'pink puffers', are able to maintain normal arterial gas tensions at the expense of a heavy respiratory work-load (Spiro *et al.*, 1975). As the disease advances, ventilation becomes progressively restricted (McNab *et al.*, 1961; Marcus *et al.*, 1971). In such patients (the 'non-fighters', or 'blue bloaters'), attempts at physical activity lead to a dramatic drop in oxygen tension (Jones, 1966) and a distressing dyspnoea.

During sub-maximal work, the heart rates are high (Spiro *et al.*, 1975), but the stroke volume is less than anticipated (Nakhjavan *et al.*, 1966; Lockhart *et al.*, 1969; Gabriel, 1972). The steady state cardiac output response to a given work-load thus shows little change (Wade & Bishop, 1962; Flenley *et al.*, 1973). The speed of adaptation to an increase of physical activity seems slow (Schrijen & Jezek, 1970; Spiro *et al.*, 1974), but much of this difference disappears if comparisons are made at a constant fraction of the individual's working capacity (Spiro *et al.*, 1974).

Ratings of perceived exertion are increased not only at a given work-load, but also at a given heart rate. This reflects the severe breathlessness. The sensation of dyspnoea limits effort in most cases of chronic obstructive lung disease (Cotes, 1965; Jones *et al.*, 1971; Gabriel, 1972). Maximum heart rates (Armstrong *et al.*, 1967; Gabriel, 1972) and blood lactate readings (Bouhuys & Pool, 1963; Cotes, 1965; Gabriel, 1972) are thus lower than the anticipated figures for healthy subjects of the same age.

Predictions of maximum oxygen intake based on the heart rate response to sub-maximum work are in substantial error because of the low maximum heart rate (Bouhuys & Pool, 1963). Alternative stratagems are (1) to report a directly measured 'symptom-limited' maximum oxygen intake, (2) to make a prediction of aerobic power based on the maximum voluntary ventilation and the ventilatory equivalent (Armstrong *et al.*, 1967), or (3) to measure the physical working capacity at a fixed heart rate, for instance the PWC_{130}.

Many authors have described an improvement in the condition of chronic chest patients in response to a programme of exercise training (Shephard, 1976). However, the majority of such studies have been uncontrolled, and it is thus difficult to separate the reported gains from the benefits of ancillary treatment such as breathing exercises, postural drainage and prompt chemotherapy for superimposed respiratory infections (Petty *et al.*, 1970; Bass, 1974). Furthermore, the groups concerned have been quite small, and the period of training has typically been three months or less. While it is conceivable that 'regulatory' changes have been induced (Holmgren, 1967b), the duration of such conditioning is plainly too brief to produce any substantial dimensional changes in the cardio-respiratory system, or indeed to assess the impact of exercise therapy on the ultimate prognosis.

There seems little dispute that symptoms are lessened by training. Physical activity is performed with greater comfort, and the patient attains greater physical independence. Exercise is often carried to a larger respiratory minute volume. This reflects partly an improvement in the mechanical efficiency of ventilation, and partly an acceptance of a greater shortness of breath by the patient (Christie, 1968). Most subjects show an improvement of their symptom-limited effort tolerance (Woolf & Suero, 1969; Bass *et al.*, 1970; Nicholas *et al.*, 1970), although occasional individuals may show no improvement despite faithful participation in an exercise programme (Mertens *et al.*, 1977). Changes of body composition occur much as in healthy subjects. In some instances, a combination of a happier mood, greater physical activity and improved appetite may lead to a gain of body weight (Paez *et al.*, 1967; Campbell *et al.*, 1975), with related increases of muscular endurance (Mertens *et al.*, 1977). On the other hand, more severely affected cases show a continuing loss of lean tissue and deterioration of muscle strength.

During sub-maximal work, there are reductions in heart rate (Miller & Taylor, 1962; Pierce *et al.*, 1965; Paez *et al.*, 1967; Alpert *et al.*, 1974; Bass, 1974; Mertens *et al.*, 1977), cardiac output (Paez *et al.*, 1967; Mertens *et al.*, 1977; but not Alpert *et al.*, 1974), respiratory minute volume (Pierce *et al.*, 1965; Paez *et al.*, 1967; Christie, 1968) and the oxygen cost of a given intensity of work (Pierce *et al.*, 1965; Alpert *et al.*, 1974), with a corresponding increase in the predicted maximum oxygen intake. Less lactate is formed during sub-maximal work (Woolf & Suero, 1969; Brundin, 1975; Mertens *et al.*, 1977), but the ability to perform work anaerobically at higher work-loads is increased.

Direct measurements of the symptom-limited maximum oxygen intake show gains of 0 to 30 per cent (Miller & Taylor, 1962; Deroanne *et al.*, 1969; Vyas *et al.*, 1971; Degré *et al.*, 1974). Apparently, there is a widening of the arterio-venous oxygen difference, without the classical increase of stroke volume and cardiac output (Degré *et al.*, 1974). The failure of cardiac output to increase is probably due to an elevated pulmonary arterial pressure (Gabriel, 1972) and associated dysfunction of the left ventricle (Baum *et al.*, 1971). Nevertheless, there is no evidence that heart failure is precipitated by training, even when the patients concerned show electrocardiographic signs of right ventricular strain (Bass *et al.*, 1970) and high pulmonary capillary pressures (Brundin, 1975).

There is general agreement that respiratory function does not improve in response to training (Shephard, 1976). There has thus been considerable discussion of possible mechanisms for the observed gains of overall condition. Part of the change may by psychological (Bass, 1974). When first seen, the patients are frightened by their shortness of breath, but with the support of an interested medical team, they are encouraged to push themselves to a larger fraction of their maximum voluntary ventilation, and thus to a higher work-load. There may also be gains of mechanical efficiency; for instance, Pierce *et al.* (1965) found a 23 per cent decrease in the oxygen cost of treadmill walking. Fear causes the patient to walk in a tense manner (Nicholas *et al.*, 1970), with stiff legs and a forward stoop (Paez *et al.*, 1967). However, repetition of the treadmill walking reduces tension; the stride becomes longer, and there is a better co-ordination of breathing and leg movements. Oxygen consumption thus falls for a given speed of walking, and better use is made of the available oxygen transport capacity. Perhaps the most important aspect of conditioning is a breaking of the vicious circle that afflicts so many patients with chronic obstructive lung disease – dyspnoea, increasing inactivity, reduction of mechanical efficiency, deterioration of physical condition, greater dyspnoea and even less enthusiasm for physical exertion (Bass *et al.*, 1970; Nicholas *et al.*, 1970; Mertens *et al.*, 1977). Other possible contributory factors are a reduction of body fat, reversal of broncho-spasm and pulmonary hypertension due to associated oxygen administration and improved bronchial hygiene due to stimulation of the cough reflex.

Implementation of a training programme is much more difficult with chest than with 'post-coronary' patients. Initially, there is no critical incident to arouse concern, and many of those with mild shortness of breath consider this as normal for their age. When the disability has become more severe, dyspnoea makes the conditioning programme quite distressing for many patients, and they have difficulty in progressing to the point where pleasure is found in the required activities. In general, patients who show an increase of arterial oxygen tension during exercise are likely to respond favourably to training, while adverse features include a low forced expiratory volume and vital capacity, an increased haemoglobin level (Vyas *et al.*, 1971; Degré *et al.*, 1974), advanced age (Longo *et al.*, 1971) and a history of previous respiratory failure (Brundin, 1975) or pulmonary hypertension (P.B. Anderson *et al.*, 1977).

Oxygen administration is sometimes helpful in the early phases of training, enabling the patient to reach an intensity of exercise where training can begin (Cotes & Gilson, 1956; Barach, 1959; Woolf, 1972; Degré *et al.*, 1974). Those benefiting most from oxygen have a large drop of arterial oxygen tension (Cotes & Gilson, 1956; Woolf & Suero, 1969) with angina or electrocardiographic signs of coronary insufficiency during effort (Brundin, 1975). There has been some interest in developing portable oxygen systems for home use (Cotes, 1965). The main problem is the essential conflict between the desired weight (< 2 kg) and capacity (> 100 litres); at present, it seems unlikely that such devices will have wide practical application.

The current consensus is that progressive endurance training does much to improve the quality of life for patients with chronic obstructive lung disease. To the extent that such activity encourages a cessation of smoking and the more complete expectoration of sputum, it may improve prognosis. However, there is little reason to suppose that exercise can restore alveolar tissue that has been destroyed. The main contribution of conditioning is thus to improve muscle tone and mechanical efficiency to the point where optimum use is made of the restricted cardio-respiratory function (Cumming & Semple, 1973).

Maturity-Onset Diabetes and Obesity

We have already considered certain aspects of insulin secretion and

physical activity (Chapter 3). In this section, we shall focus specifically
on maturity-onset diabetes and its relationship to obesity.

1. Diabetes

The British Diabetic Association distinguishes several categories of
subject: *potential diabetics*: normal glucose tolerance curve, but both
parents or an identical twin diabetic, or (in the case of a woman) birth
of a baby weighing more than ten pounds; *latent diabetics*: normal
glucose tolerance curve, but history of diabetes during pregnancy,
infection or previous obesity; *asymptomatic*: abnormal glucose
tolerance curve, but no symptoms; *clinical*: abnormal glucose tolerance
curve, with symptoms or complications of the disease. Likely
symptoms include thirst, frequent urination, muscle wasting, fatigue,
skin irritation, deterioration of vision and pain associated with
peripheral neuritis.

We have noted already the relationship between athero-sclerosis
and diabetes. Westlund (1969) compared deaths among diabetics to
the general experience of the Oslo population under the age of seventy
years; ratios were as follows:

	MEN	WOMEN
Ischaemic heart disease	4.3	8.6
Cerebro-vascular accident	3.5	4.9

Other possible clinical complications include a diabetic retinopathy
(haemorrhage and exudation into the retina), cataract, glaucoma,
diffuse sclerosis of the renal glomeruli and a neuropathy due to loss
of the myelin sheath from the peripheral nerves.

There is a striking increase in diabetes with advancing age, and
indeed by the age of 70 some 20 per cent of men and 30 per cent
of women show a diabetic glucose tolerance curve. Further, follow-up
studies of the various categories described above show a progressive
deterioration of glucose tolerance in potential, latent, asymptomatic
and clinical diabetics (Raeder, 1976). In recent years, more men have
developed diabetes in middle age (Figure 7.5), and this trend has been
blamed on a greater body weight and increased idleness (Malins, 1976).
However, there is also a strong genetic element to maturity-onset
diabetes (Table 7.9), perhaps greater than that for early-onset diabetes
(Hauge, 1976).

The inter-relationship of obesity and maturity-onset diabetes is

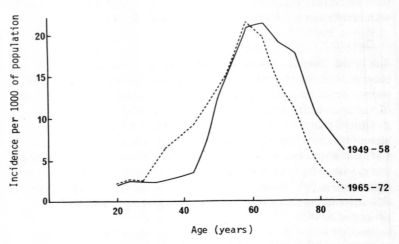

Figure 7.5   Relative incidence of newly diagnosed cases of diabetes — English males, based on data of Malins (1976) for 1949-58 and 1965-72.

Table 7.9   The risk of contracting diabetes before a specified age in the siblings and the parents of diabetic probands (data collected by Degnbol & Hansen, 1976)

Author	Siblings			Parents		
	Age 15 %	Age 30 %	Age 60 %	Age 15 %	Age 30 %	Age 60 %
Degnbol & Hansen (1976)	3.7	5.6	11.0	0.3	6.7	10.5
Harris (1950)						
early onset	2.3	4.2	—	0.2	4.2	—
late onset	0.1	0.1	5.0	0.0	2.9	8.1
Steinberg & Wilder (1952)						
early onset	2.2	4.1	—	0.3	3.3	—
late onset	—	0.4	5.8	0.0	4.2	8.9

well-recognised both clinically and experimentally. Whereas the non-obese diabetic shows a low resting insulin level, insulin values are high in the early stages of obesity-diabetes (Perley & Kipnis, 1965; Bagdade *et al.*, 1967). Burton (1976) has suggested that the responsiveness of fat cells to insulin depends upon their size; the fat person thus needs more insulin to sustain a normal carbohydrate metabolism. Studies with radioactive tracers also show that obese subjects can convert less of a given dose of ^{14}C glucose to $^{14}CO_2$ than would normal subjects (Gordon & Goldberg, 1964; Shreeve, 1965). Other metabolic changes that favour the further accumulation of fat included a reduction of phosphofructokinase activity in adipose tissue (Galton & Wilson, 1970), and a greater loss of insulin sensitivity in muscle than in adipose tissue (Stauffacher *et al.*, 1965).

When a normal subject undertakes sustained moderate exercise, blood concentrations of insulin decrease (Pruett, 1970; Wahren *et al.*, 1973). The α adrenergic receptors of the pancreatic islets are inhibited, and the rate of removal of insulin from the circulation is also increased (Brisson *et al.*, 1971; Métivier, 1975; Vranic *et al.*, 1975). The decrease of insulin in the portal circulation favours glycolysis and gluconeogenesis in the liver. The lower systemic insulin concentration may somewhat temper the greed of the muscles for glucose, conserving the blood sugar needed for cerebral function (Wahren *et al.*, 1971), although the large increase of blood flow to the active muscles effectively increases their insulin supply (Vranic *et al.*, 1975).

It is well established that an increase of physical activity is often sufficient to correct a mild case of maturity-onset diabetes. Devlin (1963) found a reduced insulin requirement with as little as fifteen days of progressive training. Grodsky & Benoit (1967) took four grossly obese individuals, and reduced them to within 20 per cent of the ideal weight by appropriate diet and training; initially, three of the four had an abnormal glucose tolerance curve, but after weight reduction only one of the four curves remained abnormal. The underlying mechanisms are less clearly understood. Short periods of moderate exercise apparently have no influence on insulin secretion or utilisation (Nikkila *et al.*, 1968), although short bursts of intermittent maximum exercise can increase plasma insulin levels (Hermansen *et al.*, 1970), possibly helping to improve glucose tolerance. There is good evidence that the obese are less sensitive to insulin than are normal subjects, and that sensitivity is restored following correction of the obesity (Perley & Kipnis, 1967). The reduced insulin response may be related in part to an increase in the thickness of the basement membranes of the muscle capillaries (Siperstein, 1970), and in part to a decrease in the number of insulin receptor sites (Soll *et al.*, 1975); there is evidence that insulin receptors are restored as the obesity is corrected (Soll *et al.*, 1975).

Activity is a particularly valuable treatment of the elderly diabetic, since as many as 30 per cent are unable to understand even the simplest attempts at a planned diet (Tunbridge & Wetherill, 1970). The general principles of exercise prescription are much as for other types of elderly patient. Body fat is reduced best by regular, sustained and not over-vigorous activity, for example a one hour daily walk at 4.5 to 5.0 km/h. Because of vulnerability to skin infections sweating should not be induced unless there is an opportunity to shower and dry the skin carefully with clean towels. Particular care is necessary if there is nerve damage. Loss of vascular reflexes can lead to postural hypotension following activity. Ill-fitting shoes with protruding nails can cause slow-healing ulcers; if there is also peripheral vascular disease, secondary infection and gangrene may develop. Lack of appreciation of the stress imposed on bones and tendons finally predisposes to musculo-skeletal injury, and radiographs of the tarsal bones may disclose one or more unsuspected fractures.

2. Obesity

Durnin (1973) commented that the disability which accounted for almost a half of the 'malnutrition' encountered by the Department of Health & Social Security, UK (1970) was obesity. Canadian statistics (Nutrition Canada, 1973) are based on the ponderal index (height in inches divided by the body weight in pounds); actuarial data have suggested an increase of mortality when the ponderal index thus defined is under 12.5, with a further sharp worsening of prognosis when values are less than 11.5. A second index that has been used in some British studies is 1,000 (weight/height^2); measuring the body weight in pounds and the height in inches, the upper limit for this index has been set at 34 units. The proportion of the population exceeding this limit and thus classed as obese rises with age (Figure 7.6), particularly in ex-smokers and non-smokers (Figure 7.7). Over the age of 65 years, 57.5 per cent of Canadian men and 43.0 per cent of Canadian women have a 'moderate' increase of risk due to obesity (ponderal index 11.6-12.5), while 8.1 per cent of men and 36.4 per cent of women have a high risk (ponderal index of less than 11.5). Having regard to the likely loss of lean tissue in the elderly (Chapter 3), the true proportion of obese subjects is probably even higher than suggested by such statistics.

As in children and younger adults, the essential pathology of the older obese person is an increase in the fat content and thus the size of adipose tissue cells (Bray, 1970; Brook *et al.*, 1972); however, the number of adipocytes drops progressively with the age of onset of

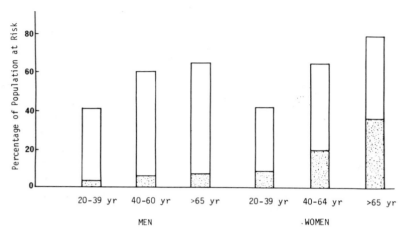

Figure 7.6 An assessment of obesity in the Canadian population. Data of Nutrition Canada (1973), showing the proportion of the population with a ponderal index of less than 12.5 (open bars) and less than 11.5 (shaded bars).

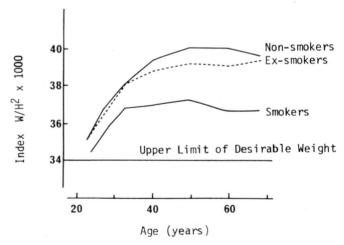

Figure 7.7 Influence of smoking habits on the obesity index weight/height^2. Based on data of Khosla & Lowe (1971) for steel-workers in South Wales.

obesity (Angel, 1974; Björntorp *et al.*, 1975), and where the condition dates from middle age the total adipocyte count may be no greater than in a person of normal body build.

The arguments for attempting to correct obesity in the senior citizen are much the same as in younger subjects. The skeleton is not well-designed to carry an excess load, and many of the orthopaedic problems of old age — flat feet, osteo-arthritis of the knees, hips and lumbar spine — are made worse by obesity. The ungainly body of a fat person cannot move quickly, and is thus more vulnerable to accidents; further, if a fall is sustained, it is much more likely to result in a fracture. Accumulation of fat around the chest and underneath the diaphragm interferes with respiration; there is a non-uniform distribution of ventilation (Dempsey *et al.*, 1966), with the possibility of carbon dioxide retention, drowsiness, and an increased predisposition to respiratory disease (Wilson & Wilson, 1969). The cardiac work-load is increased both by the physical weight to be displaced and by any associated hypertension; the obese person thus has more than normal vulnerability to angina and cardiac failure, although it is less certain that all of his cardio-vascular problems are corrected by weight reduction (Alexander & Peterson, 1972). We have already noted the association between obesity and maturity-onset diabetes; those who are overweight also have a high plasma cholesterol, and an increased risk of gall bladder and biliary tract disease. Lastly, there are often psychological problems; the obesity may initially have been a reaction to frustration and unhappiness, but an unsightly appearance, a poor body image (Chapter 4) and knowledge of increased health risks soon add to the unhappiness and depression of the fat individual (Beblinger, 1969).

As in younger individuals, the treatment of obesity involves a judicious combination of increased physical activity and dietary restriction. The importance of physical activity was emphasised by Mayer (1953). He found that experimental animals could not be made obese simply by over-feeding; however, they became fat quite quickly when they were kept in such small cages that they were unable to move about. Durnin (1971) equally showed a relationship between lack of physical activity and the development of obesity in human subjects (Table 7.10). Some authors have suggested that the placid, phlegmatic temperament of the fat person reduces his resting energy expenditure. However, Greenfield & Fellner (1969) used a special reclining chair to demonstrate that the frequency and amplitude of movements while resting were similar in normal and obese individuals.

| Late schizophrenia | 0.5 to 1.0 per cent |
| Character disorders and neuroses | 12 to 20+ per cent |

During the eighth and ninth decades, the incidence of organic psychoses increases, while functional psychiatric disorders are seen progressively more rarely. Perhaps of greater importance from the practical point of view is the proportion of disorders that prevent the subject from coping with the tasks of normal daily living. Goldberg *et al.* (1970) examined the records of 300 Londoners requesting social services (usually domestic help) and found the following psychiatric conditions:

Severe chronic organic psychoses	10 per cent
Paranoid states	3 per cent
Depressive states	1 per cent
Eccentric or alcoholic	2 per cent
Anxious/hypochondriac	2 per cent

A further 20 per cent of the sample had frequent and prolonged bouts of depression.

Neuroses

Old age has been described as the 'ultimate personality test' (Post, 1969), the many practical problems of aging bringing to light pre-existing weaknesses of personality. Certainly, neurotic and mild depressive conditions arise most frequently in relation to physical ill-health. One study found that 50 per cent of depressed patients had moderate or severe physical disability, compared with 25 per cent of a control sample of mentally healthy individuals (D. Kay *et al.*, 1964). Kavanagh *et al.* (1977b) noted that post-coronary patients often had depression scores that were two or three standard deviations higher than the population average for the test used (the Minnesota Multiphasic Personality Inventory).

Complications of such severe depression include alcoholism, the development of food fads and suicide. Alcoholism is found in some 0.5 per cent of elderly subjects in the UK, and 2.2 per cent of the elderly in the US (Rosin & Glatt, 1971). About a third of the depressed group become alcoholics late in life, and in this segment illness and emotional stresses such as bereavement frequently play a causal role. Brain damage is often a complication of alcoholism, and unfortunately the response to vitamin B_1 treatment is poor. Food fads are usually rationalised as the treatment of a digestive complaint. There may be restriction to milk, milk foods and slops, or a reliance on strength-giving foods such as eggs and meat. In a proportion of individuals, depression progresses to suicide or attempted suicide (Busse & Pfeiffer, 1969). Warning signs include severe changes in sleep and appetite, increasing agitation and bizarre hypochondriasis.

We have noted already (Chapter 4) that regular exercise can reduce manifest anxiety. 'Post-coronary' patients who have trained hard also show some reduction of depression scores (Kavanagh *et al.*, 1977b). Although the response is no greater than that yielded by mood elevating drugs, it is likely to be more permanent, since the underlying physical disability is reduced and the self-confidence of the patient is restored. Not only the activity itself, but the mental stimulation and renewed social contacts associated with an exercise class are preferable to the taking of anti-depressant medication in solitude. It is a wise precaution to check the list of drugs that are being taken, since hypotensive or sedative compounds may be contributing to the depressed state. Sedatives also provide a potential means of suicide.

Organic Disorders

Physical changes in the brain secondary to strokes and cerebral vascular degeneration can produce acute or chronic confusion. In assessing such problems, it is important to relate the scores attained on psychological tests to social background and any available information on intelligence during early adult life (Bergmann *et al.*, 1971); senile dementia may be wrongly diagnosed in a person of low basic intelligence, while functional loss may be missed in an individual who started life with an exceptionally high intelligence quotient.

Acute confusion is marked by a fluctuating level of consciousness, disorientation and an inability to retain new information. Speech is disorganised, motor activities may become stereotyped and there are sometimes visual hallucinations. The condition is often precipitated by an emotional stress such as transition from the solitude of a familiar home to the new environment and social contacts of an institution. If the condition is of recent origin, the prospects for recovery of normal mental function are quite good. Advantage must be taken of lucid intervals to maintain physical condition. There is an unfortunate tendency to treat restlessness and minimise disturbance to other patients through the prescription of large doses of hypnotics and tranquillisers. Such therapy leads to somnolence, apathy and a further rapid deterioration of cerebral function.

In persistent confusion, there are no fluctuations of awareness. The patient is perpetually puzzled, with a poor attention span. He is often apathetic, and may show an excessive response to minor stimuli. The main aim should be to allow some freedom of movement, while guarding against the risk that the patient will become lost or injured.

Other Conditions

The treatment of other psychiatric conditions is much as in younger individuals. There are advantages in maintaining physical condition through adequate physical activity, but there is no evidence that exercise influences the course of the primary disorder.

Miscellaneous Diseases

As much as a fifth of the elderly population are affected by disease to the point where they have difficulty in walking, are home-bound or are bed-ridden (Table 7.12). The commonest sources of difficulty are the psychological problems we have just discussed. Caird (1972) found that of those disabled to the point where they could not live without outside help, 48 per cent had organic brain disease and a further 22 per cent had functional psychiatric disorders. Among those unable to care for themselves, the prevalence of psycho-pathology was even higher; 93 per cent had organic brain disease, and 78 per cent were demented.

Nevertheless, there are other factors that restrict the activity and the mobility of patients, particularly rheumatoid arthritis, osteoarthrosis and other disorders of the feet. Some types of problem, such as a loss of power in an arm or a leg due to a minor stroke are usually reported to the family physician. However, other locomotor difficulties, particularly disorders of the feet, are often accepted without complaint as a normal consequence of aging (Williamson, 1966).

1. Rheumatoid Arthritis

In a proportion of the elderly who are affected by this condition, the onset dates from much earlier in life, but in others the disease first appears in old age. Unusual features of the late-onset disease (Exton-Smith, 1973) include a relatively equal number of cases in men and in women, and a tendency to an abrupt onset. The erythrocyte sedimentation rate is high, and may remain so despite subsidence of the joint inflammation. The serum also shows a high titre of rheumatoid factor. However, rheumatoid nodules are seen less frequently than in younger subjects, and with the exception of anaemia it is unusual to find signs of the disease in other body systems. As in younger

Table 7.12   Proportion of the aged showing disability while living at home, or confined to institutions. Based on data collected by Shanas (1971b)

Country	Percentage of the population over the age of 65 years			
	Difficulty in walking	Confined to home	Bed-ridden	Institutionalised
	%	%	%	%
UK	8	11	3	3.6
USA	6	6	2	3.7
Denmark	14	8	2	5.3
Israel	—	13	2	5.5
Poland	16	6	4	—

individuals, typical regions affected include the metacarpo-phalangeal, knee, shoulder, proximal inter-phalangeal, metatarso-phalangeal, ankle and elbow joints.

Rest is necessary in the acute phase of joint inflammation, but such treatment must be applied with caution in the elderly because of the high risk of developing bed sores and deep vein thromboses. Contractures are also a frequent hazard, and it may be necessary to splint vulnerable joints such as the wrist and the knees. Salicylate has a beneficial effect on the rheumatoid condition, but care is needed when prescribing large quantities of this drug, since gastro-intestinal irritation can progress to internal bleeding and anaemia. Prolonged use of the cortico-steroids has also been criticised, because normal aging increases vulnerability to complications such as osteoporosis, skin atrophy, cataract and peptic ulcer. However, it is possible to argue against this position on the basis that the short life-expectancy of the elderly makes a long course of cortico-steroids less likely than in a younger subject (Grahame, 1973). After the acute phase of the disease has passed, a careful blend of active exercises is needed to increase joint movement and to restore muscle function. Where there is substantial residual deformity, occupational therapy may also be needed to teach new approaches to industrial and domestic tasks that cannot be performed by previously learnt techniques.

2. Osteo-Arthrosis

More than 80 per cent of 60-year-old subjects have radiographic evidence of osteo-arthrosis. The affected joints are painful, stiff and sometimes deformed, but there is no sign of inflammation. Common sites of the condition are the knee, the hip and the spine. Treatment includes reducing the strain on the damaged joint by weight reduction, relief of pain by analgaesics, and active exercises to improve the range of joint movement and strengthen the surrounding muscles. In this manner it becomes possible to break the vicious cycle of a painful joint, muscle inhibition, muscle atrophy, impaired joint stability and further injury of the damaged joint surface. Where the disease process is advanced, surgical treatment such as replacement of the hip joint by a metal femoral head and a plastic socket may be contemplated. Many such operations have been advocated with initial enthusiasm but are now rejected; while the short-term results of the latest forms of arthroplasty are encouraging, further experience is needed to be sure that drastic surgical intervention improves the long-term mobility of the individual.

8 DEMOGRAPHIC TRENDS AND GOALS FOR A GERIATRIC SOCIETY

This final chapter will examine the phenomenon of the aging population, and the influence of habitual activity upon the effective age of those studied. Social implications to be discussed include national productivity, health care costs, independence and life satisfaction.

Current Population Trends

Mortality Experience

The average length of human life has increased dramatically over the past 2,000 years. Despite the mythical Methusaleh (Genesis 5:27) and the biblical promise of three score years and ten (Psalm 90:10), some authors have set the average life expectancy of Roman times at twenty to thirty years (Karpovich, 1941). By 1910, life expectancy in the United States (World Almanac, 1976) averaged 46.3 years for men and 48.3 years for women. These figures increased to 58.1 and 61.6 years in 1930, 65.6 and 71.1 years in 1950, and 67.1 and 74.6 years in 1970. By 1974, the average US male lived more than 68 years, and the average US female more than 76 years. Rather similar gains have been registered in Canada; in 1930, life-expectancy was 60.0 years for men and 62.1 years for women, but by 1971 the comparable figures were 69.3 and 76.4 years. In many nations (Table 8.1), a man may now expect to live for more than 70 years, and a woman for more than 75 years.

A large part of this trend is due to a reduction of infant mortality. For example, a twenty-year-old Canadian man had the expectation of living to 69.6 years in 1941, while in 1971 this had increased to 71.8 years; the gain for an adult man was only 2.2 years, compared with 6.4 years for a newborn child (Lalonde, 1975). Among older age groups, gains have been even smaller (Table 8.2). Substantial health benefits have resulted from control of the major communicable diseases, the development of new medical and surgical techniques, the wider availability of health care, improved programmes of public health and sanitary engineering, the closer control of working conditions, better nutrition, a higher standard of living and more general knowledge of the principles of hygiene and child care. Nevertheless, much of the

Table 8.1   Life-expectancy at birth in selected developed nations
(based in part on Schwenger, 1976)

Country	Year	Life-expectancy at birth (years)	
		Males	Females
Canada	1971	69.3	76.4
Denmark	1969-70	70.8	75.7
Iceland	1961-65	70.8	76.2
Netherlands	1970	70.7	76.5
Norway	1966-70	71.1	76.8
Sweden	1967	71.9	76.5
United States	1970	67.1	74.6

Table 8.2   Life-expectancy in Canada — A comparison of statistics for
1931 and 1971 (Schwenger, 1976)

Age at computation	1931		1971	
	Male	Female	Male	Female
Birth	60.0	62.1	69.3	76.4
65 years	13.0	13.7	13.7	17.5
75 years	7.6	8.0	8.5	10.6
85 years	4.1	4.4	4.7	5.7

potential for longevity has been dissipated through increases in
conditions such as athero-sclerosis, chronic chest disease and lung
cancer, problems created by affluence, over-nutrition, lack of exercise
and indulgence in cigarettes.

Comparative Demography

Although the main change of mortality has been among newborn
infants, the proportion of elderly people has been rising steadily in
most Western societies. In Norway, for example, the proportion of
people aged 50 to 69 years increased by 153 per cent between 1900
and 1960. Over the same time span, the proportion of the US
population aged 65 years or more also increased from 4.5 per cent to
9.2 per cent (LeCoultre, 1971).

In recent years, the world population has grown at a rate of about
1.5 per cent per annum, while the number of people over the age
of 60 years has increased by 2.5 per cent per annum. The number

of people over the age of 60 years has thus grown from about 155 million in 1952 to an estimated 300 million in 1975. The problem is particularly acute in the long-established Western democracies (Table 8.3), where the proportion of those over the age of 65 years has risen from 11.2 per cent to 12.0 per cent in a mere eight years; furthermore, a third of this group are over the age of 75 years. By way of contrast, only 6.6 per cent of Japanese (1969) and 8.2 per cent of Canadians (1971) have reached 65 years of age. However, the effects of the post-war baby boom will soon be swelling the ranks of the middle-aged and elderly in Canada. Thus, by the year 2001 AD, 11 to 12 per cent of Canadians will be 65 years and over, and by 2031 AD as many as 16 to 20 per cent of the population will be over the age of 65 years.

Table 8.3   Percentage of the population over the age of 65 in selected Western democracies, 1960-62 and 1966-69 (Paillat, 1971)

Country	Year	Percentage	Year	Percentage
Netherlands	1960	9.4	1968	10.0
Italy	1961	9.6	1967	10.2
Switzerland	1960	10.7	1968	11.3
Denmark	1960	10.9	1966	11.5
West Germany	1960	11.0	1967	12.2
Luxembourg	1960	11.1	1968	12.1
Norway	1960	11.4	1967	12.4
United Kingdom	1962	11.8	1969	12.7
France	1962	11.8	1968	12.6
Sweden	1960	12.1	1967	13.1
Belgium	1961	12.2	1967	12.1
Austria	1961	12.6	1968	13.9
Average	1960/62	11.2	1966/69	12.0

Physical Activity and Longevity

The senior citizen presents a heavy financial burden to government if he is healthy, and he becomes a financial disaster if he requires many years of institutional care. From the administrative perspective it would thus be convenient to find a life-style that kept the entire population physically and mentally alert throughout the normal working span, with a rapid and painless death following shortly thereafter. The objectives of the individual are usually quite different. He looks forward to fifteen or more years of active retirement in which he can indulge the many hobbies and pleasures for which there has been so little opportunity during his working career. Nevertheless, the senior citizen is likely to agree on the desirability of a rapid and painless termination of his sunset years, rather than a slow drift into senile degeneration. Unfortunately, there is little hard evidence regarding the impact of physical activity upon either longevity or the quality of life in the retirement years.

1. Longevity

Theoretical Considerations   There are quite a number of theoretical reasons why physical activity might increase longevity. Some relate to direct, others to less direct effects of activity. The stress imposed by vigorous physical activity is inversely related to an individual's level of cardio-respiratory fitness. A subject who has maintained his fitness through a programme of regular physical activity is known to have a lower cardiac work-load for a given external stress, and thus seems less liable to develop ventricular fibrillation or cardiac arrest if vigorous activity becomes necessary. Equally, during an acute illness such as pneumonia the individual with a large margin of oxygen transporting capacity is much less likely to succumb than the person whose cardio-respiratory function is already marginal.

Regular physical activity also plays an important role in metabolic regulation. We have seen that obesity can be reduced by an increase of daily exercise, and the association between excess weight and an increased mortality is well documented (Table 8.4). The active person is also less liable to diabetes, his blood lipids are reduced, and he may benefit from a small reduction in systemic blood pressure; all of these changes are likely to have a beneficial effect upon his life-expectancy.

Participation in an exercise class commonly makes the subject more health conscious. Not only is body weight better controlled, but the use of cigarettes (P. Morgan *et al.*, 1976) and other drugs becomes less likely. A new camaraderie and joie de vivre are discovered, and sleep is taken on a more regular basis. Among other possible benefits, there is some evidence from animal work that regular activity can enlarge the coronary arterial tree (Stevenson, 1967), increasing the collateral blood supply to parts of the heart muscle beyond coronary vascular occlusions (Eckstein, 1957); however, such responses have not always been found even in animals, and it has yet to be demonstrated that they can occur in man, particularly when exercise is initiated late in life.

Table 8.4   Mortality of grossly obese[a] men and women, classified by disease, and expressed as percentages of standard values for subjects of the same sex, aged 40 to 69 years (based on data of the Society of Actuaries, 1959)

Condition	MEN			WOMEN		
	D	E	F	D	E	F
Diabetes	197	381	—	270	247	—
Vascular diseases of brain	137	174	158	133	117	237
Heart and circulation	127	136	158	167	162	172
Pneumonia and influenza	127	121	—	160	137	—
Digestive diseases	138	190	245	143	143	—
Kidney diseases	134	215	372	92	70	—
All conditions	122	140	150	127	128	165

[a] The excess weight varies somewhat with stature; approximate averages are for the men + 24 kg (D), + 33 kg (E) and + 42 kg (F), and for the women + 28 kg (D), + 37 kg (E) and + 46 kg (F)

Epidemiological studies   Some epidemiological studies relating physical activity to the duration of life have been based on comparisons between athletes and non-athletes. We have already commented on the serious limitations of such studies (Chapter 6), particularly the initial non-random selection of the active population, and the difficulty of ensuring that activity has been sustained into later life. With the possible exception of cross-country skiers, there is little evidence that athletes live longer than the general population.

A second approach has been to compare people with active and sedentary occupations. This technique has found particular application to studies of ischaemic heart disease (Fox & Haskell, 1967). Employees in physically demanding occupations have generally shown a lower incidence of heart attacks than sedentary control groups, but again initial self-selection and subsequent attenuation of the active population restrict the interpretation of the data. Studies of leisure activity (Kannel, 1967; Morris *et al.*, 1973) also show a lesser incidence of ischaemic heart disease in active populations, but it remains difficult to rule out the possibility that the activity has led to initial selection of an unusually healthy and health-conscious segment of the community.

Experimental studies Edington *et al.* (1972) examined the longevity of rats that were exercised regularly. The life-span was extended by the added activity, but only if it was initiated before the 400th day of life (the usual life-span of the rat is about 600 days).

There are many practical problems in carrying out a comparable experiment with human subjects; indeed, it is almost inconceivable that humans could be confined to randomly assigned exercise and control groups over the course of a life-time. One possible method of reducing the scale of the necessary experiment is to start with a middle-aged population who already have an above-average risk of a heart attack due to obesity, a high blood pressure, cigarette consumption and so on. However, even with a high-risk group, the cost of the investigation has been set at the prohibitive figure of 31 million dollars (Taylor *et al.*, 1966). Furthermore, there is no guarantee that such findings would be applicable to a person with average coronary risk who had been exercising since early adulthood. We must thus conclude that while there is much suggestive evidence that physical activity may extend life-span, there is no proof of this hypothesis in human subjects, nor is a proof likely to be forthcoming in the foreseeable future.

2. Quality of Life

The quality of life is necessarily subjective, and it is therefore much harder to assess than longevity. In the context of old age, the crucial questions are whether an enhanced level of physical activity will (1) increase the duration of the 'good' years, when retirement can be enjoyed, or (2) decrease the 'bad' years of incapacity and senile degeneration.

There is little question that physical activity produces an immediate improvement of many vital functions such as maximum oxygen intake (Chapter 3). However, once this training response has been realised, functional deterioration is resumed, apparently with an unaltered slope. There is necessarily a minimum level of aerobic power compatible with a full independent life; a reasonable estimate of this limit is 1 l/min, 44.6 mM/min, equivalent to a maximum energy expenditure of some 5 kcal/min or 21 kJ/min. A typical 65-year-old has an aerobic power of some 1.5 l/min, 66.9 mM/min, with an annual functional loss of 35 ml/min, 1.56 mM/min. Within 14.3 years (age 79.3 years), his oxygen transport fails to satisfy the required standard, and thereafter retirement becomes a burden rather than a pleasure. Let us now suppose that the same individual has undertaken a training programme sufficient to augment his maximum oxygen intake by 20 per cent. He commences his retirement with the physical capacity of a person 8.6 years younger than his chronological age, and he retains this advantage as function wanes. He is therefore able to meet the minimum standard of aerobic power until he reaches the age of 87.9 years. Plainly, the 'good' years of retirement have been greatly extended.

Some 30 per cent of the population survive to the age of 79.3 years, but only about 10 per cent to the age of 87.9 years (Comfort, 1973). Thus, in the absence of any effect on longevity, one might claim that activity had brought about a three-fold reduction in the numbers of individuals who were no longer able to care for themselves on account of physiological aging. True gains are of course smaller than such calculations would suggest, since much of the burden of chronic care is attributable to pathological rather than physiological consequences of aging (Table 8.5).

Table 8.5   Percentage of the elderly population occupying various types of institution in Ontario, 1971-73 (based on data of Schwenger, 1976)

Type of institution	%
Active treatment hospitals (with psychiatric units)	1.47
Chronic treatment units or hospitals	0.89
Psychiatric hospitals and facilities for the mentally retarded	0.32
Homes for the aged and nursing homes	
extended care	4.17
other	2.30

Activity and Productivity

We have noted previously the somewhat arbitrary nature of the age of retirement. While there is substantial variation in practice from one country to another (Table 1.1), within any given jurisdiction it is administratively convenient to make pensions payable at a fixed age rather than review the fitness of the individual to continue with his work (Spitaels, 1971). In recent years, the proportion of elderly men who are economically active has shown a steady decline (Wedderburn, 1973); during the 1930s 40 to 65 per cent of those over the age of 65

Table 8.6 Percentage of elderly British men economically active in the years specified (data of Wedderburn, 1973)

Age group (years)	Year			
	1952	1956	1961	1966
60 – 64	87.5	92.0	90.0	88.7
65 – 69	48.5	53.5	44.0	37.3
Over 70	19.0	20.0	17.0	14.0

Table 8.7 Estimated changes in the Canadian population, 1971 to 2031 AD (based on data of Schwenger, 1976)

Year	Total population		Population over the age of 65 years		
	Number	Increase	Number	Percentage of total	Increase
	million	%	million	population	%
1971	20.7		1.7	8.2	
2001	28.7	40	3.3	11.5	94
2031	36.7	75	6.6	18.0	220

Table 8.8 An estimate of the possible percentage increase of older Canadians, 1971 to 2031 (based on data of Schwenger, 1976)

Age range	Percentage increase
65 – 74	232
75 – 84	280
Over 85	305
All over 65	252[a]

[a] Note that the overall increase is a little higher than predicted in Table 8.6

were still earning, but by 1966 only 37.3 per cent of those over 65 years and 14.0 per cent of those over 70 years were working. This reflects in part the wider availability of adequate pension schemes. Further, the labour force is currently increasing in North America, and the perceived problem is thus to find employment for the youth of the community. Early retirement is regarded as having social value, since it augments employment opportunities for the young (Back, 1969; Sauvy, 1970b; S.R. Parker *et al.*, 1971). However, demographers estimate that this phase in our history will have passed within twenty or thirty years, and that in the next century there will be a shortage of workers relative to those who are then seeking retirement (Tables 8.7 and 8.8). It may thus be necessary to consider an upward revision of the retirement age in the future. Relevant issues will include the wishes of the elderly, their physical ability to undertake the required work, and the actuarial implications of various possible ages of retirement.

Wishes of the Workers

It has been widely assumed that workers resent retirement. Beverfelt (1971) questioned Norwegian workers aged 60 to 70 years, and found that 90 per cent claimed to be satisfied with their jobs; 66 per cent liked their work very much and only 1 per cent expressed a strong dislike of their employment; however, there may have been some reluctance to admit dislike of a task performed for many years. Supplementary questions showed that 30 per cent found the job itself interesting and rewarding, 23 per cent regarded their employment as socially useful, 15 per cent regarded it as a means to provide for their family, 13 per cent valued the related social contacts and 9 per cent found it satisfied a need to keep active. Nevertheless, 51 per cent were looking forward to retirement, and only 26 per cent dreaded this turning point in their lives; a positive anticipation of retirement was more common in women than in men, and in the sick than in those who were healthy.

Nevertheless, fear of retirement seems in part a myth fostered by fortunate intellectuals who have a job that they enjoy (Antonini, 1971; Shanas, 1971a). It is significant that in the study of Beverfelt (1971), the proportion claiming to like their work diminished progressively with social class (77, 72, 64 and 52 per cent in the four categories distinguished). The average employee consigned to the noisy monotony of a car production line, or indeed the demanding targets and assignments of junior management may well rejoice when the age of 65 years is reached. As Shanas (1971a) puts it: 'The only deterrent to people retiring from a factory is whether they will be able to live ... in the mode or manner in which they have become accustomed.'

One useful measure of attitudes is the percentage of men who remain in the labour force after pensionable age has been reached. This is remarkably constant in the US (51 per cent), Britain (49 per cent) and Denmark (52 per cent), despite the two years higher official retirement age in Denmark (Milhøj, 1968). In Norway, Beverfelt (1971) found that 68 per cent of those retiring at age 65, but only 47 per cent of those retiring at age 70, wished to remain in the ranks of labour.

Voluntary retirement exceeds compulsory retirement at all ages (Table 8.9). By the age of retirement, about 50 per cent of the population have serious illnesses requiring medical attention. Immediately after retirement, the proportion who are sick drops to about 30 per cent. This may be partly a survivor effect, although there is also evidence that retirement leads to an improvement of health in some instances (Thompson & Streib, 1958).

Table 8.9   Reasons for retirement (Shanas *et al.*, 1968)

Reason	Age of retirement (years)		
	Under 65	65 – 69	Over 70
	%	%	%
Compulsory	20	43	16
Voluntary			
poor health	55	31	40
too tired	1	7	9
didn't want to work any longer	9	9	19
needed at home	6	5	4
other	8	5	11

The immediate cessation of work can be a traumatic experience. The manual worker may notice physiological effects from the decrease of energy expenditure, but psychological problems are more serious — feelings of loneliness, uselessness, futility, aimlessness and obsessive thoughts of old age and death (Sauvy, 1970a). Paradoxically, such reactions may be more common in the manual worker than in the intellectual, for the latter has more interests to occupy his new-found leisure. Statistics from Norway show that after the immediate shock has passed, some 60 per cent of the population enjoy retirement, and only 20 per cent describe it as something to dread (Steina, 1970). The advantages include greater opportunity for leisure activities (50 per cent) and rest (20 per cent), while negative aspects are a lack of money (32 per cent) and difficulty in passing the time (19 per cent). The three nation study (Shanas, 1968) found 48 per cent of Britons, 56 per cent of Danes and 9 per cent of US men missing 'nothing' about their work. The remainder complained of missing their friends, the feeling of being useful, the bustle of things happening around them, the intrinsic value of their work and the money that they had earned. About a half of the three nation group also complained of enjoying 'nothing' about their retirement.

The proportion of the elderly who find enjoyment in their retirement can be increased through preparatory programmes that explore the problems and the opportunities of old age. Ideally, such instruction should begin at least three years before ceasing work. Possible topics for such classes include income management, coping with ill-health in a relative or oneself, activities and hobbies suited to retirement and personal and social adjustment to increasing dependency. Demonstrations can cover home safety, nutrition and cooking (especially for men), craftwork, and tours of geriatric units and old peoples' homes (W.F. Anderson, 1973). It is also desirable that municipalities sponsor recreational centres for the elderly both inside and outside of institutions. Among other pursuits, these can provide opportunity for supervised exercise, old-time dancing, and the manufacture of toys for grandchildren and furniture for children.

Physical Ability

We have discussed previously (Chapter 3) the physical limitations of the elderly worker. Prospects for continuing employment depend on basic physical and mental endowment, the level of training and experience attained by the worker, his socio-economic status, emotional stability and physical health. The proportion of the population who are able to continue working beyond the age of 65 years varies very much from one occupation to another (Table 8.10). Edwards *et al.* (1959) concluded that much of the social class effect was health related; among men over the age of seventy, 67 per cent of those in the top two social classes but only 20 per cent of those in the lowest social class were fit to work. Other studies confirm the importance of health to continuing employment. Beverfelt (1971) commented that 40 per cent of Norwegians who wanted to work and 60 per cent of those who did not were medically incapable of carrying out their occupation. Equally, in the United Kingdom 30 to 35 per cent of manual workers and 23 per cent of non-manual workers were in poor health by the age of 65 years, so that they were glad to have the opportunity of retirement (Richardson, 1964; D. Kay *et al.*, 1964).

Demographic Trends 279

Table 8.10 Proportion of the elderly population still employed
(based on data of Sequeira [Lessa, 1971])

Occupation	Men	Women	All subjects
Primary			
Agriculture, forestry, hunting, fishing	71.3	45.6	67.1
Mining	0.2	0.0	0.2
Secondary			
Manufacturing	9.5	12.2	9.9
Construction	4.5	0.1	3.7
Public services	0.1	0.0	0.1
Tertiary			
Commerce, banking, insurance, real estate	6.8	7.7	6.9
Transport, shops, communications	1.4	0.4	1.3
Domestic services	5.3	33.3	9.9

If health remains good, the potential and even the actual level of attainment of many skills shows little decline up to and beyond the normal age of retirement (Thomae & Lehr, 1968). However, in demanding physical work, the average load for an eight-hour day begins to exceed the fatigue threshold (40 per cent of aerobic power). If the task is unpaced, problems first appear in the late fifties or the early sixties, while if the work is paced difficulty may be encountered in the late forties (Fulgraff, 1971). Paced work is usually of the unskilled variety, since the required rate of performance then has little influence on the quality of the finished product. Unfortunately, this means that the older person has little opportunity to compensate for a decline of speed through his greater experience of the task.

Problems may also arise from the introduction of new machinery. Six months after completion of an automation programme, one firm found that production ratings were negatively correlated with age; it was judged that the older workmen were slower on the uptake and less profitable to retain (Chown, 1961). Certainly, the current speed of technical change prevents the accumulation of specific job experience which was once the strength of the elderly worker. Retraining may also take longer than in a younger person, due partly to loss of memory and learning ability, and partly to a fear of failure (Eisdorfer, 1969). However, the apparent additional cost of retraining the elderly may be illusory, since the young are more apt to change their employment after training has been completed. Moreover, many aging workers retain the advantages of greater diligence, accuracy and experience, and partly for these reasons they have a low accident rate despite the handicaps of failing hearing and sight.

There is still considerable discussion regarding the loss of intelligence among those employed at desk jobs. Wechsler (1958) found from a cross-sectional study that scores on the Adult Intelligence Scale peaked at about 24 years, with a steady decline from 30 to 60 years, and a steeper rate of loss thereafter. However, verbal performance was preserved better than the ability to manipulate symbols.

In management, the main effect of aging is on personality. The young are generally more adaptable than older staff, who are afraid to take initiatives and seek only to take life quietly until their service has been completed. On the other hand, older managers are sometimes valued for the attributes of emotional stability and seasoned judgement that help them to cope with difficult personal and social situations.

Much of the current difficulty in finding employment for the older person is economic. In manual work, a standard union salary is demanded, but productivity may be lower than in a younger man. In office work, regular annual increments of salary produce a situation where a 50- or 55-year-old worker is paid far more than he is worth in terms of ability and usefulness. If alternative employment becomes necessary, it is often necessary for an employee to accept a substantial reduction in both salary and status. One interesting long-range suggestion (Sauvy, 1970b) has been to alter pay structure so that all employees receive a subsistence salary, supplemented by an equitably determined bonus, based on the current worth of the individual. Such a plan would avoid many of the heart-breaking dismissals of older employees, and at the same time would provide a useful incentive to all workers to maintain their productivity through regular courses of advanced training. Some redistribution of tasks already occurs among the labour force, particularly in the socialist economies (Figure 8.1). Hard physical work and modern skilled tasks are allocated to the young, while the more traditional pursuits and declining industries are staffed by the elderly. Spitaels (1971) has suggested that all companies should make a regular and systematic analysis of all jobs, with a view to reapportioning them among staff on the basis of their age and skills. Reclassification of elderly workers would depend on the extent of their senescence, as medically determined. In some

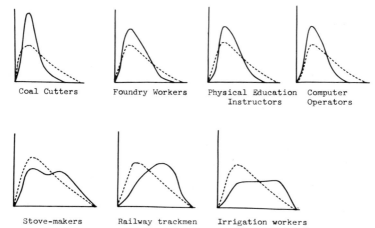

Figure 8.1 Age distribution of Russian workers in specific occupations (solid lines) compared with the total labour force (interrupted lines). Based on data of Sachuk (1971).

cases, the problem might be solved by allowing a slower rhythm of work or part-time employment, but in other instances a less demanding occupation would be necessary. Where organic disability was discovered, occupational therapy and a sheltered workshop could be of value in bringing the individual back into the labour force.

A further useful development would be to modify the initial training of workers and to increase opportunities for their subsequent retraining. Teaching should aim not merely at imparting knowledge that will soon be out-dated, but also at imparting attitudes, particularly the ability to cope with unfamiliar processes and situations. Unfortunately, many large industrial organisations regard it as uneconomic to attempt the retraining of older workers. However, they can be taught new skills (Belbin, 1963), particularly if there is an appropriate modification of teaching techniques (Shephard, 1974b).

Arguments can also be advanced for more flexibility in the age of retirement. Heavy, dirty and dangerous trades may merit early super-annuation, although care must be taken that the privilege is removed if technical advances later make the work more congenial. One instance where adjustment has not been made is on the French Railways; footplate engineers are still entitled to retire at the age of fifty, although their work is plainly much less tough and tedious than was the case in the days of steam traction. Women also have some justification for early retirement, because (1) they generally start work at an earlier age than men, (2) they have a lower physiological work capacity, and (3) they commonly have to cope with both their employment and household chores. It seems significant that whereas housewives live much longer than men, this is not the case for elderly women who are employed.

Actuarial Considerations

The ever-increasing proportion of senior citizens who make no formal contribution to national economies raises serious actuarial problems. Where there is reliance on private pension plans, high premium payments become a significant factor in dissuading employers from hiring workers over the age of 45 years (Sheppard, 1971). Where pensions are met from government revenues, a static production with a rising money supply due to increased pension payments inevitably leads to inflation, and (unless pensions are indexed to the cost of living) an increase in the poverty of the elderly.

If the needs of children and of the elderly are set at 70 per cent of figures for the working adult, the percentage of the earnings of active people that must be allocated to pension funds can be calculated as follows:

$$P = \frac{0.7E}{0.7C + A + A_i + 0.7E}$$

where E is the number of inactive elderly, C is the number of inactive children, A is the number of active adults and A_i is the number of inactive adults (Paillat, 1971). Actual contributions to superannuation, and the required contributions for more adequate pension payments (50 and 75 per cent of working salaries) are illustrated in Table 8.11. Some countries, such as Switzerland, fare quite well in this analysis because they have a substantial proportion of transient foreign workers who fail to collect any pension. The figures presented refer to the early 1960s, and there has already been a substantial increment in costs due to aging of the population. In France, for example, the values of P_1, P_2 and P_3 had increased to 9.5, 14.8 and 22.2 per cent by 1968. Equally, the United States had 73 citizens of non-working age for every 100 workers in 1950, but by 1970 this 'dependency ratio' had risen to 93 (Sheppard, 1971).

A second factor augmenting costs is a progressive lowering of the retirement age. In the United States, for example, it is possible to apply for early social security benefits between the ages of 62 and 64

Table 8.11   Actual and theoretical pension costs for selected
European countries. P_1 is the actual proportion of salaries applied to
pensions, P_2 the contribution required for a 50 per cent pension, and
P_3 the contribution required for a 75 per cent pension. Based on
data of Paillat (1971)

Country and year		Pension (as % of salaries of active workers)	P_1	P_2	P_3
Austria,	1961	35.4	8.6	12.1	18.1
Belgium	1961	29.8	9.0	15.1	22.7
Denmark	1960	35.3	6.7	9.9	14.9
France	1962	33.3	8.2	12.3	18.4
West Germany	1961	36.5	7.2	9.9	14.9
Italy	1961	29.9	5.4	10.7	16.0
Luxembourg	1960	31.4	7.1	11.3	17.0
Norway	1960	30.6	6.9	11.3	17.0
Netherlands	1960	28.6	6.1	10.7	16.1
Sweden	1960	33.5	7.9	11.8	17.7
Switzerland	1960	35.8	6.0	8.4	12.6
United Kingdom	1960	36.6	8.1	11.1	16.6

years. The proportion of men who choose to work full-time thus drops
from 73 per cent at ages 60-61 years to 60 per cent for the period
62-64 years, and 27 per cent for the period 65-69 years. Taking account
also of part-time work, the corresponding figures are 88, 81 and 55
per cent. The effect of varying the working period has been calculated
for the French labour force as follows:

School-leaving age (years)	Retirement age (years)	Relative dependency ratio
15	65	100
20	65	118
15	60	185
20	60	195

Given a school-leaving age of 15, a reduction of the retirement age
from 65 to 60 years changes the coefficients P_1, P_2 and P_3 from 9.5,
14.8 and 22.2 per cent to 15.0, 25.2 and 38.0 per cent. It is
particularly interesting to see that the cost of a 50 per cent pension
at age 60 is greater than that of a 75 per cent pension at age 65 years.

It is plain from Table 8.11 that even the rather inadequate 50 per cent pension is not being met in any European country, and many senior citizens are at or below the poverty line (Wedderburn, 1973). The priority should thus be to press for more adequate pension payments at age 65, rather than to seek any reduction in the pensionable age.

The optimum solution to the increasing costs of the aging population would be to increase the gross national product through such devices as automation, more effective training of the labour force, a decrease in under-employment and unemployment, increased use of women workers, and (where an entire nation has aged) immigration. In the past twenty years, many Western nations have in fact succeeded in making large gains in their productivity, so that all citizens (the elderly generally included) have enjoyed a higher standard of living. However, it is less certain that this trend can continue with the progressive exhaustion of non-renewable resources. A second option is a detailed review of national expenditures, with a diversion of money from non-productive areas such as national defence, or (as is currently happening in some Western democracies) a general reduction of social services. A third and less palatable alternative is to increase the burden on some segment of society — to impose a special levy on the rich, to increase taxes or to reduce the effective value of pensions through inflation. Although this last remedy has been used in the past, it is becoming less practicable from a political point of view, since the elderly form a powerful and growing block of voters. Significantly, the proportion of the population who exercise their franchise actually increases with age, at least to 75 years (Sheppard, 1971; Shephard & LaBarre, 1978).

Activity and Health Care Costs

The vast costs of health care for the elderly (Rice, 1967; US Senate, 1972) can be gauged from Tables 8.12 and 8.13. In the United States, the average annual per capita cost for 1970 was $791 for persons over 65 years of age, compared with $296 for those aged 19-64 years. Some $534 of the expense of the elderly was met by health insurance plans, leaving an average of $257 to be taken from the individual's meagre resources. Figures for Canada seem roughly comparable. By 1975, the cost of institutional care alone amounted to some $1,897 million, or $1,116 per senior citizen.

Unfortunately, there is no direct evidence regarding savings that might result from a programme of physical conditioning for the elderly. Through its probable impact on cardio-vascular and respiratory disease,

Table 8.12 Annual cost of health care in the elderly. Per capita expenditures for the United States, 1970, including all persons over the age of 65 years (based on data of US Senate report, 1972)

Hospital care	$ 372
Physicians' services	136
Other professional services	32
Drugs	84
Nursing home care	129
Miscellaneous	37
Total	791

Table 8.13 Approximate costs of institutional care for the elderly in Canada, 1975 (capital cost of facilities not included)

Type of care	Per cent of elderly	Population	Daily costs (per person)[a]	Annual cost ($ millions)
Active treatment	1.47	24,990	$ 110	$ 1,003
Chronic treatment	0.89	15,130	30	166
Mental care	0.32	5,440	30	60
Extended care	4.17	70,890	17	440
Other residential care	2.30	39,100	16[b]	228
TOTAL				1,897

[a] Estimates of Sidney (unpublished) for London, Ontario, 1975
[b] Includes $10/day charge to patient for occupation of ambulatory care residence, plus an amount that varies with the nursing care required

physical activity could conceivably reduce the costs of acute and chronic treatment by at least a third. A decrease of anxiety and an elevation of mood might also yield a 10 per cent reduction in the costs of mental care. However, the biggest saving would likely come from a reduced use of extended care and residential homes. As we have seen, a 20 per cent gain of cardio-respiratory fitness could extend the period of independence by as much as 8.6 years, and reduce the number of people requiring residential care by as much as two thirds. Accepting these rather crude estimates, the total reduction in health care costs would be as follows:

Active and chronic care	$ 1,169 million	× 1/3	= $ 386 mn
Mental care	60 million	× 1/10	= 6 mn
Extended care	668 million	× 2/3	= 445 mn
Total			$ 837 mn

Against this must be set the costs of a physical activity programme. As discussed elsewhere (Shephard, 1977d), both motivation and implementation can be quite expensive items. However, estimates for London, Ontario (Sidney, 1975, unpublished) suggest that a simple programme could be arranged for about $120 per person-year. Sidney allowed three one-hour classes per week (the minimum to maintain cardio-respiratory fitness), with twenty subjects per class. Individual sessions cost eight dollars ($3 for rental of a school gymnasium to a non-profit group, and $5 honorarium to an undergraduate fitness instructor); assuming that the class operated for fifty weeks of the year, the cost of this facility was then $60 per person. To this must be added a minimum of $60 for four fitness tests a year, the tests playing a role in both motivation and the safe prescription of physical activity on an individual basis. If all of the elderly population were to join such classes, the annual cost would be $204 million, and the net saving in health care costs would be $633 million, or $372 per senior citizen. The money thus saved could be spent in many different ways, but one rather appealing suggestion would be to augment the pension of each elderly couple by $744 per year, a sum that would do much to alter the balance between survival and happiness.

Implications for Independence and Life Satisfaction

Unfortunately, many physicians are bemused by the goal of longevity, and modern medicine has rightly been accused of converting acute terminal conditions into long-term disablement. While the resulting statistics may look impressive in medical and surgical journals, the true objective of any geriatric programme should not be longevity or a reduction of health care costs, but rather an increase in the well-being and life satisfaction of the senior citizen. Often, this is linked to his physical independence.

Maslow (1962) has provided a convenient framework for the discussion of life satisfaction through his description of a hierarchy of human needs, physiological, sociological and psychological.

Table 8.14 Marital status of men and women in the United Kingdom (based on data of Shanas *et al.*, 1968)

Age (years)	MEN			WOMEN		
	Married	Widowed	Single	Married	Widowed	Single
	%	%	%	%	%	%
65 – 66	82	14	4	54	33	12
67 – 69	75	20	4	46	42	12
70 – 74	71	24	4	31	53	15
75 – 79	58	36	6	27	56	17
Over 80	60	36	4	18	68	13

Physiological Needs

For many senior citizens, even some of the fundamental physiological needs — food and a sexual relationship — are not fully met. Few elderly people suffer the acute pangs of hunger, but often income is inadequate to provide nutritious food. Calculations may 'prove' that a wisely spent pension could provide an acceptable minimum diet, but the budget is frequently upset by 'unnecessary' expenditures such as the rental of a television set that provides an old person with some external focus of interest. Problems may also arise because of difficulty in shopping or in the preparation of meals. The period of independent living can often be extended through such services as 'meals on wheels', preparation of food by neighbours or arrangement of a home help. Alternatively, lunches can be provided at day-care centres. This last approach is particularly valuable in encouraging mobility and social contact.

A surprisingly small percentage of senior citizens are still married (Table 8.14). In the United Kingdom, only two of every ten women and six of every ten men over the age of 75 years have a spouse who is still alive. Furthermore, intercourse has ceased in many marriages (Chapter 3). Nevertheless, interest in a sexual relationship persists on the part of many older people. This leads to much frustration, particularly for women who accept the traditional female role, and find any form of liaison with a younger man the subject of fierce taboos (Weg, 1975). Possible alternatives to the traditional attempts at sublimation (Weg, 1975) include: treatment of a marital partner with sexual dysfunction; maximisation of potential by undertaking sexual activity early in the day; research to increase the vigour of older men and to equalise the life span of men and women; encouragement of dating and marriage between older women and younger men; and masturbation by those who have no appropriate marriage partners. Other morally less acceptable suggestions include more lenient attitudes towards homosexuality and polygamy.

Social Needs

Yearning for love, affection and a sense of belonging are at the next level in Maslow's hierarchy, to be sought once physiological needs have been largely satisfied.

A substantial segment of the elderly population have no immediate family. Shanas *et al.* (1968) reported that in Britain 16 per cent of those over the age of 65 years had no spouse and no surviving children, while a further 7 per cent were married but had no children; of this 23 per cent, 4 per cent had no close relatives. Nevertheless, where there were children, contact had generally remained close. About 70 per cent of elderly parents had seen at least one of their children within the preceding 48 hours, and 86 per cent had encountered one of their children during the previous week. Excluding those who were actually living with their children, the percentages were still 50 and 87 per cent. In California (Burch & Collot, 1972), contacts were a little less frequent; 36 per cent saw their relatives daily, and 29 per cent weekly, while 4 per cent saw friends daily and 48 per cent weekly. Differences seem an expression of travelling distances; a study in suburban Paris (Burch & Collot, 1972) observed that 43 to 55 per cent of family living in the same town paid daily visits to their aging parents, but this figure dropped to 19 to 35 per cent when the children lived in a neighbouring town, and to 10 to 19 per cent when they were living further away. Such contacts play an important role in sustaining the independence of the elderly. When there are no surviving children, it is common for substitute relationships to develop with more remote kin or with neighbours (Rosow, 1971). Such individuals not only help with shopping and preparing meals, but in many instances even care for those who are bed-ridden and incontinent. Indeed, Isaacs (1971) commented that 31 per cent of admissions to geriatric wards were for the relief of strain on the part of those caring for the elderly in their homes.

Shanas *et al.* (1968) estimated that 2 to 3 per cent of the elderly in Britain were severely isolated, in that they lived alone, had received no visitors in the previous week and had made no human contacts on the previous day. Tunstall (1966) used a more elaborate method of scoring

isolation, and concluded that 21 per cent of old people were isolated,
4 per cent of them extremely so. Loneliness is not quite the same
thing as isolation. Shanas *et al.* (1968) have defined it as a sensation of
lack or loss of companionship. These authors found 7 per cent of old
people were often lonely and a further 21 per cent were sometimes
lonely. The problem was particularly frequent in widows, the recently
bereaved and those in poor health. As Abel-Smith & Titmus (1956)
have put it: 'Marriage and its survival into old age appears to be a
powerful safeguard against admission to hospitals in general and to
mental and "chronic" hospitals in particular.' Nevertheless, a
surprisingly large proportion of the elderly are well-integrated into
society; Burch & Collot (1972) noted that 75 to 81 per cent of those
living in Paris, and 83 per cent of those living in California felt a part
of their respective communities.

Psychological Needs

At the highest level in Maslow's hierarchy stands the needs of the ego
– the regard of significant others, a sense of self-respect engendered by
feelings of competence and control over one's destiny, and the
ultimate goal of self-actualisation, with its sense of growth to
maturity and realisation of potential.

The elderly often equate self-respect with independence. Stehouwer
(1970) comments that 'a high degree of contact and especially living
together with children have by no means always a positive effect on the
morale of elderly parents. The optimum arrangement is seen to live for
as long as possible in one's own house.' We have already observed that
in Canada 9.15 per cent of the elderly are institutionalised (Table 8.13),
2.36 per cent being in general hospitals, 0.32 per cent in psychiatric
institutions and 6.47 per cent in residential institutions. Perhaps
because of the smaller distances separating parents from their children,
the proportion who are institutionalised is somewhat lower in Britain.
Wedderburn (1973), for example, found that 5.2 per cent of the elderly
were living in institutions (2 per cent in hospitals, 1.6 per cent in
mental hospitals and 1.6 per cent in residential care). Between a third
and a half of this group were over the age of 80 years. Furthermore, 53
per cent of those in institutions and 20 per cent of those receiving
domiciliary services were bed-ridden or severely incapacitated, compared
with only 7 per cent of the elderly population in general. The majority
were poor, and came from manual occupations. A high proportion had
also been living alone and had no children. A. Harris (1968) estimated
that at least 20 per cent of senior citizens would not have needed

admission to an institution if suitable housing had been available. Munnichs & Bigot (1973) reported slightly different statistics for England and Wales in 1970; at this time, 6.1 per cent of the elderly were in some form of institution, 3.8 per cent in geriatric and mental hospitals and 2.3 per cent in residential homes. A further 7.7 per cent were receiving home nursing and 6.2 per cent had been provided with home help.

Nevertheless, formal care is not always available to the most needy cases. Townsend (1972) estimated that more of the bed-ridden and severely incapacitated were living at home than in institutions. The 'availability of children, particularly of daughters, is a strong protection against admission to hospital' (Townsend, 1957). While a daughter often seems willing to care for physical disability, mental confusion, restless or disturbed behaviour and incontinence are usually regarded as insupportable burdens (D. Kay *et al.*, 1970).

Once hospital admission has occurred, the prognosis is not good. Isaacs (1971) found that over a three-month period, only 21 per cent of elderly patients were discharged; 33 per cent died, and the remaining 38 per cent were still in hospital, as much from a problem of disposition as from continuing illness (Edge & Nelson, 1964). Often, hard-pressed relatives see hospital admission as an opportune moment to resign from their responsibilities. Nisbet (1970) questioned 50 elderly women who were about to be discharged from hospital, and found that only 15 were really happy to be leaving, and that only 9 of their relations were genuinely pleased to see them return. Brocklehurst & Shergold (1968) also commented that 21 per cent of old people were not welcomed by their families after discharge from hospital.

Accepting continued independence as the desired goal of the elderly, we have already seen that an increase in the level of physical fitness can contribute as much as 8-9 years of the required cardio-respiratory power. Other possible techniques for a further extension of the independent years include assistance with domestic work (home helps, meals on wheels), increase of social contact (golden age clubs, with provision of suitable transportation), improved design of homes (non-slip floors, hand-grips in bathrooms, central heating and an absence of stairs), and subsequent provision of sheltered housing, with a warden or friend to provide a daily monitoring of physical condition. Given such assistance, perhaps we may all face advancing years with the spirit of John Diefenbaker, former prime minister of Canada. Summoned to an eightieth birthday party 'at the mid-point in his political career', he made the swift response 'while there's snow on the roof, it doesn't mean the fire has gone out in the furnace!'

REFERENCES

1. Abel-Smith, B. & R.M. Titmuss. *The cost of the National Health Service in England and Wales.* London: Cambridge University Press, 1956.
2. Abramson, J.H. The Cornell Medical Index as an epidemiological tool. *Amer. J. Publ. Health* 56: 287-98, 1966.
3. Abramson, J.H., L. Terespolsky, J.G. Brook, & S.L. Kark. Cornell Medical Index as a health measure in epidemiological studies. A test of the validity of a health questionnaire. *Brit. J. Prev. Soc. Med.* 19: 103-10, 1965.
4. Acheson, J. & E.C. Hutchinson. The natural history of 'focal cerebral vascular disease'. *Quart. J. Med.* 40: 15-23, 1971.
5. Adams, D.L. Analysis of a life satisfaction index. *J. Geront.* 24: 470-4, 1969.
6. Adams, G.M. & H.A. DeVries. Physiological effects of an exercise training regimen upon women aged 52 to 79. *J. Geront.* 28: 50-55, 1973.
7. Adams, W.C. Influence of age and body weight on energy expenditure of bicycle riding. *J. Appl. Physiol.* 22: 539-45, 1967.
8. Adams, W.C., M.M. McHenry & E.M. Bernauer. Multistage treadmill walking performance and associated cardiorespiratory responses of middle-aged men. *Clin. Sci.* 42: 355-70, 1972.
9. Adelman, R.C. An age-dependent modification of enzyme regulation. *J. Biol. Chem.* 245: 1032-5, 1970.
10. Adler, W.H. An 'auto-immune' theory of aging. In *Theoretical aspects of aging,* ed. M. Rockstein. New York: Academic Press, 1974.
11. Aitken, G.T. The geriatric amputee. A report on a conference sponsored by the National Res. Council Committee on Prosthetics Res. & Devt. NAS-NRC Publ. 919: 1961.
12. Albanese, A.A., R.A. Higgins, L.A. Orto & D.N. Zavarotto. Protein and amino-acid needs of the aged in health and convalescence. *Geriatrics* 12: 465-75, 1957.
13. Albert, N.R., H.H. Gale & N. Taylor. The effect of age on contractile protein ATPase activity and the velocity of shortening. In *Factors influencing myocardial contractility,* ed. R.D. Tanz, F. Kavaler & J. Roberts. New York: Academic Press, 1967.
14. Alexander, J.K. & K.L. Peterson. Cardiovascular effects of weight reduction. *Circulation* 45: 310-18, 1972.
15. Alexander, P. The role of DNA lesions in processes leading to aging in mice. *Symp. Soc. Exp. Biol.* 21: 29-50, 1967.
16. Alexander, P. & D.I. Connell. Differences between radiation induced life-span shortening in mice and normal aging as revealed by serial killing. In *Cellular basis and aetiology of late somatic effects of ionizing radiations,* ed. R.J.C. Harris, pp. 277-83. New York: Academic Press, 1963.
17. Allen, J.G. Aerobic capacity and physical fitness of Australian men. *Ergonomics* 9: 485-94, 1966.
18. Allen, T.H., E.C. Anderson & W.H. Langham. Total body potassium and gross body composition in relation to age. *J. Geront.* 15: 348-57, 1960.
19. Allman, F.L. Conditioning for sports. In *Sports Medicine,* ed. A.J. Ryan & F.L. Allman. New York: Academic Press, 1974.
20. Alpert, J.S., H. Bass, M.M. Szues, J.S. Banas, J.E. Dalen & L. Dexter. Effects of physical training on hemodynamics and pulmonary function at rest

and during exercise in patients with chronic obstructive pulmonary disease. *Chest* 66: 647-51, 1974.

21. American Thoracic Society. Chronic bronchitis, asthma and pulmonary emphysema. (Definitions and classification of chronic bronchitis, asthma and pulmonary emphysema). *Amer. Rev. Resp. Dis.* 85: 762-9, 1962.

22. Amundsen, L.R. & B. Balke. Glucocorticoid response to acute and chronic physical exercise. Paper presented at the annual meeting Amer. College Sports Med., *Med. Sci. Sports* 5. 59, 1973.

23. Andersen, K.L. *Respiratory recovery from muscular exercise of short duration.* Oslo: Oslo Univ. Press, 1959.

24. Andersen, K.L. Physical fitness – studies of healthy men and women in Norway. In *International research in sport & physical education*, ed. E. Jokl & E. Simon. Springfield, Ill.: C.C. Thomas, 1964.

25. Anderson, K.L., R.J. Shephard, H. Denolin, E. Varnauskas & R. Masironi. *Fundamentals of exercise testing.* Geneva: World Health Org., 1971.

26. Anderson, P.B., S.R. Brennan & P. Howard. Posture, exercise and pulmonary arterial pressure in chronic obstructive airways disease. *Clin. Sci. Mol. Biol.* 50: 22P, 1977.

27. Anderson, T.W. The vulnerable myocardium. *Lancet* (2), 1084-5, 1973.

28. Anderson, T.W., J.R. Brown, J.W. Hall & R.J. Shephard. The limitations of linear regressions for the prediction of vital capacity and forced expired volume. *Respiration* 25: 140-58, 1968.

29. Anderson, T.W. & R.J. Shephard. Physical training and exercise diffusing capacity. *Int. Z. angew. Physiol.* 25: 198-209, 1968a.

30. Anderson, T.W. & R.J. Shephard. The effects of hyperventilation and exercise upon the pulmonary diffusing capacity. *Respiration* 25: 465-84, 1968b.

31. Anderson, W.F. In *Practical management of the elderly*, p. 129. Oxford: Blackwell Scientific, 1967.

32. Anderson, W.F. Preventive medicine in old age. In *Textbook of geriatric medicine & gerontology*, ed. J.C. Brocklehurst, pp. 718-26. Edinburgh: Churchill-Livingstone, 1973.

33. Anderson, W.F. & N.R. Cowan. Arterial blood pressure in healthy older people. *Geront. Clin.* 14: 129-36, 1972.

34. Anderson, W.G. Further studies in the longevity of Yale athletes. *Medical Times* 44: 75-6, 1916.

35. Andres, R. The study of aging in man: practical and theoretical problems. In *Theoretical aspects of aging*, ed. M. Rockstein. New York: Academic Press, 1974.

36. Andrew, W. The fine structural and histochemical changes in aging. In *The biological basis of medicine*, vol. 1. New York: Academic Press, 1968.

37. Andrews, J., M. Brook & M.A. Allen. Influence of abode and season on the Vitamin C status of the elderly. *Geront. Clin.* 8: 257-66, 1966.

38. Angel, A. Pathophysiology of obesity. *Canad. Med. Ass. J.* 110: 540-48, 1974.

39. Anthonisen, N.R., J. Danson, P.C. Robertson & W.R.D. Ross. Airway closure as a function of age. *Resp. Physiol.* 8: 58-65, 1969-70.

40. Antonini, F. Some reflections on the anthropology and biology of work. In *Work & aging*, ed. J.A. Huet, pp. 13-20. Paris: International Centre of Social Gerontology, 1971.

41. Armaly, M.F. On the distribution of applanation tension. *Arch. Ophthalmol.* 73: 11-18, 1965.

42. Armstrong, B.W., J.M. Workman, H.H. Hurt & W.R. Roemich. Clinico-physiologic evaluation of physical working capacity in persons with pulmonary disease; rationale and application of a method based on estimating maximal

294   *References*

oxygen consuming capacity from MBC and O_2 V_e. *Amer. Rev. Resp. Dis.* 93: 223-33, 1967.

43.   Arnold, J.S. Quantification of mineralization of bone as an organ and tissue in osteoporosis. *Clin. Orthop.* 17: 167-75, 1960.

44.   Arnold, J.S., M.H. Bartley, S.S. Tont & D.P. Jenkins. Skeletal changes in aging and disease. *Clin. Orthop.* 49: 17-38, 1966.

45.   Asano, K., S. Ogawa & Y. Furuta. Aerobic work capacity in middle and old-aged runners. *Proc. int. congress of physical activity sciences,* Quebec City, Canada, 1976.

46.   Aslan, A. Theoretical and practical aspects of chemotherapeutic techniques in the retardation of the aging process. In *Theoretical aspects of aging,* ed. M. Rockstein. New York: Academic Press, 1974.

47.   Ashley, F.W. & W.B. Kannel. Relation of weight change to changes in atherogenic traits: the Framingham study. *J. Chr. Dis.* 27: 103-14, 1974.

48.   Asmussen, E. Muscular exercise. In *Handbook of physiology,* Section 3, *Respiration,* part 2, ed. W. Fenn & H. Rahn. Washington D.C.: Amer. Physiol. Soc., 1964.

49.   Asmussen, E. & K. Heebøll-Nielsen. Isometric muscle strength of adult men and women. Communications from the Testing and Observation Institute. *Danish Nat. Ass. Infantile Paralysis.* Hellerup, Denmark, 11: 1961.

50.   Asmussen, E. & P. Mathiasen. Some physiologic functions in physical education students re-investigated after 25 years. *J. Amer. Geriatric Soc.* 10: 379-87, 1962.

51.   Asmussen, E. & S.V. Molbech. Methods and standards for evaluation of the physiological working capacity of patients. *Comm. Test. Obs. Inst.* Hellerup, Denmark 4: 1959.

52.   Asmussen, E. & E. Poulsen. Energy expenditure in light industry. Its relation to age, sex and aerobic capacity. *Communications from Danish Nat. Assoc. for Infantile Paralysis.* Hellerup, Denmark, 13: 3-13, 1963.

53.   Åstrand, I. The physical work capacity of workers 50-64 years old. *Acta Physiol. Scand.* 42: 73-86, 1958.

54.   Åstrand, I. Aerobic work capacity in men and women with special reference to age. *Acta Physiol. Scand.* 49, Suppl. 169: 1-92, 1960.

55.   Åstrand, I. Exercise electrocardiograms recorded twice with an 8 year interval in a group of 204 women and men 48-63 years old. *Acta Med. Scand.* 178: 27-39, 1965a.

56.   Åstrand, I. Blood pressure during physical work in a group of 221 women and men 48-63 years old. *Acta Med. Scand.* 178: 41-6, 1965b.

57.   Åstrand, I. Aerobic work capacity. Its relation to age, sex, and other factors. *Circulat. Res.* 20 (Suppl. 1): 211-17, 1967a.

58.   Åstrand, I. Degree of strain during building work as related to individual work capacity. *Ergonomics* 10: 293-303, 1967b.

59.   Åstrand, I. (Chairwoman). The Scandinavian Committee on ECG classification: 'The Minnesota Code' for ECG classification. Adaptation to CR leads and modification of the code for ECG's recorded during and after exercise. *Acta Med. Scand. Suppl.* 481: 1967c.

60.   Åstrand, I. Electrocardiographic changes in relation to the type of exercise, the work load, age and sex. In *Measurement in exercise electrocardiography,* ed. H. Blackburn, pp. 309-21. Springfield, Illinois: C.C. Thomas, 1969.

61.   Åstrand, I., P.O. Åstrand, I. Hallbäck & A. Kilbom. Reduction in maximal oxygen uptake with age. *J. Appl. Physiol.* 35: 649-54, 1973.

62.   Åstrand, I., P.O. Åstrand & K. Rodahl. Maximal heart rate during work in older men. *J. Appl. Physiol.* 14: 562-6, 1959.

63.   Åstrand, P.O. *Experimental studies of physical working capacity in*

relation to sex and age. Copenhagen: Munksgaard, 1952.
64.   Åstrand, P.O. Measurement of maximal aerobic capacity. In Proc.
International Symposium on Physical Activity & Cardiovascular Health. *Canad.*
Med. Ass. J. 96. 732-5, 1967.
65.   Åstrand, P.O. Physical performance as a function of age. *J. Amer. Med.*
Ass. 205: 729-33, 1968.
66.   Åstrand, P.O. The age factor in sport: sport in the modern world –
chances & problems. Paper presented at the World Congress of Sports Medicine:
Munich, 1972.
67.   Åstrand, P.O. & I. Ryhming, A nomogram for calculation of aerobic
capacity (physical fitness) from pulse rate during submaximal work. *J. Appl.*
Physiol. 7. 218-21, 1954.
68.   Back, K.W. The ambiguity of retitrement. In *Behaviour and adaptation*
in late life, ed. E.W. Busse and E. Pfeiffer. Boston: Little Brown, 1969.
69.   Bagdade, J.D., E.L. Bierman & D. Porte. The significance of basal insulin
levels in the evaluation of the insulin response to glucose in diabetic and non
diabetic subjects. *J. Clin. Invest.* 46: 1549-56, 1967.
70.   Bailey, D.A., R.J. Shephard, R.L. Mirwald & G.A. McBride. A current
view of cardiorespiratory fitness levels of Canadians. *Canad. Med. Ass. J.* Ill:
25-30, 1974.
71.   Bailey, D.A., R.J. Shephard & R.L. Mirwald. Validation of a self-
administered home test of cardio-respiratory fitness. *Can. J. Appl. Sports Sci.*
1: 67-78, 1976.
72.   Bakerman, S. Distribution of the alpha and beta components in human
skin collagen with age. *Biochem. Biophys. Acta* 90: 621-3, 1964.
73.   Bakerman, S. *Ageing life processes,* p. 10. Springfield, Ill.: C.C.
Thomas, 1969.
74.   Balke, B. Optimale korperliche Leistungsfahigkeit, ihre Messung und
Veränderung infolge Arbeitsmüdung. *Int. Z. angew. Physiol.* 15: 311-23, 1954.
75.   Bang, J.O., J. Dyerberg & A.B. Nielsen. Plasma lipid and lipoprotein
pattern in Greenlandic West Coast Eskimos. *Lancet* i: 1143-5, 1971.
76.   Barach, A.L. Ambulatory oxygen therapy; oxygen inhalation at home
and out of doors. *Dis. Chest.* 35: 229-41, 1959.
77.   Bard, G. Energy expenditure of hemiplegic subjects during walking.
Arch. Phys. Med. Rehab. 44: 368-70, 1963.
78.   Barr, S.A. & R.M. Glaser. Physiological responses to wheelchair and
bicycle activity. *Fed. Proc.* 36: 580, 1977.
79.   Barrows, C.H. Enzymes in the study of biological aging. In *Perspectives*
in experimental gerontology, ed. N.W. Shock. Springfield, Ill.: C.C. Thomas,
1966.
80.   Barrows, C.H. & R.E. Beauchene. Aging and nutrition. In *Newer*
methods of nutritional biochemistry, ed. A.A. Albanese, vol. 4. New York:
Academic Press, 1970.
81.   Barrows, C.H., J.A. Falzone & N.W. Shock. Age differences in the
succin-oxidase activity of homogenates and mitochondria from the liver and
kidney of rats. *J. Gerontol.* 15: 130-3, 1960.
82.   Barry, A.J., J.W. Daly, E.D.R. Pruett, J.R. Steinmetz, H.F. Page, N.C.
Birkhead & K. Rodahl. The effects of physical conditioning on older individuals.
I. Work capacity, circulatory-respiratory function, and work electrocardiogram.
J. Geront. 21: 182-91, 1966.
83.   Bartlett, R.G. & V.C. Bohr. Physiologic responses during coitus in the
human. *Fed. Proc.* 15: 10, 1956.
84.   Bass, H. Exercise and respiratory disease. In *Sports medicine,* ed. A.J.
Ryan & F.L. Allman. San Francisco: Academic Press, 1974.

85.   Bass, H., J.F. Whitcomb & R. Forman. Exercise training: therapy for patients with chronic obstructive pulmonary disease. *Dis. Chest* 57: 116-21, 1970.

86.   Bassey, E.J. & P.H. Fentem. Extent of deterioration in physical condition during post-operative bed rest and its reversal by rehabilitation. *Brit. Med. J.* iv: 194-6, 1974.

87.   Batata, M., G.H. Spray, F.G. Bolton, G. Higgins & L. Wollner. Blood and bone marrow changes in elderly patients, with particular reference to folic acid, Vitamin B_{12}, iron and ascorbic acid. *Brit. Med. J.* ii: 667-9, 1967.

88.   Bates, D.V., N.G. Boucot & A.E. Dormer. The pulmonary diffusing capacity in normal subjects. *J. Physiol.* 129: 237-52, 1955.

89.   Baum, G.L., A. Schwartz, R. Llamas & C. Castillo. Left ventricular function in chronic obstructive lung disease. *New Engl. J. Med.* 285: 361-5, 1971.

90.   Beblinger, K.W. Obesity and psychologic stress. In *Obesity*, ed. N.L. Wilson. Philadelphia: F.A. Davis, 1969.

91.   Becklake, M.R., H. Frank, G.R. Dagenais, G.L. Ostiguy & G.A. Guzman. Influence of age and sex on exercise cardiac output. *J. Appl. Physiol.* 20: 938-47, 1965.

92.   Bedell, G.N. & R.W. Adams. Pulmonary diffusing capacity during rest and exercise. A study of normal persons and persons with atrial septal defect, pregnancy and pulmonary disease. *J. Clin. Invest.* 41: 1908-14, 1962.

93.   Bedford, P.D. & L. Wollner. Occult intestinal bleeding as a cause of anaemia in elderly people. *Lancet* i: 1144-47, 1958.

94.   Begin, R., A.D. Renzetti, A. Bigler & S. Watanabe. Flow and age dependence of airway closure and dynamic compliance. *J. Appl. Physiol.* 38: 199-207, 1975.

95.   Belbin, E. Some studies of training older people. 6th International Congress of Gerontology, Copenhagen, 1963. Cited by Roth, M. Mental health problems of aging and the aged with some comments on the role of World Health and other International Organizations. In *Work & aging,* ed. J.A. Huet. Paris: Int. Centre of Social Gerontology, 1971.

96.   Belloc, N.B. & L. Breslow. Relationship of physical health status and health practices. *Prev. Med.* 1: 409-21, 1972.

97.   Belloc, N.B., L. Breslow & J.R. Hockstim. Measurement of physical health in a general population survey. *Amer. J. Epidemiol.* 93: 328-36, 1971.

98.   Bender. A.E. Recent advances in protein synthesis. *Lancet* 265: 1142-3, 1953.

99.   Benditt, E.P. & J.M. Benditt. Evidence for a monoclonal origin of human atherosclerotic plaques. *Proc. Nat. Acad. Sci. (U.S.A.)* 70: 1753-6, 1973.

100.   Benestad, A.M. Trainability of old men. *Acta Med. Scand.* 178: 321-7, 1965.

101.   Bennett, G.A., W. Waine & W. Bauer. *Changes in the knee joint at various ages.* New York: Commonwealth Fund, 1942.

102.   Berglund, E., G. Birath, J. Bjure, G. Grimby, I. Kjellmer, I. Sandqvist & B. Söderholm. Spirometric studies in normal subjects. I. Forced expirograms in subjects between 7 and 70 years of age. *Acta Med. Scand.* 173: 185-92, 1963.

103.   Bergman, M. Hearing and aging. Implications of recent research findings. *Audiology* 10: 164-70, 1971.

104.   Bergmann, K., D.W.K. Kay, E.M. Foster, A.A. McKechnie & M. Roth. Follow-up study of randomly selected community residents to assess the effects of chronic brain syndrome and cerebrovascular disease. 5th World Congress of Psychiatry. Mexico City, 1971.

105.   Berry, W.T.C. Protein status of the elderly. *Proc. Nutr. Soc.* 27: 191-6, 1968.

106.   Bertolini, A.M. Aging in red cells. In *Perspectives in experimental gerontology*, ed. N.W. Shock. Springfield, Ill.: C.C. Thomas, 1966.
107.   Beverfeldt, E. Psychic behaviour of the worker facing old age. In *Work and aging*, ed. J.A. Huet, pp. 135-46. Paris: International Centre of Social Gerontology, 1971.
108.   Bickert, F.W. Einfluss des Wettkampfmassig betriebenen Sports auf die Lebensdauer und Todesursache. *Deutsche Med. Wschr.* 55: 23-5, 1929.
109.   Biörck, G. *Report of symposium on society, stress, and disease.* Stockholm: 1972.
110.   Birath, G., I. Kjellmer & L. Sandqvist. Spirometric studies in normal subjects. II. Ventilatory capacity tests in adults. *Acta Med. Scand.* 173: 193-8, 1963.
111.   Birath, G., T. Wessel-Aas, K.N. Rasmussen, P. Bonnevie, A.E. Korrekangas, S. Bjorkman, K. Larsen & B. Simonsson. Chronic bronchitis. In Proceedings of the 21st Scand. Congress of Pneumology. *Acta Tuberc. Pneumol. Scand.* Suppl. 56: 56-84, 1964.
112.   Birren, J.E. Age changes in speed of behavior: its central nature and physiological correlates. In *Behaviour, aging and the nervous system*, ed. A.T. Welford and J.E. Birren, pp. 191-216. Springfield, Ill.: C.C. Thomas, 1965.
113.   Birren, J.E. & J. Botwinick. Age differences in finger, jaw and foot reaction time to auditory stimuli. *J. Gerontol.* 10: 429-32, 1955.
114.   Birren, J.E., R.N. Butler, S.W. Greenhouse, L. Sokoloff & M.R. Yarrow. *Human aging.* Washington: US Government Printing Office, 1963.
115.   Birren, J.E. & P.D. Wall. Age changes in conduction velocity, refractory period, number of fibers, connective tissue, space, and blood vessels in sciatic nerves of rats. *J. Comp. Neutrol.* 104: 1-16, 1956.
116.   Bjelke, E. Variation in height and weight in the Norwegian population. *Brit. J. Prev. Soc. Med.* 25: 192-202, 1971.
117.   Bjorksten, J. Cross-linkage and the aging process. In *Theoretical aspects of aging*, ed. M. Rockstein. New York: Academic Press, 1974.
118.   Björntorp, P., G. Carlgren, B. Isaksson, M. Krotkiewski, B. Larsson & L. Sjöstrom. Effect of an energy-reduced dietary regimen in relation to adipose tissue cellularity in obese women. *Amer. J. Clin. Nutr.* 28: 445-52, 1975.
119.   Björntorp, P., M. Fahlén, J. Holm, T. Scherstén & J. Stenberg. Changes in the activity of skeletal muscle succinic oxidase after training. In *Coronary heart disease and physical fitness*, ed. O.A. Larsen & R.O. Malmborg, pp. 138-42. Copenhagen: Munksgaard, 1971.
120.   Blackburn, H. The exercise electrocardiogram. Technological, procedural, and conceptual developments. In *Measurement in exercise electrocardiography*, ed. H. Blackburn, pp. 220-57. Springfield, Illinois: C.C. Thomas, 1969a.
121.   Blackburn, H. (editor). *Measurement in exercise electrocardiography.* Springfield, Ill.: C.C. Thomas, 1969b.
122.   Blomqvist, G. The Frank lead exercise electrocardiogram. A quantitative study based on averaging technique and digital computer analysis. *Acta Med. Scand.* 178. Suppl. 440, pp. 1-98, 1965.
123.   Blomqvist, G. Variations of the electrocardiographic response to exercise under different experimental conditions; deconditioning, reconditioning, and high altitude. In *Measurement in exercise electrocardiography*, ed. H. Blackburn. Springfield, Ill.: C.C. Thomas, 1969.
124.   Bloor, K. The natural history of arteriosclerosis of the lower extremities. *Ann. Roy. Coll. Surg. Engl.* 28: 36-52, 1961.
125.   Blumberger, K.J. & M. Sigisbert. Studies of cardiac dynamics. In *Cardiology, and encyclopaedia of the cardiovascular disease*, ed. A.A. Luisada, vol. 2, chapter 14, 4-372 to 4-377. New York: McGraw-Hill, 1959.

126.   Blumenthal, H.T. Athero-arteriosclerosis as an aging phenomenon. In *The physiology and pathology of human aging*, ed. R. Goldman & M. Rockstein. New York: Academic Press, 1975.

127.   Boas, E.P. & E.F. Goldschmidt. *The heart rate*. Springfield, Illinois: C.C. Thomas, 1932.

128.   Bobath, B. *Adult hemiplegia; evaluation and treatment*. London: Heinemann, 1970.

129.   Bogert, L.J., G.M. Briggs & D.H. Calloway. *Nutrition and physical fitness*, 8th ed. Philadelphia: Saunders, 1966.

130.   Bonjer, F.H. Relationship between working time, physical work capacity and allowable caloric expenditure. In *Muskelarbeit und Muskeltraining*, ed. W. Rohmert, pp. 86-99. Stuttgart: A.W. Gentner Verlag, 1968.

131.   Bookwalter, K.W. Grip strength norms for males. *Res. Quart.* 21: 249-73, 1950.

132.   Boren, H., R.C. Kory & J.C. Syner. The Veterans Administration − Army cooperative study of pulmonary function. II. Lung volume and its subdivisions in normal men. *Amer. J. Med.* 41: 96-114, 1966.

133.   Borg, G. *Physical performance and perceived exertion*. Lund: Gleerup, 1962.

134.   Borg, G. The perception of physical performance. In *Frontiers of Fitness*, ed. R.J. Shephard, pp. 280-94. Springfield, Illinois: C.C. Thomas, 1971.

135.   Borg, G. & H. Linderholm. Perceived exertion and pulse rate during exercise in various age groups. *Acta Med. Scand. Suppl.* 472: 194-206, 1967.

136.   Bose, S.K., J. Andrews & P.D. Roberts. Haematological problems in a geriatric unit with special reference to anemia. *Geront. Clin.* 12: 339-46, 1970.

137.   Botwinik, J. Theories of antecedent conditions of speed of response. In *Behaviour, aging and the nervous system*, ed. A.T. Welford & J.E. Birren, pp. 67-87. Springfield, Ill.: C.C. Thomas, 1965.

138.   Boucher, C.A. Accidents among old persons. *Geriatrics* 14: 293-300, 1959.

139.   Bouhuys, A. & J. Pool. Physical working capacity in pulmonary disease. *Amer. Rev. Resp. Dis.* 88: 103-4, 1963.

140.   Bourlière, F. Ecology of human senescence. In *Textbook of geriatric medicine and gerontology*. Edinburgh: Churchill-Livingstone, 1973.

141.   Bourlière, F. & S. Parot. Le vieillissement de deux populations blanches vivant dans des conditions écologiques très différentes, etude comparative. *Rev. Fr. Etud. Clin. Biol.* 7: 629-35, 1962.

142.   Bramwell, J.C. Arterial elasticity in man. *Quart. J. Med.* 17: 225-43, 1924.

143.   Brandfonbrener, M., M. Landowne & N.W. Shock. Changes in cardiac output with age. *Circulation* 12: 557-66, 1955.

144.   Bray, G.A. Measurement of subcutaneous fat cells from obese patients. *Ann. Int. Med.* 73: 565-9, 1970.

145.   Brin, M. Biochemical methods and findings in the USA surveys. In *Vitamins in the elderly*, ed. A.N. Exton-Smith & D.L. Scott, pp. 25-33. Bristol: J. Wright, 1968.

146.   Brinley, J.F. Cognitive sets, speed and accuracy of performance in the elderly. In *Behaviour, aging and the nervous systems*, ed. A.T. Welford & J.E. Birren, pp. 114-49. Springfield, Ill.: C.C. Thomas, 1965.

147.   Brisson, G.R., F. Malaisse-Laque & W.J. Malaisse. Effect of Phentolamine upon insulin secretion during exercise. *Diabetologia* 7: 223-6, 1971.

148.   British Medical Journal, Editorial. Intermittent claudication. *Brit. Med. J.* 6019: 1165-6, 1976.

149.   Broadbent, D.E. & A. Heron. Effects of a subsidiary task on perfor-

mance involving immediate memory by younger and older men. *Brit. J. Psychol.* 53: 189-98, 1962.
150. Brocklehurst, J.C. Geriatric services and the day hospital. In *Textbook of geriatric medicine & gerontology,* ed. J.C. Brocklehurst, pp. 673-91. Edinburgh: Churchill-Livingstone, 1973.
151. Brocklehurst, J.C. & M. Shergold. What happens when geriatric patients leave hospital? *Lancet* ii: 1133-5, 1968.
152. Brodman, K., A.J. Erdmann, I. Lorge & H.G. Wolff. The Cornell Medical Index – Health Questionnaire VI. The relation of patients' complaints to age, sex, race and education. *J. Gerontol.* 8: 339-42, 1953.
153. Brodman, K., A.J. Erdmann & H.G. Wolff. *Medical index – health questionnaire manual.* New York: Cornell University Medical College, 1956.
154. Brody, H. Organization of the cerebral cortex III. A study of aging in the human cerebral cortex. *J. Comp. Neurol.* 102: 511-56, 1955.
155. Brook, C.G.D., J.K. Lloyd & O.H. Wolf. Relationship between age of onset of obesity and size and number of adipose cells. *Brit. Med. J.* (ii): 25-7, 1972.
156. Brooks, A.L., D.K. Mead & R.F. Peters. Effect of aging on the frequency of metaphase chromosome aberrations in the liver of the Chinese hamster. *J. Gerontol.* 28: 452-4, 1973.
157. Brown, J.R. & G.P. Crowden. Energy expenditure ranges and muscular work grades. *Brit. J. Indust. Med.* 20: 277-83, 1963.
158. Brown, J.R. & R.J. Shephard. Some measurements of fitness in older female employees of a Toronto department store. *Canad. Med. Ass. J.* 97: 1208-13, 1967.
159. Bruce, R.A. Evaluation of functional capacity in patients with cardiovascular disease. *Geriatrics* 12: 317-28, 1957.
160. Bruce, R.A. Comparative prevalence of segmental ST depression after maximal exercise in healthy men in Seattle and Taipei. In *Physical activity and the heart,* ed. M.J. Karvonen & A.J. Barry, pp. 144-58. Springfield, Ill.: C.C. Thomas, 1967.
161. Bruce, R.A., E.R. Alexander, Y.B. Li, N. Chiang & T.R. Hornsten. Electrocardiographic responses to maximal exercise in American and Chinese population samples. In *Measurement in exercise electrocardiography,* ed. H. Blackburn, pp. 413-44. Springfield, Illinois: C.C. Thomas, 1969.
162. Brundin, A. Physical training in severe chronic obstructive lung disease. 1. Clinical course, physical working capacity and ventilation. 2. Observations on gas exchange. *Scand. J. Resp. Dis.* 55: 25-36, 37-46, 1975.
163. Brunner, B.C. Personality and motivating factors influencing adult participation in vigorous physical activity. *Res. Quart.* 40: 464-9, 1969.
164. Brunner, D. Active exercise for coronary patients. *Rehab. Rec.* 9: 29-31, 1968.
165. Brunnstrom, S. *Movement therapy in hemiplegia in a neurophysiological approach.* New York: Harper & Row, 1971.
166. Büchi, E.C. Änderung der Korperform beim erwachsenen Menschen. Eine Untersuchung nach der Individual-Methode. *Anthropol. Forsch.* 1: 1-44, 1950.
167. Buckler, J.M. The effect of age, sex and exercise on the secretion of growth hormone. *Clin. Sci.* 37: 765-74, 1969.
168. Buist, A.S. & B.B. Ross. Predicted values for closing volumes using a modified single breath nitrogen test. *Amer. Rev. Resp. Dis.* 107: 744-52, 1973.
169. Burch, G.E., A.E. Cohn & C. Neumann. A study of the rate of water loss from the surfaces of the finger tips and toe tips of normal and senile subjects and patients with arterial hypertension. *Amer. Heart J.* 23: 185-96, 1942.
170. Burch, G. & C. Collot. *Elderly people in their towns.* Paris: Int. Centre of Social Gerontology, 1972.

171.   Burch, P.R.J. Auto-immunity; some aetiological aspects. *Lancet* i: 1253-7, 1963.

172.   Burnet, F.M. *Clonal selection.* London: Croonian Lecture, Royal College of Physicians, 1959.

173.   Burr, H.T. *Psychological functioning of older people.* Springfield, Ill.: C.C. Thomas, 1971.

174.   Burry, H.C. Soft tissue injury. *Exercise & Sport Sci. Rev.* 3: 275-301, 1975.

175.   Burton, B.T. *Human nutrition,* 3rd ed. New York: McGraw-Hill, 1976.

176.   Buskirk, E.R., D. Harris, J. Mendez & J. Skinner. Comparison of two assessments of physical activity and a survey method for caloric intake. *Amer. J. Clin. Nutr.* 24: 1119-25, 1971.

177.   Busse, E.W. & E. Pfeiffer. Functional psychiatric disorders in old age. In *Behaviour and adaptation in late life,* ed. E.W. Busse & E. Pfeiffer, Boston: Little, Brown, 1969.

178.   Buzina, R.A., A. Keys, I. Mohacek, M. Marinkovic, A. Hahn & H. Blackburn. Coronary heart disease in seven countries. V. Five year follow-up in Dalmatia and Slavonia. *Circulation.* 41: Suppl. 1: 40-51, 1970.

179.   Caird, F.I. (1972). Cited by W.F. Anderson. Preventive medicine in old age. In *Textbook of geriatric medicine & gerontology,* ed. J.C. Brocklehurst, pp. 718-26. Edinburgh: Churchill-Livingstone, 1973.

180.   Caird, F.I., G.R. Andrews & R.D. Kennedy. Effect of posture on blood pressure in the elderly. *British Heart J.* 35: 527-30, 1973.

181.   Caird, F.L. Cited by Fitzgerald, M.G. Diabetes. In *Textbook of geriatric medicine and gerontology,* ed. J.C. Brocklehurst, pp. 458-75. Edinburgh: Churchill-Livingstone, 1973.

182.   Calloway, N.O. A general theory of senescence. *J. Amer. Geriatr. Soc.* 12: 856-62, 1964.

183.   Campbell, R.H.A., H.L. Brand, J.R. Cox & P. Howard. Body weight and body water in chronic cor pulmonale. *Clin. Sci. Mol. Biol.* 49: 323-35, 1975.

184.   Carrel, A. On the permanent life of tissues outside the organism. *J. Exp. Med.* 15: 516-28, 1912.

185.   Carswell, S. Changes in aerobic power in patients undergoing elective surgery. *J. Physiol.* 251: 42-3P, 1975.

186.   Carter, J.E.L. The somatotype of athletes – a review. *Human Biol.* 42: 535-9, 1970.

187.   Cartlidge, N.E.F., M.M. Black, M.R.P. Hall & R. Hall. Pituitary function in the elderly. *Geront. Clin.* 12: 65-70, 1970.

188.   Cattell, R.B. Theory of fluid and crystallized intelligence; a critical experiment. *J. Educ. Psychol.* 54: 127-36, 1963.

189.   Chapman, E.A., H.A. DeVries & R. Swezey. Joint stiffness: effects of exercise on young and old men. *J. Gerontol.* 27: 218-21, 1972.

190.   Charlesworth, D. & R.H. Baker. Surgery in old age. In *Textbook of geriatric medicine & gerontology,* ed. J.C. Brocklehurst, pp. 656-7. Edinburgh: Churchill-Livingstone, 1973.

191.   Charlton, J.M. & R. Van Heyningen. An investigation into the loss of proteins of low molecular size from the lens in senile cataract. *Exp. Eye Res.* 7. 47-55, 1968.

192.   Cheraskin, E. & W.M. Ringsdorf. Predictive medicine. X. Physical activity. *J. Amer. Geriatric Soc.* 19: 969-73, 1971.

193.   Cheraskin, E. & W.M. Rinsgdorf. *Predictive medicine. A study in strategy.* California: Pacific Press Publishing Ass., 1973.

194.   Chiang, B.N., H.J. Montoye & D.A. Cunningham. Treadmill exercise – study of healthy males in a total community – Tecumseh, Michigan: Clinical

and electrocardiographic characteristics. *Amer. J. Epidemiol.* 91: 368-77, 1970.
195.   Choquette, G. & R. Ferguson. Blood pressure reduction in 'borderline' hypertensives following physical training. *Canad. Med. Assoc. J.* 108: 699-793, 1973.
196.   Chown, I. Adaptability to technological change. Cited by Roth, M. In *Mental health problems of ageing and the aged with some comments on the role of World Health and other International Organizations.* International Labour Office 1962. Report of the Director General: Part I. Old People — work and retirement. Geneva: Int. Labour Office, 1962.
197.   Chrastek, J. & J. Adimirova. Höher Blütdruck und Korperliche Ubungen. *Sportarzt und Sportmedizin* 3: 61-6, 1970.
198.   Christie, D. Physical training in chronic obstructive lung disease. *Brit. Med. J.* 5598: 150-1, 1968.
199.   Christie, S.B.M., N. Conway & H.E.S. Pearson. Observations on the performance of standard exercise test by claudicants taking γ-linoleic acid. *J. Atherosclerosis Res.* 8: 83-90, 1968.
200.   Chung, E.B. Ageing in human joints. I. Articular cartilage. *J. Nat. Med. Ass.* 58: (2), 87, 1966a.
201.   Chung, E.B. Ageing in human joints. II. Joint capsule. *J. Nat. Med. Ass.* 58: (4), 254-60, 1966b.
202.   Citizens Board of Inquiry into Hunger and Malnutrition in the United States. (W.P. Reuther, Chairman). *Hunger USA,* pp. 1-100. Washington D.C.: Citizens Crusade Against Poverty, 1968.
203.   Clarke, S.W. Letter to the Editor. *Lancet* i: 369, 1973.
204.   Clarke-Williams, M.J. The management of aged amputees. In *Textbook of geriatric medicine & gerontology,* ed. J.C. Brocklehurst, pp. 524-7. Edinburgh: Churchill-Livingstone, 1973.
205.   Clausen, J.P. Effects of physical conditioning. *Scand. J. Clin. Lab. Invest.* 24. 305-13, 1969.
206.   Clausen, J.P. Muscle blood flow during exercise and its significance for maximal performance. In *Limiting factors of physical performance,* ed. J. Keul. Stuttgart: Georg Thieme, 1973.
207.   Clausen, J.P., K. Klausen, B. Rasmussen & J. Trap-Jensen. Central and peripheral circulatory changes after training of the arms and legs. *Amer. J. Physiol.* 225: 665-82, 1973.
208.   Clausen, J.P. & N.A. Lassen. Muscle blood flow during exercise in normal men studied by the Xe^{133} clearance method. *Cardiovasc. Res.* 5: 245-54, 1971.
209.   Cochrane, A.L. The detection of pulmonary tuberculosis in a community. *Brit. Med. Bull.* 10: 91-8, 1954.
210.   Cohn, J.E., D.G. Carroll, B.W. Armstrong, R.H. Shepard & R.L. Riley. Maximal diffusing capacity of the lung in normal male subjects of different ages. *J. Appl. Physiol.* 6: 588, 1954.
211.   Cohn, J.E. & H.D. Donoso. Mechanical properties of lung in normal men over 60 years old. *J. Clin. Invest.* 42: 1406-10, 1963.
212.   Cole, T.J. The influence of height on the decline in ventilatory function. *Int. J. Epidemiol.* 3: 145-52, 1974.
213.   Coleman, A.E., C.L. Burford & P. Kreuzer. Aerobic capacity of relatively sedentary males. *J. Occup. Med.* 15: 628-32, 1973.
214.   Colin, W., S. Degré, R. Messin, P. Vandermoten & H. Denolin. Evolution de quelques grandeurs respiratoires et circulatoires au cours du travail professionel chez des patients atteints de pneumopathies chroniques. *Int. Z. für angew. Physiol.* 30: 142-50, 1972.
215.   Comfort, A. *Ageing. The biology of senescence,* 2nd ed. New York:

Holt, Rinehart & Winston, 1964.

216. Comfort, A. Test-battery to measure ageing rate in man. *Lancet,* ii: 411-14, 1969.

217. Comfort, A. Theories of aging. In *Textbook of geriatric medicine & gerontology,* ed. J.C. Brocklehurst. Edinburgh: Churchill-Livingstone, 1973.

218. Commoner, B., J.J. Heise, B.B. Lippincot, R.E. Norberg, J.V. Passoneau & J. Townsend. Biological activity of free radicals. *Science* 126: 57-63, 1957.

219. Consolazio, C.F., L.O. Matoush, H.L. Johnson, H.J. Krzywicki, G.T. Isaac & N.F. Witt. Metabolic aspects of calorie restriction: nitrogen and mineral balances and vitamin excretion. *Amer. J. Clin. Nutr.* 21: 803-12, 1968.

220. Cooper, K.H. A means of assessing maximal oxygen intake. *J. Amer. Med. Ass.* 203: 201-14, 1968a.

221. Cooper, K.H. *Aerobics,* pp. 1-253. New York: Evans, 1968b.

222. Cooper, L., J. O'Sullivan & E. Hughes. Athletics and the heart: an electrocardiographic and radiological study of the response of the healthy and diseased heart to exercise. *Med. J. Austral.* 1: 569-79, 1937.

223. Corcoran, P.J. Energy expenditure during ambulation. In *Physiological basis of rehabilitation medicine,* ed. J.A. Downey & R.C. Darling. Philadelphia: Saunders, 1971.

224. Corcoran, P.J. & G.L. Brengelmann. Oxygen uptake in normal and handicapped subjects in relation to speed of walking beside a velocity controlled cart. *Arch. Phys. Med. Rehab.* 51: 78-87, 1970.

225. Corcoran, P.J., R.H. Jebsen, G.L. Brengelmann & B.C. Simons. Effects of plastic and metal leg braces on speed and energy cost of hemi-paretic ambulation. *Arch. Phys. Med. Rehab.* 51: 69-77, 1970.

226. Coronary Drug Research Group. Prognostic importance of premature beats following myocardial infarction. Experience in the coronary drug project. *J. Amer. Med. Assoc.* 223: 1116-24, 1973.

227. Costello, T.Y. Subclinical adenoma of the pituitary gland. *Amer. J. Path.* 12: 205-15, 1936.

228. Costill, D.L., G.E. Branam, J.C. Moore, K. Sparks & C. Turner. Effects of physical training in men with coronary heart disease. *Med. Sci. Sports* 6: 95-100, 1974.

229. Cotes, J.E. *Lung function. Assessment and application in medicine.* Oxford: Blackwell Scientific, 1965.

230. Cotes, J.E. & J.C. Gilson. The effect of oxygen on exercise ability in chronic respiratory insufficiency. Use of portable apparatus. *Lancet* 6928: 872-9, 1956.

231. Cotes, J.E., A.M. Hall, G.R. Johnson, P.R.M. Jones & A.V. Knibbs. Decline with age of cardiac frequency during submaximal exercise on healthy women. *J. Physiol.* 238: 24-45P, 1973.

232. Court-Brown, W.M. & R. Doll. Expectation of life and mortality from cancer among British radiologists. *Brit. Med. J.* ii: 181-9, 1958.

233. Cumming, E. & W.E. Henry. *Growing old: The process of disengagement.* New York: Basic Books, 1961.

234. Cumming, G.R. Current levels of fitness. In Proc. International Symposium on Physical Activity and Cardiovascular Health. *Canad. Med. Ass. J.* 96: 868-82, 1967.

235. Cumming, G.R. Yield of ischaemic exercise electrocardiograms in relation to exercise intensity in a normal population. *Brit. Heart J.* 34: 919-23, 1972.

236. Cumming, G.R. Exercise e.c.g. tests prior to exercise programs in well persons. *Canad. J. Appl. Sports Sci.* 1: 205-9, 1976.

237. Cumming, G.R. & L.M. Borysyk. Criteria for maximum oxygen intake

in men over 40 in a population survey. *Med. Sci. Sports* 4: 18-22, 1972.

238. Cumming, G.R., L.M. Borysyk & C. Dufresne. The maximal exercise ECG in asymptomatic men. *Canad. Med. Ass. J.* 106: 649-53, 1972.

239. Cumming, G.R., C. Dufresne & J. Samm. Exercise e.c.g. changes in normal women. *Canad. Med. Ass. J.* 109: 108-11, 1973a.

240. Cumming, G.R., C. Dufresne, L. Kich & J. Samm. Exercise electrocardiogram patterns in normal women. *Brit. Heart J.* 35: 1055-66, 1973b.

241. Cumming, G.R., D. Goulding & G. Baggley. Working capacity of deaf and visually and mentally handicapped children. *Arch. Dis. Childh.* 46: 490-4, 1971.

242. Cumming, G. & S.G. Semple. *Disorders of the respiratory system.* Oxford: Blackwell, 1973.

243. Cunningham, D.A. & J.S. Hill. Effect of training on cardiovascular response to exercise in women. *J. Appl. Physiol.* 39: 891-5, 1975.

244. Cunningham, D.A., H.J. Montoye, H.L. Metzner & J.B. Keller. Active leisure time activities as related to age among males in a total population. *J. Gerontol.* 23: 551-6, 1968.

245. Cunningham, D.A., H.J. Montoye, H.L. Metzner & J.B. Keller. Physical activity at work and active leisure as related to occupation. *Med. Sci. Sports* 1: 165-70, 1969.

246. Dalderup, L., V.A. Opdam-Stockmann & H. Rechsteiner-de Vos. Basal metabolic rate, anthropometric, electrocardiographic & dietary data relating to elderly persons. *J. Gerontol.* 21: 22-6, 1966.

247. Daly, J.W., A.J. Barry & N.C. Birkhead. The physical working capacity of older individuals. *J. Gerontol.* 23: 134-9, 1968.

248. Daly, M.B. & H.A. Tyroler. Cornell Medical Index response as a predictor of mortality. *Brit. J. Prev. Soc. Med.* 26: 159-64, 1972.

249. Damon, A., S.T. Damon, H. Harpending & W.B. Kannel. Predicting coronary heart disease from body measurements of Framingham males. *J. Chron. Dis.* 21: 781-804, 1969.

250. Damon, A., C.C. Seltzer, H.W. Stoudt & B. Bell. Age and physique in healthy white veterans at Boston. *J. Gerontol.* 27: 202-8, 1972.

251. Danowski, T.S., C.T. Tsai, C.R. Morgan, J.C. Sieracki, R.A. Alley, T.J. Robbins, G. Sabeh & J.H. Sunder. Serum growth hormone and insulin in females without glucose intolerance. *Metabolism* 18: 811-20, 1969.

252. Das, B.C. An examination of variability of blood chemistry, hematology and proteins in relation to age. *Gerontologia* 15: 275-87, 1969.

253. Dasco, M.M., A.K. Luczak, A. Hass & H.A. Rusk. Bracing and rehabilitation training: effect on the energy expenditure of the elderly hemiplegic: preliminary report. *Post Grad. Med.* 34: 42-7, 1963.

254. Davidson, S., R. Passmore & J.F. Brock. *Human nutrition and dietetics,* 5th ed. Edinburgh: Churchill-Livingstone, 1972.

255. Davies, C.T.M. Limitations to the prediction of maximum oxygen intake from cardiac frequency measurements. *J. Appl. Physiol.* 24: 700-6, 1968.

256. Davies, C.T.M. The oxygen transporting system in relation to age. *Clin. Sci.* 42: 1-13, 1972.

257. Davies, C.T.M. & A.V. Knibbs. The training stimulus: the effects of intensity, duration and frequency of effort on maximum aerobic power output. *Int. Z. angew. Physiol.* 29: 299-305, 1971.

258. Davies, C.T.M., W. Tuxworth & J.M. Young. Physiological effects of repeated exercise. *Clin. Sci.* 39: 247-58, 1970.

259. Davies, D.R. & S. Griew. Age and vigilance. In *Behaviour, aging and the nervous system,* ed. A.T. Welford & J.E. Birren, pp. 54-9. Springfield, Ill.: C.C. Thomas, 1965.

260.   Davison, W. Anaemia in the elderly with special reference to iron deficiency. *Geront. Clin.* 9: 393-400, 1967.

261.   Dawber, T.R., F.E. Moore & G.V. Mann. Coronary heart disease in the Framingham study. *Amer. J. Publ. Health.* 47: 4-64, 1957.

262.   Dayton, S., S.D. Hashimoto, W.J. Dixon & W. Tomiyasu. A controlled clinical trial of a diet high in unsaturated fat in preventing complications of athero-sclerosis. *Circulation* 40: Suppl. II: 1-63, 1969.

263.   Degré, S., R. Sergysels, R. Messin, P. Vandermoten, P. Salhadin, H. Denolin & A. de Coster. Hemodynamic response to physical training in patients with chronic lung disease. *Amer. Rev. Resp. Dis.* 110: 395-402, 1974.

264.   Degnbol, B. & A.G. Hansen. Prevalence of diabetes mellitus among near relatives to 187 probands with early onset diabetes. *Nordic Council Arct. Med. Res. Rep.* 15: 16-18, 1976.

265.   Dehn, M.M. & R.A. Bruce. Longitudinal variations in maximal oxygen intake with age and activity. *J. Appl. Physiol.* 33: 805-7, 1972.

266.   Delhez, L., A. Botton-Thonon & J.M. Petit. Influence de l'entrainment sur la force maximum des muscles respiratoires. *Societé Medicale Belgique d'Education Physique* 20: 52-63, 1967.

267.   Dempsey, J.A., W. Reddan, J. Rankin & B. Balke. Alveolar-arterial gas exchange during muscular work in obesity. *J. Appl. Physiol.* 21: 1807-14, 1966.

268.   Denolin, H., R. Messin, S. Degré, P. Vandermoten & A. de Coster. Influence of age on the behaviour of normal subjects during exercise. In *Physical activity and aging*, ed. D. Brunner & E. Jokl, pp. 309-15. Basel: Karger, 1970.

269.   Department of Health & Social Security (DHSS). First report by the panel on nutrition of the elderly. *Reports on public health & medical subjects,* 123. London: HMSO, 1970.

270.   Department of Health and Social Security (UK). Recommended intakes of nutrients for the United Kingdom. *Report on public health & medical subjects,* 120. London: HMSO, 1969.

271.   Department of Health and Social Security (UK). Nutrition survey of the elderly. *Report on public health & medical subjects,* 3. London: HMSO, 1972.

272.   Deroanne, R., J.M. Petit, A. Salmon & P. Hereng. Influence de la réadaptation au travail sur l'aptitude physique de handicapés pulmonaires et de chomeurs handicapés. *Acta tuberc. Pneumol. Belg.* 60: 66-78, 1969.

273.   Detry, J.M. & R.A. Bruce. Effects of physical training on exertional ST segment depression in coronary heart disease. *Circulation* 44: 390-6, 1971.

274.   Devlin, J. The effect of training and acute physical exercise on plasma insulin-like activity. *Irish J. Med. Sci.* 6: 423-5, 1963.

275.   DeVries, H.A. Physiological effects of an exercise training regimen upon men aged 52 to 88. *J. Gerontol.* 25: 325-36, 1970.

276.   DeVries, H.A. Exercise intensity threshold for improvement of cardio-vascular-respiratory function in older men. *Geriatrics* 26: 94-101, 1971.

277.   DeVries, H.A. & G.M. Adams. Comparison of exercise responses in old and young men. I. The cardiac effort/total body effort relationship. *J. Gerontol.* 27: 344-8, 1972a.

278.   DeVries, H.A. & G.M. Adams. Comparison of exercise responses in old and young men. II. Ventilatory mechanics. *J. Gerontol.* 27: 349-52, 1972b.

279.   Dickinson, R.L. & L.E. Beam. *A thousand marriages.* Baltimore: Williams & Wilkins, 1931.

280.   Dill, D.B., S. Robinson & J.C. Ross. A longtitudinal study of 16 champion runners. *J. Sports Med.* 7: 4-32, 1967.

281.   DiPrampero, P.E. Anaerobic capacity and power. In *Frontiers of Fitness,* ed. R.J. Shephard. Springfield, Ill.: C.C. Thomas, 1971.

282.   Doan, A.E., D.R. Peterson, J.R. Blackmon & R.A. Bruce. Myocardial

ischemia after maximal exercise in healthy men. *Amer. Heart J.* 69: 11-21, 1965.
283.   Döbeln, W. von, I. Åstrand & Å. Bergström. An analysis of age and other factors related to maximal oxygen uptake. *J. Appl. Physiol.* 22: 934-8, 1967.
284.   Dock, W. How some hearts age. *J. Amer. Med. Assoc.* 195: 442-4, 1966.
285.   Donevan, R.E., W.H. Palmer, C.J. Varvis & D.V. Bates. Influence of age on pulmonary diffusing capacity. *J. Appl. Physiol.* 14: 483-92, 1955.
286.   Dormandy, J.A., E. Hoare, A.H. Khattab, D.E. Arrowsmith & T.L. Dormandy. Prognostic significance of rheological and biochemical findings in patients with intermittent claudication. *Brit. Med. J.* (iv): 581-3, 1973.
287.   Dotter, C.T. & I. Steinberg. The angiocardiographic measurement of the great vessels. *Radiology* 52: 353-7, 1949.
288.   Draper, H.H. Nutritional research in circumpolar populations. In *Circumpolar health*, ed. R.J. Shephard & S. Itoh. Toronto: University of Toronto Press, 1976.
289.   Dublin, L.I. Longevity of college athletes. *Harper* 157: 229-38, 1928.
290.   Dublin, L.I. College honor men long-lived. *Statistical Bulletin of the Metropolitan Life Insurance Company.* 13: 5-7, 1932.
291.   Dublin, L.I., A.J. Lotka & M. Spiegelman. *Length of life, a study of the life table*, chapter 6. New York: Ronald Press, 1949.
292.   Dubois, E.F. *Basal metabolism in health and disease.* Philadelphia: Lea & Febiger, 1927.
293.   Durnin, J.V.G.A. The dietary intake of the elderly. In *Current achievements in geriatrics*, ed. W.F. Anderson & B. Isaacs, pp. 41-6. London: Cassel, 1964.
294.   Durnin, J.V.G.A. Age, physical activity and energy expenditure. *Proc. Nutr. Sci.* 25: 107-13, 1966.
295.   Durnin, J.V.G.A. Activity patterns in the community. In Proc. of International Symposium on Physical Activity and Cardiovascular Health. *Canad. Med. Ass. J.* 96: 882-6, 1967.
296.   Durnin, J.V.G.A. Energy expenditure in relation to age, sex, body weight and physical activity. *Excerpta Med. Internat. Congress Series* #213. Proc. 8th Internat. Cong. Nutr., Prague: 1969.
297.   Durnin, J.V.G.A. The regulation of energy balance. *Brit. J. Hosp. Med.* (May) 5: 649-64, 1971.
298.   Durnin, J.V.G.A. Nutrition. In *Textbook of geriatric medicine and gerontology.* ed. J.C. Brocklehurst, pp. 384-404. Edinburgh: Churchill-Livingstone, 1973.
299.   Durnin, J.V.G.A., E.C. Blake, M.K. Allan, E.J. Shaw & S. Blair. Food intake and energy expenditure of elderly women with varying size families. *J. Nutr.* 75: 73-6, 1961a.
300.   Durnin, J.V.G.A., E.C. Blake, M.K. Allan, E.J. Shaw, E.A. Wilson, S. Blair & S.A. Yuill. The food intake and energy expenditure of some elderly men working in heavy and light engineering. *Brit. J. Nutr.* 15: 587-91, 1961b.
301.   Durnin, J.V.G.A., E.C. Blake & J.M. Brockway. The energy expenditure and food intake of middle-aged Glasgow housewives and their adult daughters. *Brit. J. Nutr.* 11: 85-94, 1960.
302.   Durnin, J.V.G.A., E.C. Blake, J.M. Brockway & E.A. Drury. The food intake and energy expenditure of elderly women living alone. *Brit. J. Nutr.* 15: 499-506, 1961c.
303.   Durnin, J.V.G.A., J.M. Brockway & H.N. Whitcher. Effects of a short period of training of varying severity on some measurements of physical fitness. *J. Appl. Physiol.* 15: 161-5, 1960.

304. Durnin, J.V.G.A. & V. Mikulic. Influence of graded exercises on the oxygen consumption, pulmonary ventilation and heart rate of young and elderly men. *Quart. J. Exp. Physiol.* 41: 442-52, 1956.

305. Durnin, J.V.G.A. & R. Passmore. *Energy, work and leisure.* London: Heinemann, 1967.

306. Durnin, J.V.G.A. & M.M. Rahaman. The assessment of the amount of fat in the human body from measurements of skinfold thickness. *Brit. J. Nutr.* 21: 681-9, 1967.

307. Durnin, J.V.G.A. & J. Womersley. Body fat assessed from total body density and its estimation from skinfold thickness: measurements on 481 men and women aged from 16-72 years. *Brit. J. Nutr.* 32: 77-97, 1974.

308. Durusoy, F.P., E.J. Klaus, D. Clasing & W. Niemann. Herz-kreislauf-untersuchungen bei 68 über 60 jährigen altersturnern in ruhe. *Sportarzt und Sportmedizin* 19: 443-6, 1968.

309. Eckstein, R.W. Effect of exercise and coronary artery narrowing on coronary collateral circulation. *Circulation Res.* 5: 230-5, 1957.

310. Edelman, N.H., C. Mittman, A.H. Norris & N.W. Shock. Effects of respiratory pattern on age differences in ventilation uniformity. *J. Appl. Physiol.* 24: 49-53, 1968.

311. Edge, J.R., F.J.C. Millard, L. Reid & G. Simon. The radiographic appearance of the chest in persons of advanced age. *Brit. J. Radiol.* 37: 769-74, 1964.

312. Edge, J.R. & I.D.M. Nelson. Survey of arrangements for the elderly in Barrow in Furness. *Medical Care* 2: 7-23, 1964.

313. Edington, D.W., A.C. Cosmas & W.B. McCafferty. Exercise and longevity: evidence for a threshold age. *J. Gerontol.* 27: 341-3, 1972.

314. Edington, D.W. & V.R. Edgerton. *The biology of physical activity.* Boston: Houghton Mifflin, 1976.

315. Edwards, D.A.W. Difference in the distribution of subcutaneous fat with sex and maturity. *Clin. Sci.* 10: 305-15, 1951.

316. Edwards, J.N. & D.L. Klemmack. Correlates of life satisfaction: a reexamination. *J. Gerontol.* 28: 299-502, 1973.

317. Edwards, F., T. McKeown & A.G.W. Whitfield. Incidence of disease and disability in elderly men. *Brit. J. Prev. Soc. Med.* 13: 51-8, 1959.

318. Eisdorfer, C. Intellectual and cognitive changes in the aged. In *Behaviour and adaptation in late life*, ed. E.W. Busse & E. Pfeiffer. Boston: Little Brown, 1969.

319. Ekblöm, B. Effects of physical training on oxygen transport systems in man. *Acta Physiol. Scand. Suppl.* 328: 9-45, 1969.

320. Ekblöm, B., P.O. Åstrand, B. Saltin, J. Stenberg & B. Wallstrom. Effect of training on circulatory response to exercise. *J. Appl. Physiol.* 24: 518-28, 1968.

321. Ekblöm, B. & A.N. Goldbarg. The influence of physical training and other factors on the subjective rating of perceived exertion. *Acta. Physiol. Scand.* 83: 399-406, 1971.

322. Elden, H.R. Aging in collagen. In *Perspectives in experimental gerontology*, ed. N.W. Shock. Springfield, Illinois: C.C. Thomas, 1966.

323. Eldridge, F. Blood lactate and pyruvate in pulmonary insufficiency. *New Engl. J. Med.* 274: 878-82, 1966.

324. Elgrishi, I., P. Ducimetière & J.L. Richard. Reproducibility of analysis of the electrocardiogram in epidemiology using the 'Minnesota Code'. *Brit. J. Prev. Soc. Med.* 24: 197-200, 1970.

325. Ellerstad, M.H. Stress testing – principles and practice. Philadelphia: F.A. Davis, 1975.

References 307

326. Ellerstad, M.H. Paper presented at Symposium on Coronary Rehabilitation. Toronto Rehabilitation Centre, 1975. Toronto: Toronto Rehabilitation Centre, 1977.
327. Elwood, P.C. Epidemiological aspects of iron deficiency in the elderly. *Geront. Clin.* 13: 2-11, 1971.
328. Emirgil, C., B.J. Sobol, S. Campodonico, W.H. Herbert & R. Mechkati. Pulmonary circulation in the aged. *J. Appl. Physiol.* 23: 631-40, 1967.
329. Epshtein, E.V. Effect of muscle activity on the phosphate metabolism in skeletal muscles of animals of different age. Misheihnaya deyatel' nost'i Funktsü organisma pri starenü (Muscle activity and organic functions in aging. *Kiev: Akad. Med. Nauk. SSSR*, pp. 63, 1968 (Russ.). Cited by E. Simonson, *Physiology of work capacity and fatigue.* Springfield, Ill.: C.C. Thomas, 1971.
330. Erdman, W.J., T. Hettinger & F. Saeg. Comparative work stress for above-knee amputees using artificial legs or crutches. *Amer. J. Phys. Med.* 39: 225-32, 1960.
331. Ericsson, P. Total hemoglobin and physical work capacity in elderly people. *Acta Med. Scand.* 188: 15, 1970.
332. Ericsson, P. & L. Irnell. Spirometric studies of ventilatory capacity in elderly people. *Acta Med. Scand.* 185: 179-84, 1969a.
333. Ericsson, P. & L. Irnell. Physical work capacity and static lung volumes in elderly people. *Acta Med. Scand.* 185: 185-91, 1969b.
334. Eriksson, B.O., B. Persson & J.I. Thorell. The effects of repeated prolonged exercise on plasma growth hormone, insulin, glucose, free fatty acids, glycerol, lactate and β -hydroxybutyric acid in 13 year old boys and in adults. *Acta Paediat. Scand. Suppl.* 217: 142-6, 1971.
335. Evans, D.M.D. Haematological aspects of iron deficiency in the elderly. *Geront. Clin.* 13: 12-30, 1971.
336. Evans, D.M.D., M.S. Pathy, N.G. Sanerkin & J.J. Deeble. Anaemia in geriatric patients. *Geront. Clin.* 10: 228-41, 1968.
337. Exton-Smith, A.N. Musculo-skeletal system. Bone aging and metabolic bone disease. In *Textbook of geriatric medicine & gerontology*, ed. J.C. Brocklehurst, pp. 476-91. Edinburgh: Churchill-Livingstone, 1973.
338. Exton-Smith, A.N. The problems of sub-clinical malnutrition in the elderly. In *Vitamins in the elderly*, ed. A.N. Exton-Smith & D.L. Scott. Bristol: J. Wright, 1968.
339. Exton-Smith, A.N. *Care of the elderly: meeting the challenge of dependency*, ed. A.N. Exton-Smith & J.G. Evans. London: Academic Press, 1977.
340. Exton-Smith, A.N., P.H. Millard, P.H. Payne & E.F. Wheeler. Pattern of development and loss of bone with age. *Lancet* ii: 1154-7, 1969.
341. Exton-Smith, A.N., B.R. Stanton, M. Newman & M. Ramsey. *Report on an investigation into the dietary habits of elderly women living alone.* London: King Edward's Hospital Fund, 1965.
342. Failla, G. The aging process and somatic mutations. A.I.B.S. Symposium – "The Biology of Aging". *A.I.B.S. publ.* 6: 170-5, Washington, D.C., 1960.
343. Fazekas, I.G. & G. Jobba. Beitrag zur morphologie der senilen hypophyse. *Acta Morphol. Acad. Sci. Hung.* 18: 74-89, 1970.
344. Feldman, R.M. & S.N. Roger. Relations among hearing, reaction time and age. *J. Speech Hear. Res.* 10: 479-95, 1967.
345. Filley, G.F. Pulmonary ventilation and the oxygen cost of exercise in emphysema. *Amer. Clin. Climatol. Assoc. J.* 70: 193-203, 1958.
346. Finch, C.E., J.R. Foster & A.E. Mirsky. Ageing and the regulation of cellular activities during exposure to cold. *J. Gen. Physiol.* 54: 690-712, 1969.
347. Finkle, A.L. Sexual potency in aging males. *J. Amer. Med. Assoc.*

170: 1391-3, 1959.

348. Fisch, L. Special senses: the aging auditory system. In *Textbook of geriatric medicine and gerontology*, ed. J.C. Brockiehurst, pp. 265-79. Edinburgh: Churchill-Livingstone, 1973.

349. Fischer, A., J. Parizkova & Z. Roth. The effect of systematic physical activity on maximal performance and functional capacity in senescent men. *Int. Z. angew. Physiol.* 21: 269-304, 1965.

350. Fisher, M.B. & J.E. Birren. Age and strength. *J. Appl. Psychol.* 31: 490-7, 1947.

351. Fisher, R.F. The significance of the shape of the lens and the capsular energy changes in accommodation. *J. Physiol.* 201: 21-47, 1969.

352. Fisher, R.H. The urinary excretion of 4-hydroxy 3-methoxy mandelic acid in the elderly. *Geront. Clin.* 13: 257-60, 1971.

353. Fitzgerald, M.G., J.M. Malins, D.J. O'Sullivan & M. Wall. The effect of sex & parity on the incidence of diabetes mellitus. *Quart. J. Med.* 15: 57-70, 1961.

354. Flenley, D.C., H.C. Miller, A.J. King, B.J. Kirby & A.L. Muir. Oxygen transport in acute pulmonary oedema and in acute exacerbations of chronic bronchitis. *Brit. Med. J.* 5845: 78-81, 1973.

355. Fletcher, C.M., N.L. Jones, B. Burrows & A.H. Niden. American emphysema and British bronchitis. A standardized comparative study. *Amer. Rev. Resp. Dis.* 90: 1-13, 1964.

356. Folkins, C.H., S. Lynch & M.M. Gardner. Psychological fitness as a function of physical fitness. *Arch. Phys. Med. Rehab.* 53: 503-8, 1973.

357. Forbes, G.B., J. Gallup & J.B. Hursh. Estimation of total body fat from potassium[40] content. *Science* 133: 101-2, 1961.

358. Forbes, G.B. & J.B. Hursh. Age and sex trends in lean body mass calculated from K[40] measurements with a note on the theoretical basis for the procedure. *Ann. N.Y. Acad. Sci.* 110: 255-63, 1963.

359. Forbes, G.B. & J.C. Reina. Adult lean body mass declines with age: some longitudinal observations. *Metabolism* 19: 653-63, 1970.

360. Foss, M.L., R.M. Lampman, E. Watt & D.E. Schteingart. Initial work tolerance of extremely obese patients. *Arch. Phys. Med. Rehab.* 57: 63-7, 1975.

361. Fox, R.H., R. MacGibbon, L. Davies & P.M. Woodward. Problem of the old and the cold. *Brit. Med. J.* i: 21-4, 1973.

362. Fox, S.M. & W.L. Haskell. Population studies. *Canad. Med. Ass. J.* 96: 806-11, 1967.

363. Frank, N.R., J. Mead & B.G. Ferris. The mechanical behaviour of the lungs in healthy elderly persons. *J. Clin. Invest.* 36: 1680-9, 1957.

364. Frantz, A.G. & M.T. Rabkin. Effects of estrogen and sex difference on secretion of human growth hormone. *J. Clin. Endocrinol.* 25: 1470-80, 1965.

365. Franzblau, C., F.M. Sinex & B. Faris. Chemistry and maturation of elastin. In *Perspectives in experimental gerontology*, ed. N.W. Shock. Springfield, Illinois: C.C. Thomas, 1966.

366. Freeman, E. The respiratory system. In *Textbook of geriatric medicine and gerontology*, ed. J.C. Brocklehurst, pp. 405-25. Edinburgh: Churchill-Livingstone, 1973.

367. Frenkl, R., L. Csalay & G. Csakvary. A study of the stress reaction elicited by muscular exertion in trained and untrained man and rats. *Acta Physiol. Sci. Hung.* 36: 365-70, 1969.

368. Frick, M.H., A. Konttinen & S.H.S. Sarajas. Effects of physical training on circulation at rest and during exercise. *Amer. J. Cardiol.* 12: 142-7, 1963.

369. Fried, T. & R.J. Shephard. Deterioration and restoration of physical fitness after training. *Canad. Med. Assoc. J.* 100: 831-7, 1969.

370. Fried, T. & R.J. Shephard. Assessment of a lower extremity training programme. *Canad. Med. Assoc. J.* 103: 260-6, 1970.

371. Friedman, M., R.H. Rosenman & A.E. Brown. The continuous heart rate in men exhibiting an overt behavior pattern associated with increased incidence of clinical coronary artery disease. *Circulation* 28: 861-8, 1963.

372. Friedsam, H.J. & H.W. Martin. A comparison of self and physicians' health ratings in an older population. *J. Health Social Behavior* 4: 179-83, 1963.

373. Friis-Hansen, B. Hydrometry of growth and aging. In *Human body composition. Approaches and applications. Symposia of the society for the study of human biology*, ed. J. Brozek, vol. 7, pp. 191-209. Oxford: Pergamon Press, 1965.

374. Frisch, R. & R. Revelle. Variation in body weights and the age of the adolescent growth spurt among Latin American populations in relation to calorie supplies. *Human Biol.* 41: 185-212, 1969.

375. Frolkis, V.V. Regulatory processes in the mechanism of aging. *Exp. Gerontol.* 3: 113-23, 1968.

376. Fry, P., L.R. Harkness & R.D. Harkness. Mechanical properties of the collagenous framework of skin in rats of different ages. *Amer. J. Physiol.* 206: 1425-9, 1964.

377. Fukui, T. & T. Morioka. The blink method as an assessment of fatigue. In *Methodology in human fatigue assessment*, ed. K. Hashimoto, K. Kogi & E. Grandjean. London: Taylor & Francis, 1971.

378. Fulgraff, B. Possible substitutes for work as the productive activity decreases (in the case of flexible retirement). In *Work & aging*, ed. J. Huet. Paris: International Centre of Social Gerontology, 1971.

379. Gabbato, F & A. Media. Analysis of the factors that may influence the duration of isotonic systole in normal conditions. *Cardiologia* 29: 114-31, 1956.

380. Gabriel, S.K. Respiratory and circulatory investigations in obstructive and restrictive lung disease. *Acta Med. Scand. Suppl.* 546: 1-91, 1972.

381. Galton, J.D. (1884). *Age and strength*. Cited by Fisher & Birren, 1947.

382. Galton, D.J. & J.P. Wilson. Glycolytic enzymes in adipose tissue of adult diabetics. *Brit. Med. J.* (iii): 444-5, 1970.

383. Gardiner, E. Reflex muscular responses to stimulation of articular nerves in the cat. *Amer. J. Physiol.* 161: 133-41, 1950.

384. Garn, S.M. Bone loss and aging. In *The physiology and pathology of aging*, ed. R. Goldman & M. Rockstein. New York: Academic Press, 1975.

385. Gershon, H. & D. Gershon. Detection of inactive enzyme molecules in ageing organisms. *Nature (Lond.)* 227: 1214-17, 1970.

386. Gershon-Cohn, I., H. Schraer & N. Blumberg. Bone density measurements of osteoporosis in the aged. *Radiology* 65: 416-19, 1955.

387. Getchell, L.H. & J.C. Moore. Physical training: comparative responses of middle-aged adults. *Arch. Phys. Med. Rehabil.* 56: 250-4, 1975.

388. Gillespie, J.A. Future place of lumbar sympathectomy in obliterative vascular disease of lower limbs. *Brit. Med. J.* ii: 1640-2, 1960.

389. Gillet, M.C., W.P. Morgan & B. Balke. Influence of acute physical activity on state anxiety. Cited by W.P. Morgan (1973).

390. Gillum, H.L. & A.F. Morgan. Nutritional status of the ageing. *J. Nutr.* 55: 265-88, 1955.

391. Gillum, H.L., A.F. Morgan & D.W. Jerome. Nutritional status of the ageing. *J. Nutr.* 55: 449-68, 1955a.

392. Gillum, H.L., A.F. Morgan & F. Sailer, Nutritional status of the ageing. *J. Nutr.* 55: 655-70, 1955b.

393. Gillum, H.L., A.F. Morgan & R.I. Williams. Nutritional status of the ageing. *J. Nutr.* 55: 289-303, 1955c.

394. Girandola, R.N. Body composition changes in women: effects of high and low exercise intensity. *Arch. Phys. Med. Rehab.* 57: 297-300, 1976.

395. Girdwood, R.H., A.D. Thomson & J. Williamson. Folate status in the elderly. *Brit. Med. J.* ii: 670-72, 1967.

396. Glagov, S., D.A. Rowley, D.B. Gramer & R.G. Page. Heart rates during 24 hours of usual activity for 100 normal men. *J. Appl. Physiol.* 29: 799-805, 1970.

397. Glaser, R.M., R.E. Young & A.G. Suryaprasad. Reducing cost and cardiopulmonary stresses during wheelchair activity. *Fed. Proc.* 36: 580, 1977.

398. Glendy, R.E., S.A. Levine & P.D. White. Coronary disease in youth. *J. Amer. Med. Assoc.* 109: 1775-81, 1937.

399. Glick, S.M., J. Roth, R.S. Yalow & S.A. Berson. The regulation of growth hormone secretion. *Rec. Progr. Horm. Res.* 21: 241-83, 1965.

400. Goldbarg, A.N., J.F. Moran, R.W. Childers & H.T. Ricketts. Results and correlations of multistage exercise tests in a group of clinically normal business executives. *Amer. Heart J.* 79: 194-200, 1970.

401. Goldberg, A.L. Work-induced growth of skeletal muscle in normal and hypophysectomized rats. *Amer. J. Physiol.* 213: 1193-8, 1967.

402. Goldberg, A.L. & H.M. Goodman. Relationship between growth hormone and muscular work in determining muscle size. *J. Physiol.* 200: 655-66, 1967.

403. Goldberg, M.E., A. Mortimer, M. Speak & B. Williams. *Helping the aged: a field experiment in social work.* London: Allen & Unwin, 1970.

404. Goldie, I. Epicondylitis lateralis humeri. *Acta Chir. Scand. Suppl.* 339: 7-114, 1964.

405. Goldman, H.I. & M.R. Becklake. Respiratory function tests. Normal values at median altitudes and the prediction of normal results. *Amer. Rev. Resp. Dis.* 79: 475, 1959.

406. Goldsmith, R. & T. Hale. Relationship between habitual physical activity and physical fitness. *Amer. J. Clin. Nutr.* 24: 1489-93, 1971.

407. Gollnick, P.D. & L. Hermansen. Biochemical adaptions to exercise: anaerobic metabolism. In *Exercise & sport science reviews,* ed. J.H. Wilmore, vol. 1, p. 1. New York: Academic Press, 1973.

408. Gompertz, B. On the nature of the function expressive of the law of human mortality and a new mode of determining the value of life contingencies. *Philosoph. Trans. R. Soc., London., A.* 115: 513-85, 1825.

409. Goode, R.C., J.B. Firstbrook & R.J. Shephard. Effects of exercise and a cholesterol-free diet on human serum lipids. *Canad. J. Physiol. Pharm.* 44: 575-80, 1966.

410. Gordon, E.E. Physiological approach to ambulation in paraplegia. *J. Amer. Med. Assoc.* 161: 686-8, 1956.

411. Gordon, E.E. & K.H. Kohn. Evaluation of rehabilitation methods in the hemiplegic patient. *J. Chron. Dis.* 19: 3-16, 1966.

412. Gordon, E.S. & M. Goldberg. Studies of energy metabolism compounds. I. Effect of sex, state of nutrition and body weight. *Metabolism* 13: 775-90, 1964.

413. Gordon, P. Free radicals and the aging process. In *Theoretical aspects of aging,* ed. M. Rockstein. New York: Academic Press, 1974.

414. Grahame, R. Diseases of the joints. In *Textbook of geriatric medicine & gerontology,* ed. J.C. Brocklehurst. Edinburgh: Churchill-Livingstone, 1973.

415. Granath, A., B. Jonsson & T. Strandell. Studies on the central circulation. Studies by right heart catheterization at rest and during exercise in supine and sitting positions in older men. *Acta Med. Scand.* 169: 125-6, 1961.

416. Granath, A., B. Johnson & T. Strandell. Circulation in healthy old men

studied by right heart catheterization at rest and during exercise in supine and sitting position. *Acta Med. Scand.* 176: 425-46, 1964.

417.   Greene, R. A remedy for aging. *Lancet* i: 786, 1959.

418.   Greenfield, N.S. & C.H. Fellner. Resting level of physical activity in obese females. *Amer. J. Clin. Nutr.* 22: 1418-19, 1969.

419.   Greenway, J.C. & I.V. Hiscock. Mortality among Yale men. Editorial. *J. Amer. Med. Assoc.* 87: 175, 1926.

420.   Gregerman, R.L., G.W. Gaffney & N. Shock. Thyroxin turnover in euthyroid man with special reference to changes with age. *J. Clin. Invest.* 41: 2065-74, 1962.

421.   Greifenstein, F.E., R.M. King, S.S. Latch & J.H. Comroe. Pulmonary function studies in healthy men and women 50 years and older. *J. Appl. Physiol.* 4: 641-8, 1952.

422.   Griew, S. & D.R. Davies. The effect of aging on auditory vigilance performance. *J. Gerontol.* 17: 88-90, 1962.

423.   Griffiths, H.J.L., W.J. Nicholson & P. Gorman. A haematological study of 500 elderly females. *Geront. Clin.* 12: 18-32, 1970.

424.   Grimby, G., J. Bjure, M. Aurell, B. Ekstrom-Jodal, G. Tibblin & L. Wilhelmsen. Work capacity and physiologic responses to work. Men born in 1913. *Amer. J. Cardiol.* 30: 37-42, 1972.

425.   Grimby, G., N.J. Nilsson & B. Saltin. Cardiac output during sub-maximal and maximal exercise in active middle-aged athletes. *J. Appl. Physiol.* 21: 1150-6, 1966.

426.   Grimby, G. & B. Saltin. A physiological analysis of physically well-trained middle-aged and old athletes. *Acta Med. Scand.* 179: 513-26, 1966.

427.   Grimby, G. & B. Soderholm. Energy expenditure of men in different age groups during level walking and bicycle ergometry. *Scand. J. Clin. Lab. Invest.* 14: 321-8, 1962.

428.   Grimby, G. & J. Stiksa. Flow-volume curves and breathing patterns during exercise in patients with obstructive lung disease. *Scand. J. Clin. Lab. Invest.* 25: 303-13, 1970.

429.   Grodsky, G.M. & F. Benoit. Effect of massive weight reduction on insulin secretion in obese subjects. *International Diabetes Symposium,* Stockholm, 1967.

430.   Gwinup, G. Effect of exercise alone on the weight of obese women. *Arch. Int. Med.* 135: 676-80, 1975.

431.   Hall, D.A. The aging of connective tissue. *Exptl. Gerontol.* 3: 77-89, 1968.

432.   Hall, D.A. Metabolic and structural aspects of aging. In *Textbook of geriatric medicine & gerontology,* ed. J.C. Brocklehurst. Edinburgh: Churchill-Livingstone, 1973.

433.   Hall, D.A. & H. Saxl. Studies of human and tunicate cellulose and their relation to reticulin. *Proc. Roy. Soc. B* 155: 202-17, 1961.

434.   Hall, M.R.P. Hypophyso-adrenal axis. In *Textbook of geriatric medicine and gerontology,* ed. J.C. Brocklehurst, pp. 431-2. Edinburgh: Churchill-Livingstone, 1973.

435.   Hammer, W.M. A comparison of differences in manifest anxiety in university athletes and non-athletes. *J. Sports Med.* 7: 31-4, 1967.

436.   Hammett, V.B.O. Psychological changes with physical fitness training. *Canad. Med. Assoc. J.* 96: 764-9, 1967.

437.   Hammond, E.C. & L. Garfinkel. Coronary heart disease, stroke and aortic aneurysm. Factors in the etiology. *Arch. Env. Health* 19: 167-82, 1969.

438.   Hanson, J.S. & W.H. Nedde. Preliminary observations on physical training for hypertensive males. *Circ. Research.* 36/37 Suppl. I: 49-53, 1970.

439.   Hanson, J.S. & B.S. Tabakin. Carbon monoxide diffusing capacity in normal male subjects aged 20-60, during exercise. *J. Appl. Physiol.* 15: 402-4, 1960.

440.   Hanson, J.S., B.S. Tabakin & A.M. Levy. Comparative exercise cardio-respiratory performance of normal men in the third, fourth and fifth decades of life. *Circulation* 37: 345-60, 1968a.

441.   Hanson, J.S., B.S. Tabakin, A.M. Levy & W. Nedde. Long-term physical training and cardiovascular dynamics in middle-aged men. *Circulation* 38: 783-9, 1968b.

442.   Harlan, W.R., A. Graybiel, R.E. Mitchell, A. Oberman & R.K. Osborne. Serial electrocardiograms: their reliability and prognostic validity during a 24-hour period. *J. Chron. Dis.* 20: 853-67, 1967.

443.   Harris, A. *Government social survey: old people in Lewisham.* London: King Edward Hosp. Trust Fund, 1962.

444.   Harris, A.I. *Social welfare for the elderly.* London: HMSO, 1968.

445.   Harris, D.V. Physical activity history and attitudes of middle-aged men. *Med. Sci. Sports* 2: 203-8, 1970.

446.   Harris, E.A. & J.G. Thomson. The pulmonary ventilation and heart rate during exercise in healthy old age. *Clin. Sci.* 17: 349-59, 1958.

447.   Harrison, B.J. & R. Holliday. Senescence and the fidelity of protein synthesis in Drosophila. *Nature (Lond.)* 213: 990-2, 1967.

448.   Harrison, T.R., K. Dixon, R.O. Russell, P.S. Bidwai & H.N. Coleman. The relation of age to the duration of contraction, ejection and relaxation of the normal human heart. *Amer. Heart J.* 67: 189-99, 1964.

449.   Harrison, T.R. & T.J. Reeves. *Principles and problems of ischemic heart disease.* Chicago: Year Book Publishers, 1968.

450.   Hartley, L.H., G. Grimby, Å. Kilböm, N.J. Nilsson, I. Åstrand, J. Bjure, B. Ekblom & B. Saltin. Physical training in sedentary middle-aged and older men. III. Cardiac output and gas exchange at submaximal and maximal exercise. *Scand. J. Clin. Lab. Invest.* 24: 335-44, 1969.

451.   Hartley, L.H., J.W. Mason, R.P. Hogan, L.G. Jones, T.A. Kotchen, E.H. Mougey, F.E. Wherry, L.L. Pennington & P.T. Ricketts. Multiple hormonal responses to graded exercise in relation to physical training. *J. Appl. Physiol.* 33: 602-6, 1972a.

452.   Hartley, L.H., J.W. Mason, R.P. Hogan, L.G. Jones, T.A. Kotchen, E.H. Mougey, F.E. Wherry, L.L. Pennington & P.T. Ricketts. Multiple hormonal responses to prolonged exercise in relation to physical training. *J. Appl. Physiol.* 33: 607-10, 1972b.

453.   Hartley, P.H.S. & G.F. Llewellyn. The longevity of oarsmen. A study of those who rowed in the Oxford and Cambridge boat race from 1829 to 1928. *Brit. Med. J.* i: 657-62, 1939.

454.   Haskell, W. Personal communication, 1976.

455.   Hass, G.E. Elastic tissue (iii): Relation between the structure of the ageing aorta and the properties of the isolated aortic elastic tissue. *Arch. Path.* 35: 29-45, 1943.

456.   Hass, G.M. Studies of cartilage (iv). A morphological and clinical analysis of aging human costal cartilage. *Arch. Path.* 35: 275-84, 1943.

457.   Hassler, R. Extrapyramidal control of the speed of behaviour and its change by primary age processes. In *Behaviour, aging and the nervous system,* ed. A.T. Welford and J.E. Birren, pp. 67-87. Springfield, Ill.: C.C. Thomas, 1965.

458.   Hauge, M. The genetics of diabetes. *Nordic Council Arctic Med. Res. Rep.* 15: 26-8, 1976.

459.   Hayflick, L. Cytogerontology. In *Theoretical aspects of aging,* ed. M. Rockstein. New York: Academic Press, 1974.

460. Heidrick, M.L. & T. Makinodan. Nature of cellular deficiences in age-related decline of the immune system. *Gerontologia* 18: 305-20, 1972,

461. Heikkinen, E. & E. Kulonen. Age factor in the maturation of collagen. Intramolecular linkages in mildly denatured collagen. *Experientia* 20: 310-12, 1964.

462. Hedlund, S. & J.B. Pørje. Cirkulationstörningar hos äldre. Synpunkter på fysiologi och fysisk träning som terapiform. *Svenska Läk – Tidn.* 61: 2970-85, 1964.

463. Heinzelmann, F. Social and psychological factors that influence the effectiveness of exercise programs. Paper presented at 1st Canadian Congress on Sport and Physical Activity, Montreal, 1973.

464. Heinzelmann, F. & R. Baggley. Response to physical activity programs and their effects on health behavior. *Publ. Health Rep.* 85: 905-11, 1970.

465. Hellerstein, H.K. & E.H. Friedman. Sexual activity and the post-coronary patient. *Medical Aspects of Human Sexuality* 3: 70, 1969.

466. Hellon, R.F., A.R. Lind & J.S. Weiner. The physiological reactions of men of two age groups to a hot environment. *J. Physiol.* 133: 118-31, 1956.

467. Henry, F.M. Stimulus complexity, movement complexity, age and sex in relation to reaction latency and speed in limb movement. *Res. Quart.* 32: 353-66, 1961.

468. Henschel, A. Physical fitness in old age. Occupational Health Program. U.S. Public Health Service. A working paper for the Scientific Group on the Optimal Levels of Physical Performance Capacity for Adults, Geneva, Switzerland, Oct. 1968. Cited by Simonson (1971).

469. Hermansen, L., E.D.R. Pruett & F.A. Gière. Blood glucose and plasma insulin response to maximal exercise and glucose infusion. *J. Appl. Physiol.* 29. 13-16, 1970.

470. Hettinger, T.H. *Physiology of strength,* pp. 44-53. Springfield, Illinois: C.C. Thomas, 1961.

471. Hill, A.B. Cricket and its relation to the duration of life. *Lancet* (ii): 949-50, 1927.

472. Hinchcliffe, R. The threshold of hearing of a random sample rural population. *Acta Otolaryngol.* 50: 411-22, 1959a.

473. Hinchcliffe, R. Correction of pure tone audiograms for advancing age. *J. Laryng. Otol.* 73. 830-2, 1959b.

474. Hirai, M. Muscle blood flow measured by Xe^{133} clearance method and peripheral vascular diseases. Part I. Standard exercise method – with special reference to work load and volume injected. *Jap. Circ. J.* 38: 655-9, 1974.

475. Hirschberg, C.G. & H.J. Ralston. Energy cost of stair-climbing in normal and hemiplegic subjects. *Amer. J. Phys. Med.* 44: 165-8, 1965.

476. Hobson, W. & J. Pemberton. *The health of the elderly at home.* London: Butterworth, 1955.

477. Hodgkins, J. Reaction time and speed of movements in males and females of various ages. *Res. Quart.* 34: 335-43, 1963.

478. Holland, W.W., D.D. Reid, R. Seltzer & R.W. Stone. Respiratory disease in England and the United States. *Arch. Env. Health* 10: 338-43, 1965.

479. Hollmann, W. Changes in the capacity for maximal and continuous effort in relation to age. In *International research in sport and physical education,* ed. E. Jokl and E. Simon, pp. 369-71. Springfield, Illinois: C.C. Thomas, 1964.

480. Hollmann, W. *Körperliches Training als Prävention von Herz-Kreislauf Krankheiten.* Stuttgart: Hippokrates Verlag, 1965.

481. Hollmann, W. Diminution of cardiopulmonary capacity in the course of life and its prevention by participation in sports. In: *Proc. of intern. congress of sports sciences, Tokyo,* 3-8 Oct. 1964, ed. K. Kato. pp. 91-3. Tokyo: Japanese

Union of Sports Sciences, 1966.
482.   Hollmann, W., W. Barg, G. Weyer & H. Heck. Der alterseinfluss auf spiroergometrische messgrössen im submaximalen arbeitsbereich. *Die Medizinische Welt*, Stuttgart, 17 July 1970. Nr. 28 Sonderdruck.
483.   Hollmann, W. & H. Liesen. Der Trainingseinfluss auf die Leistungsfahigkeit von Herz, Kreislauf und Stoffwechsel im Alter. *Munch. Med. Wschr.* 114: 1336-42, 1972.
484.   Holloszy, J.O., J.S. Skinner *et al.* Effects of a six month programme of endurance exercise on the serum lipids of middle-aged man. *Amer. J. Cardiol.* 14: 753-60, 1964.
485.   Holmdahl, D.E. & B.E. Inglemark. Der Bau des Gelenkknorpels unter verschiedenen funktionellen verhaltnissen. *Acta Anat.* 6: 309, 1949.
486.   Holmgren, A. On the reproducibility of steady-state DL, CO measurements during exercise in man. *Scand. J. Clin. Lab. Invest.* 17: 110-16, 1965.
487.   Holmgren, A. Cardiorespiratory determinants of cardiovascular fitness. In Proc. international symposium on physical activity & cardiovascular health. *Canad. Med. Assoc. J.* 96: 697-705, 1967a.
488.   Holmgren, A. Commentary. In Proc. international symposium on physical activity & cardiovascular health. *Canad. Med. Ass. J.* 96: 794, 1967b.
489.   Holmgren, A. & T. Strandell. Relationship between heart volume, total hemoglobin and physical work capacity in former athletes. *Acta Med. Scand.* 163: 146-60, 1959.
490.   Holter, N.J. Radioelectrocardiography: a new technique for cardiovascular studies. *Ann. N.Y. Acad. Sci.* 65: 913, 1957.
491.   Holter, N.J. New Method for heart studies. *Science* 134: 1214-20, 1961.
492.   Horwitt, M.K. Dietary requirements of the aged. *J. Amer. Diet. Assoc.* 29: 443-8, 1953.
493.   Hotcin, J. & E. Sikova. Long-term effects of virus infection on behaviour and aging in mice. *Proc. Soc. Exp. Biol. Med.* 134: 204-9, 1970.
494.   Hughes, A.L. & R.F. Goldman. Energy cost of hard work. *J. Appl. Physiol.* 29: 570-2, 1970.
495.   Hult, L. Cervical, dorsal and lumbar spinal syndromes. *Acta Orthop. Scand. Suppl.* 17: 7-102, 1954.
496.   Hultman, E. Muscle glycogen stores and prolonged exercise. In *Frontiers of Fitness,* ed. R.J. Shephard. Springfield, Ill.: C.C. Thomas, 1971.
497.   Hurdle, A.D.R. & A.J. Rosin. Red cell volume and red cell survival in normal aged people. *J. Clin. Path.* 15: 343-5, 1962.
498.   Hutchinson, A.O., R.A. McCance & E.M. Widdowson. Serum cholinesterase. In Studies of Undernutrition, Wuppertal, 1946-9. *Spec. Rep. Ser. Med. Res. Council, Lond.* 285: London: HMSO, 1951.
499.   Hyams, D.E. The blood. In *Textbook of geriatric medicine & gerontology,* ed. J.C. Brocklehurst, pp. 528-92. Edinburgh: Churchill-Livingstone, 1973.
500.   Hyatt, R.E. Reaction to Dr Shephard's paper. Ventilatory mechanics during exercise in health and disease. In *Fitness and exercise,* ed. J.F. Alexander, R.C. Serfass & C.M. Tipton. Chicago: Athletic Institute, 1972.
501.   Illsley, R.A., A. Finlayson & B. Thompson. The motivation and characteristics of internal migrants. *Millbank Memorial Fund Quarterly* 41: 217-48, 1963.
502.   Inglis, J. Immediate memory, age and brain function. In *Behaviour, aging and the nervous system,* ed. A.T. Welford & J.E. Birren, pp. 88-113. Springfield, Ill.: C.C. Thomas, 1965.
503.   Irvine, R.E. Thyroid disease in old age. In *Textbook of geriatric medicine & gerontology,* ed. J.C. Brocklehurst, pp. 435-58. Edinburgh: Churchill-

Livingstone, 1973.

504. Isaacs, B. *Studies of illness and death in the elderly in Glasgow.* Edinburgh: Scottish Home & Health Department, 1971.

505. Isaacs, B. Stroke. In *Textbook of geriatric medicine & gerontology*, ed. J.C. Brocklehurst. Edinburgh: Churchill-Livingstone, 1973.

506. Isacsson, S.O. Venous occlusion plethysmography in 55 year old men. *Acta Med. Scand. Suppl.* 537: 1-62, 1972.

507. Jackson, D.S. *Connective tissue, thrombosis and atherosclerosis*, ed. I.H. Page. New York: Academic Press, 1959.

508. Jalavisto, E. The role of simple tests measuring speed of performance in the assessment of biological vigour: a factorial study in elderly women. In *Behaviour, Aging and the Nervous System*, ed. A.T. Welford and J.E. Birren, pp. 353-65. Springfield, Ill.: C.C. Thomas, 1965.

509. James, U. Oxygen uptake and heart rate during prosthetic walking in healthy male unilateral above-knee amputees. *Scand J. Rehab. Med.* 5: 71-80, 1973.

510. Jamison, P.L. Growth of Wainwright Eskimos: stature and weight. *Artic Anthropology* 7: 86-94, 1970.

511. Jansen, L.H. & P.B. Rottier. Some mechanical properties of human abdominal skin measured in excised strips. *Dermatologia* 117: 65, 1958.

512. Jelinek, M.V. & B. Lown. Exercise stress testing for exposure of cardiac arrhythmia. *Progr. Cardiovasc. Dis.* 16: 497-522, 1974.

513. Jéquier, J.C., R. LaBarre, M. Rajic, C. Beaucage, R.J. Shephard & H. Lavallée. The assumption of normality in longitudinal studies. In *Frontiers of physical activity and child health*, ed. H. Lavallée and R.J. Shephard. Quebec: Editions du Pélican, 1977.

514. Jerham, V.J., V.C. Lavides & J.V.G.A. Durnin. A nutrition survey on crofters in North West Scotland. *Nutrition (Lond.)* 23: 159-64, 1969.

515. Johnson, H.D., L.D. Kintner & H.H. Kibler. Effects of 48°F (8.9°C) and 83°F (28.4°C) on longevity and pathology of male rats. *J. Gerontol.* 18: 29-36, 1961.

516. Jokl, E. *The clinical physiology of physical fitness and rehabilitation.* Springfield, Illinois: C.C. Thomas, 1958.

517. Jokl, E., M. Jokl-Ball, P. Jokl & L. Frankel. Notation of exercise. In *Medicine and sport*, vol. 4, *Physical Activity and Aging*, ed. D. Brunner and E. Jokl, pp. 2-18. Basel: Karger, 1970.

518. Jones, N.L. Pulmonary gas exchange during exercise in patients with chronic airway obstruction. *Clin. Sci.* 31: 39-50, 1966.

519. Jones, N.L., G. Jones & R.H.T. Edwards. Exercise tolerance in chronic airway obstruction. *Amer. Rev. Resp. Dis.* 103: 477-91, 1971.

520. Joseph, J.J. The relationship of selected physical fitness test scores to the chronic complaints and ailments of adult males. *J. Sports Med.* 7: 83-94, 1967.

521. Julius, S., A. Amery, L.S. Whitlock & J. Conway. Influence of age on the hemodynamic response to exercise. *Circulation* 36: 222-30, 1967.

522. Kaiser, H. The importance of the locomotor system in geroprophylaxis. In *First International Course in Gerontology*, ed. J.A. Huet, pp. 137-46. Paris: International Centre of Social Gerontology, 1970.

523. Kalk, W.J., A.I. Vinik, B.L. Pimstone & W.P.U. Jackson. Growth hormone response to insulin hypoglycemia in the elderly. *J. Gerontol.* 28: 431-3, 1970.

524. Kallman, F.J. & G. Sander. Twin studies on ageing and longevity. *J. Hered.* 39: 349-57, 1948.

525. Kaltreider, N.L., W.W. Fray & H. Van Zile Hyde. The effects of age on

the total pulmonary capacity and its sub-divisions. *Amer. Rev. Tuberc.* 37: 662-89, 1938.

526.   Kannel, W.B. Habitual level of physical activity and risk of coronary heart disease. The Framingham Study. In Proc. int. symp. on physical activity and cardiovascular health. *Canad. Med. Assoc. J.* 96: 811-2, 1967.

527.   Kannel, W.B. Current status of the epidemology of brain infarction associated with occlusive arterial disease. *Stroke* 2: 295-318, 1971.

528.   Kannel, W.B. & M. Fanlieb. Natural history of angina pectoris in Framingham Study. *Amer. J. Cardiol.* 29: 154-63, 1972.

529.   Karlsson, J., P.O. Åstrand & B. Ekblöm. Training of the oxygen transport system in man. *J. Appl. Physiol.* 22: 1061-5, 1967.

530.   Karpovich, P.V. Longevity and athletics. *Res. Quart.* 12: 451-5, 1941.

531.   Karvonen, M.J. Problems of training the cardiovascular system. *Ergonomics* 2. 207-15, 1959.

532.   Karvonen, M.J., E. Kentala & O. Mustala. The effects of training on heart rate. A longitudinal study. *Ann. Med. Exp. Biol. Fenn.* 35: 307, 1957.

533.   Karvonen, M.J., H. Klemola, J. Virkajarvi & A. Kekkonen. Longevity of endurance skiers. *Med. Sci. Sports* 6: 49-51, 1974.

534.   Kasser, I.S. & R.A. Bruce. Comparative effects of ageing and coronary heart disease on submaximal and maximal exercise. *Circulation* 39: 759-74, 1969.

535.   Kataria, M.S., D.B. Rao & R.C. Curtis. Vitamin C levels in the elderly. *Geront. Clin.* 7: 189-90, 1965.

536.   Kattus, A. & J. Grollman. Patterns of coronary collateral circulation in angina pectoris: relation to exercise training. In *Changing concepts in cardiovascular disease*, ed. H.I. Russek & B.L. Zohman. Baltimore: Williams & Wilkins, 1972.

537.   Kavanagh, T. A cold weather 'jogging mask' for angina patients. *Canad. Med. Assoc. J.* 103: 1290-1, 1970.

538.   Kavanagh, T. *Heart attack! Counter attack!* Toronto: Van Nostrand-Reinhold, 1976.

539.   Kavanagh, T., V. Pandit & R.J. Shephard. The application of exercise testing to the elderly amputee. *Canad. Med. Assoc. J.* 108: 314-7, 1973a.

540.   Kavanagh, T. & R.J. Shephard. Maintenance of hydration in post-coronary marathon runners. *Brit. J. Sports Med.* 9: 130-5, 1957a.

541.   Kavanagh, T. & R.J. Shephard. Conditioning of post-coronary patients: Comparison of continuous and interval training. *Arch. Phys. Med. Rehabil.* 56: 72-6, 1975b.

542.   Kavanagh, T. & R.J. Shephard. Sexual activity after myocardial infarction. *Canad. Med. Assoc. J.* 116: 1250-3, 1977a.

543.   Kavanagh, T. & R.J. Shephard. On the frequency of exercise sessions for post-coronary patients. *Arch. Phys. Med. Rehab.* In press, 1978.

544.   Kavanagh, T. & R.J. Shephard. The effects of continued training on the aging process. *Ann. N.Y. Acad. Sci.* 301: 656-70, 1977b.

545.   Kavanagh, T. & R.J. Shephard. Are the benefits of exercise in ischemic heart disease an artefact of patient selection? *Int. Congr. Cardiol.* Hamburg, 1977c.

546.   Kavanagh, T., R.J. Shephard, H. Doney & V. Pandit. Intensive exercise in coronary rehabilitation. *Med. Sci. Sports* 5: 34-9, 1973b.

547.   Kavanagh, T., R.J. Shephard & J. Kennedy. Characteristics of post-coronary marathon runners. *Ann. N.Y. Acad. Sci.* 301: 455-65, 1977a.

548.   Kavanagh, T., R.J. Shephard & J.A. Tuck. Depression following myocardial infarction — the effects of distance running. *New York Acad. Sci.* 301: 1029-38, 1977b.

References 317

549.   Kay, C. & R.J. Shephard. On muscle strength and the threshold of anaerobic work. *Int. Z. angew. Physiol.* 27: 311-28, 1969.
550.   Kay, D.W.K., P. Beamish & M. Roth. Old age mental disorders in Newcastle-upon-Tyne. Part I – a study of prevalence. *Brit. J. Psychiatr.* 110: 146-58, 1964.
551.   Kay, D.W.K., K. Bergmann, E. Foster, A.A. McKechnie & M. Roth. Mental illness and hospital usage in the elderly: a random sample follow-up. *Comprehensive Psychiatry (New York)*, 2: 26-35, 1970.
552.   Kellgren, J.H. & J.S. Lawrence. Radiological assessment of osteoarthrosis. *Ann. Rheum. Dis.* 16: 494-502, 1957.
553.   Kemsley, W.F.F., W.Z. Billewicz & A.M. Thomson. A new weight-for-height standard based on British Anthropometric Data. *Brit. J. Prev. Soc. Med.* 16: 189-95, 1962.
554.   Kenyon, G.S. Six scales for assessing attitude toward physical activity. *Res. Quart.* 39: 566-74, 1968.
555.   Kenyon, G.S. *Values held for physical activity by selected urban secondary school students in Canada, Australia, England and the United States.* Univ. of Winsconsin: US Office of Education Contract S-376, 1961.
556.   Keys, A., J.T. Anderson & F. Grande. Serum cholesterol in man: diet fat and intrinsic responsiveness. *Circulation* 19: 201-14, 1959.
557.   Keys, A., C. Aravanis, H. Blackburn, F.S.P. Van Buchem, R. Buzina, B.S. Djordjevic, F. Fidanza, M.J. Karvonen, A. Menotti, V. Puddu & H.L. Taylor. Coronary heart disease: overweight and obesity. *Ann. Int. Med.* 77: 15-27, 1972.
558.   Khosla, T. & C.R. Lowe. Indices of obesity derived from body weight and height. *Brit. J. Prev. Soc. Med.* 21: 122-8, 1967.
559.   Khosla, T. & C.R. Lowe. Obesity and smoking habits. *Brit. Med. J.* 4: 10-13, 1971.
560.   Kiessling, K.H., L. Pilström, A-Ch. Bylund, B. Saltin & K. Piehl. Enzyme activities and morphometry in skeletal muscle of middle-aged men after training. *Scand. J. Clin. Lab. Invest.* 33: 63-9, 1974.
561.   Kilböm, Å. Physical training in women. *Scand. J. Clin. Lab. Invest.* 28: Suppl. 119: 1-34, 1971.
562.   Kilböm, Å. & I. Åstrand. Physical training with submaximal intensities in women. II. Effect on cardiac output. *Scand. J. Clin. Lab. Invest.* 28: 163-75, 1971.
563.   Kilböm, Å., L.H. Hartley, B. Saltin, J. Bjure, G. Grimby & I. Åstrand. Physical training in sedentary middle-aged and older men. I. Medical evaluation. *Scand. J. Clin. Lab. Invest.* 24: 315-28, 1969.
564.   Kinsey, A.C., W.B. Pomeroy & C.E. Martin. *Sexual behaviour in the human male.* Philadelphia: W.B. Saunders, 1948.
565.   Kinsey, A.C., W.B. Pomeroy, C.E. Martin & P.H. Gebgard. *Sexual behaviour in the human female.* Philadelphia: W.B. Saunders, 1953.
566.   Kitamura, K. The role of sports activities in the prevention of cardiovascular malfunction. In *Proceeding of international congress of sports science, Tokyo*, ed. K. Kato. Tokyo: Japanese Union of Sports Sciences, 1966.
567.   Klasen, H.J. & J.C.C. Swiersta. Rupture of the Achilles tendon. *Arch. Chir. Neerl.* 23: 249-58, 1971.
568.   Klumbies, G. & H. Kleinsorge. Circulatory dangers and prophylaxis during orgasm. *Int. J. Sexol.* 10: 97, 1930.
569.   Knoll, W. Welches Lebens alter erreichen die Ruderer von 'Oxford-Cambridge?' (Eine Richtigstellung). *Med. Klin.* 34: 464-6, 1938.
570.   Kny, W. Über die Verteilung des Lipofuscins in der Skeletmuskulatur in ihrer Beziehung zur Funktion. *Virchows Arch. (Pathol. Anat.)* 299: 468-78, 1937.

318   *References*

571.   Kohm, R.R. Human aging and disease. *J. Chron. Dis.* 16: 5-21, 1963.
572.   Korenchevsky, V. *Physiological and pathological ageing,* ed. G.H. Bourne, pp. 40-4, 311-15. Basel: Karger, 1961.
573.   Kral, V.A. Senescent forgetfulness. Benign and malignant. *Canad. Med. Assoc. J.* 86: 257-60, 1962.
574.   Kraus, H. Effects of training on skeletal muscle. In *Coronary heart disease and physical fitness,* ed. O.A. Larsen & R.O. Malmborg, pp. 134-7. Copenhagen: Munksgaard, 1971.
575.   Kreitler, H. & S. Kreitler. Movement and aging: A psychological approach. In *Medicine and sport,* vol. 4, *Physical activity and aging,* ed. D. Brunner and E. Jokl, pp. 302-6. Basel: Karger, 1970.
576.   Kritchevsky, D., B.V. Howard & V.J. Cristofalo. Biochemical studies on aging diploid cells. In *Physical activity and aging,* ed. D. Brunner & E. Jokl. Basel: Karger, 1970.
577.   Kuhlen, R.G. Personality change with age. In *Personality change,* ed. P. Worchel & D. Byrne. New York: John Wiley, 1964.
578.   Kunze. (1933). Cited by Comfort, 1964.
579.   Kutal, I., J. Pǎřizková & J. Dycka. Muscle strength and lean body mass in old men of different physical activity. *J. Appl. Physiol.* 29: 168-71, 1970.
580.   Lalonde, M. *A new perspective on the health of Canadians.* Ottawa: Govt. of Canada, 1974.
581.   Lamb, D.R. Androgens and exercise. *Med. Sci. Sports* 7: 1-5, 1975.
582.   Landowne, M., M. Brandfonbrener & N.W. Shock. The relation of age to certain measures of performance of the heart & the circulation. *Circulation* 12: 567-76, 1955.
583.   Lansing, A.I. Some physiological aspects of ageing. *Physiol. Rev.* 31: 274-84, 1951.
584.   Lansing, A.I. Elastic tissue. In *The arterial wall,* pp. 136-60. Baltimore: Williams & Wilkins, 1959.
585.   Largey, G. Athletic activity and longevity. *Lancet* ii: 286, 1972.
586.   Laron, Z., M. Doron & B. Amikam. Plasma growth hormone in men & women over 70 years of age. In *Medicine and sport,* vol. 4, *Physical activity and aging,* ed. D. Brunner & E. Jokl, pp. 126-31. Basel: Karger, 1970.
587.   Laros, G.S., C.M. Tipton & R.R. Cooper. Influence of physical activity on ligament insertions in the knees of dogs. *J. Bone Joint Surg., Amer.* 53: 275-86, 1971.
588.   Larsen, K. & Th., Skulason. The normal electrocardiogram. I. Analysis of the extremity deviations from 100 normal persons whose ages range from 30 to 50 years. *Amer. Heart J.* 22: 625, 1941.
589.   Larsen, O.A. & N.A. Lassen. Effect of daily muscular exercise in patients with intermittent claudication. *Lancet* ii: 1093-6, 1966.
590.   Lawson, I.R. Anaemia in a group of elderly patients. *Geront. Clin.* 2: 87-101, 1960.
591.   Lawson, I.R. Anaemia in the elderly with special reference to iron deficiency. *Geront. Clin.* 9: 393-400, 1967.
592.   Lawrence, J.S., R. De Graff & V.A.I. Laine. Degenerative joint disease in random samples and occupational groups. In *The epidemology of chronic rheumatism,* ed. J.H. Kellgren, M.R. Jeffrey & J. Ball, vol. 1. Oxford: Blackwell Scientific, 1963.
593.   LeBlanc, P., F. Ruff & J. Milic Emili. Effects of age and body position on 'airway closure' in man. *J. Appl. Physiol.* 28: 448-51, 1970.
594.   LeCoultre, D. Employment of older workers — economic aspects. In *Work and aging,* 2nd International course in social gerontology. Paris: International Centre of Social Gerontology, 1971.

595. Lee, M.M.C. & G.W. Lasker. The thickness of subcutaneous fat in elderly men. *Amer. J. Phys. Anthropol.* 16: 125-34, 1959.

596. Leeming, J.T. Skeletal disease in the elderly. *Brit. Med. J.* (iv): 472-4, 1973.

597. Lehman, H.C. Chronological age vs. proficiency in physical skills. *Amer. J. Physiol.* 44: 161-87, 1951.

598. Leighton, D.A. Special senses: Aging of the eye. In *Textbook of geriatric medicine and gerontology*, ed. J.C. Brocklehurst. Edinburgh: Churchill-Livingstone, 1973.

599. Leinhos, R. Die Altersabhängigkeit des Augenpupillendurchmessers. *Optik* 16: 669-71, 1959.

600. Lempert, S.M. *Report on the survey of the aged in Stockport.* Stockport: County Borough of Stockport, 1958.

601. Lepeschkin, E. Physiological factors influencing the electrocardiographic response to exercise. In *Measurement in exercise electrocardiography*, ed. H. Blackburn, pp. 363-87. Springfield, Illinois: C.C. Thomas, 1969.

602. Lesher, S., R.J. Fry & H.I. Kohn. Aging and the generation cycle of intestinal epithelial cells in the mouse. *Gerontologia* 5: 176-81, 1961.

603. Lesher, S. & G.A. Sacher. Effects of age on cell proliferation in mouse duodenal crypts. *Exptl. Gerontol.* 3: 211-7, 1968.

604. Lessa, A. Evolution of the worker's physiological abilities according to his age and activity. In *Work and aging*, ed. J. Huet, pp. 221-42. Paris: Internat. Centre of Social Gerontology, 1971.

605. Lester, F.M., L.T. Sheffield & T.J. Reeves. Electrocardiographic changes in clinically normal older men following maximal and near-maximal exercise. *Circulation* 36: 5-14, 1967.

606. Lester, F.M., L.T. Sheffield, P. Trammell & T.J. Reeves. The effect of age and athletic training on maximal heart rate during muscular exercise. *Amer. Heart J.* 76: 370-6, 1968.

607. Leusink, J.A. A comparison of the body composition estimated by densitometry and total body potassium measurement in trained and untrained subjects. *Pflüg. Archiv.* 348: 357-62, 1974.

608. Leveille, G.A. & D.R. Romsos. Meal eating and obesity. *Nutrition Today* (Nov/Dec.) 4-9, 1974.

609. Levison, H. & R.M. Cherniack. Ventilatory cost of exercise in chronic obstructive pulmonary disease. *J. Appl. Physiol.* 25: 21-7, 1968.

610. Li, Y.B., N. Ting, B.N. Chiang, E.R. Alexander, R.A. Bruce & T. Grayston. Electrocardiographic response to maximal exercise. Treadmill and double Master exercise tests in middle-aged Chinese men. *Amer. J. Cardiol.* 20: 541-8, 1967.

611. Liburd, E.M., A.S. Russell & J.B. Dossetor. Spleen cell cytotoxicity in New Zealand and black mice (NZB) with autoimmune disease. *J. Immunol. Illinois:* 1288-91, 1973.

612. Likoff, W., B.L. Segal & H. Kasparian. Paradox of normal selective coronary arteriograms in patients considered to have unmistakable coronary heart disease. *New Engl. J. Med.* 276: 1063-6, 1967.

613. Lind, A.R. & G.W. McNicol. Muscular factors which determine the cardiovascular responses to sustained and rhythmic exercise. In Proc. int. symposium on physical activity and cardiovascular health. *Canad. Med. Assoc. J.* 96: 706-12, 1967.

614. Lindsay, S. & I.L. Chaikoff. Naturally occurring arteriosclerosis in animals: a comparison with experimentally induced lesions. In *Atherosclerosis and its origin*, ed. M. Sandler & G.H. Browne. New York: Academic Press, 1963.

615. Linn, B.S. Chronologic versus biologic age in geriatric patients. In *The*

physiology and pathology of human aging, ed. R. Goldman & M. Rockstein, pp. 9-18. New York: Academic Press, 1975.

616.   Ljunggren, H. Sex difference in body composition. In *Human body composition*, ed. J. Brozek, pp. 129-38. Oxford: Pergamon Press, 1963.

617.   Lloyd, B. Presidential address. Section 1. (Physiology and Biochemistry). British Association. In *Advancement of sciences*, pp. 515-30, 1966.

618.   Lockhart, A., M. Tzareva, F. Nader, P. LeBlanc, F. Schrijen & P. Sadoul. Elevated pulmonary artery wedge pressure at rest and during exercise in chronic bronchitis. *Brit. Med. J.* 5845: 78-81, 1973.

619.   Lodenkamper, H. & G. Steinen. Beitrag zum Problem des Alterns. *Dtsch. Med. Wschr.* 79: 739-41, 1954.

620.   Loeb, J. & J.H. Northrup. On the influence of food and temperature upon the duration of life. *J. Biol. Chem.* 32: 103-21, 1917.

621.   Lombard, W.P. & O.M. Cope. The duration of systole in man. *Amer. J. Physiol.* 77: 263-95, 1926.

622.   Longo, A.M., K.M. Moser & P.C. Luchsinger. The role of oxygen therapy in the rehabilitation of patients with chronic obstructive pulmonary disease. *Amer. Rev. Resp. Dis.* 103: 690-7, 1971.

623.   Lopez, M.G., P. Runge, D.C. Harrison & J.C. Schroeder. Comparison of 24 hour ambulatory electrocardiographic monitoring in detection of ST-T changes. *Brit. Heart J.* 36: 90-95, 1974.

624.   Malhotra, M.S., S.S. Ramaswamy, G.L. Dua & J. Sengupta. Physical work capacity as influenced by age. *Ergonomics* 9: 305-16, 1966.

625.   Malins, J.M. The definition of the diabetic population. *Nordic Council Artic Med. Res. Rep.* 15: 5-8, 1976.

626.   Mann, G.V., L.H. Garrett, A. Farlie, H. Murray & F.T. Billings. Exercise to prevent coronary heart disease. *Amer. J. Med.* 46: 12-27, 1969.

627.   Mann, G.V., R.D. Shaffer, R.S. Anderson & H.H. Sandstead. Cardiovascular disease in the Masai. *J. Atherosclerosis Res.* 4: 289-312, 1964.

628.   Mann, G.V., K. Teel, O. Hayes, A. McNally & D. Bruno. Exercise in the disposition of dietary calories. *New Engl. J. Med.* 253: 349-55, 1955.

629.   Marcus, J.H., R.H. Ingram & R.L. McLean. The threshold of anaerobic metabolism in chronic obstructive pulmonary disease. *Amer. Rev. Resp. Dis.* 104: 490-8, 1971.

630.   Margaria, R. Energy production for muscular work in the aged. *Proc. 7th International Congr. on Gerontology*, Vienna, Austria, 1966a.

631.   Margaria, R. An outline for setting significant tests of muscular performance. In *Human adaptability and its methodology*, ed. H. Yoshimura & J.S. Weiner. Tokyo: Society for the Promotion of Sciences, 1966b.

632.   Margaria, R., P. Aghemo & E. Rovelli. Indirect estimation of maximal oxygen consumption in man. *J. Appl. Physiol.* 20: 1070-3, 1965.

633.   Margolis, J.R., R.F. Gillum, M. Feinleib, R.C. Brasch & R.B. Fabsitz. Community surveillance for coronary heart disease: the Framingham cardiovascular disease survey. Methods and preliminary results. *Amer. J. Epidemiol.* 100: 425-36, 1974.

634.   Marquardsen, J. The natural history of acute cerebrovascular disease: a retrospective study of 769 patients. *Acta Neurol. Scand.* 45: Suppl. 38: 9-188, 1969.

635.   Martens, R. Trait and state anxiety. In *Ergogenic aids and muscular performance*, ed. W.P. Morgan, pp. 35-66. New York: Academic Press, 1972.

636.   Martin, G.M. & C.A. Sprague. Symposium on in vitro studies of hyperplastoid cell lines from aorta and skin. *Exp. Mol. Pathol.* 18: 125-41, 1973.

637.   Maslow, A. *Towards a psychology of being*. Princeton, N.J.: Van Nostrand, 1962.

638. Mason, R.E., I. Likar, R.O. Biern & R.S. Ross. Correlation of graded exercise electrocardiographic response with clinical and coronary cinearteriographic findings. In *Measurement in exercise electrocardiography*, ed. H. Blackburn. Springfield, Illinois: C.C. Thomas, 1969.

639. Massie, J.F. & R.J. Shephard. Physiological and psychological effects of training. *Med. Sci. Sports* 3: 110-17, 1971.

640. Master, A.M. The Master two-step test. Some historical highlights and current concepts. *J.S. Carol. Med. Ass.* 65: Suppl. 1: 12-17, 1969.

641. Master, A.M., R. Friedman & S. Dack. The electrocardiogram after standard exercise as a functional test of the heart. *Amer. Heart J.* 24: 777-93, 1942.

642. Master, A.M., R.P. Lasser & H.L. Jaffe. Blood pressure in white people over 65 years of age. *Ann. Int. Med.* 48: 284-99, 1958.

643. Master, A.M., E.J. Van Liere, H.A. Lindsay & W.S. Hartroft. Arterial blood pressure. In *Biology data book,* ed. P.L. Altman, & D.S. Dittmer. Washington, D.C.: Fed. Amer. Soc. Exp. Biol., 1964.

644. Matarazzo, R.G., J.D. Matarazzo & G. Saslow. The relationship between medical and psychiatric symptoms. *J. Abnorm. Soc. Psychol.* 62: 55-61, 1961.

645. Mattingly, T.W. The post-exercise electrocardiogram. Its value in the diagnosis and prognosis of cornary arterial disease. *Amer. J. Cardiol.* 9: 395-409, 1962.

646. Matzker, J. & E. Springborn. Richtungshören und Lebensalter. *Ztschr. Laryngol.* 37: 737-45, 1958.

647. Mayer, J. Multiple origins of obesity. *Nutr. News* 17 (2), 1953.

648. Mayer, J. *Proc. Amer. Acad. Arts Sci.* 93, 830, 1964. Cited by Davidson *et al.* 1972.

649. Mayer, J. *Overweight: causes, cost and control.* Englewood Cliffs, NJ: Prentice-Hall, 1968.

650. Maynard-Smith, J. A theory of aging. *Nature (Lond.)* 184: 956-68, 1959.

651. Mazer, M. & J.A. Reisinger. An electrocardiographic study of cardiac aging based on records at rest and after exercise. *Ann. Int. Med.* 21: 645-52, 1944.

652. Mazess, R.B. & J.R. Cameron. In *International conference on bone mineral measurement*, ed. R.B. Mazess, pp. 228-338. US Dept. Health, Education Welfare. Pub. No. (NIH) 75-683, 1973.

653. Mazzarella, J.A., J.S. Skinner & T.O. Evans. Effects of interval training on the exercise electrocardiogram. *Circulation* 34: (Suppl. 3) 165-6, 1966.

654. McDonough, J.R. & R.A. Bruce. Maximal exercise testing in assessing cardiovascular function. *J. S. Carol. Med. Assoc.* 65: Suppl. 1: 26-33, 1969.

655. McFarland, R.A. Experimental evidence of the relationship between ageing and oxygen want: in search of a theory of ageing. *Ergonomics* 6: 339-66, 1963.

656. McGavak, T.H. *The thyroid*, p. 111. St. Louis: Mosby, 1951.

657. McNab, G.R., W.S. Grove & S. Nariman. A comparison of physiological and pathological findings in chronic bronchitis and emphysema, with special reference to response to exercise. *Thorax* 16: 56-64, 1961.

658. McNeill, K.G. & R.M. Green. Measurements with a whole body counter. *Canad. J. Physics* 37: 683-9, 1959.

659. McNeill, K.G., H.A. Kostalis & J.E. Harrison. Effects of body thickness on in vivo neutron activation analysis. In preparation, 1978.

660. McNeill, K.G., B.J. Thomas, W.C. Sturtridge & J.E. Harrison. In vivo neutron activation analysis for calcium in man. *J. Nucl. Med.* 14: 502-6, 1973.

661. McPherson, B.D., A. Paivio, M.S. Yuhasz, P.A. Rechnitzer, H.A. Pickard

322   *References*

& N.M. Lefcoe. Psychological effects of an exercise program for post-infarct and normal adult men. *J. Sports Med.* 7: 95-102, 1967.

662. McPherson, B.D. & M.S. Yuhasz. An inventory for assessing men's attitudes toward exercise and physical activity. *Res. Quart.* 39: 218-20, 1968.

663. Medalie, J.H. Current developments in the epidemiology of atherosclerosis in Israel. In *Atherosclereosis: proc. 2nd int. symp.*, ed. R.J. Jones, New York: Springer, 1970.

664. Medawar, P.B. *The uniqueness of the individual.* London: Methuen, 1957.

665. Mertens, D.J., T. Kavanagh & R.J. Shephard. Exercise rehabilitation for chronic obstructive lung disease. *Respiration.* In press, 1978.

666. Métivier, G. The effects of long-lasting physical exercise and training on hormonal regulation. In *Metabolic adaptation to prolonged exercise,* ed. H. Howald & J.R. Poortmans, pp. 276-92. Basel: Birkhauser Verlag, 1975.

667. Métivier, G., J. Poortmans, R. Vanroux, P. Leclercq & G. Copinschi. Arterial blood plasma cortisol and human growth hormone changes in male trained subjects submitted to various physical work intensity levels. Paper presented at the annual meeting Amer. College Sports Med., *Med. Sci. Sports* 3: g, 1971.

668. Meyer, W.W. Die Lebenswandlung der Struktur von Arterien und Venen. *Verhandl. Deutsch Ges. Kreislaufforsch.* 24: 15-40, 1958.

669. Meylan, G.L. Harvard Univeristy Oarsmen. *Harvard Grad. Magazine* 9: 362-76, 1904.

670. Miall, W.E., M.T. Ashcroft, H.G. Lovell & F. Moore. A longitudinal study of the decline of adult height with age in two Welsh communities. *Human Biol.* 39: 445-54, 1967.

671. Milch, R.A. Aging of connective tissues. In *Perspective in experimental gerontology*, ed. N.W. Shock. Springfield, Illinois: C.C. Thomas, 1966.

672. Miles, W.R. In *Problems of aging*, ed. E.V. Cowdry. Baltimore: Williams & Wilkins, 1942.

673. Milhøj, P. Work and retirement. In *Old people in three industrial societies*. London: Routledge, 1968.

674. Miller, W.F., R.L. Johnson & N. Wu. Relationships between fast vital capacity and various timed expiratory capacities. *J. Appl. Physiol.* 14: 157-63, 1959.

675. Miller, W.F. & H.F. Taylor. Exercise training in the rehabilitation of patients with severe respiratory insufficiency due to pulmonary emphysema: The role of oxygen breathing. *Southern Med. J.* 55: 1216-21, 1962.

676. Mills, J.N. Variability of the vital capacity of the normal human subject. *J. Physiol.* 110: 76-82, 1949.

677. Milne, J.S., M.E. Lonergan, J. Williamson, F.M.L. Moore, R. McMaster & N. Percy. Leucocyte ascorbic acid levels and vitamin C intake in older people. *Brit. Med. J.* (iv) 383-6, 1971a.

678. Milne, J.S., M.M. Maule & J. Williamson. Method of sampling in a study of older people with a comparison of respondents and non-respondents. *Brit. J. Prev. Soc. Med.* 25: 37-41, 1971b.

679. Minot, C.S. *The problem of age, growth and death.* New York: Putnam.

680. Mithoefer, J.C. & M.S. Karetzky. The cardiopulmonary system in the aged. In *Surgery of the aged and debilitated patient,* ed. J.H. Powers, pp. 140-64. Philadelphia: W.B. Saunders Co., 1968.

681. Molbech, S. Energy cost in level walking in subjects with an abnormal gait. Hellerup, Denmark: Rept. Danish National Soc. for Infantile Paralysis 22: 1966.

682. Molen, N.H. Energy/speed relationship in amputees. *Int. Z. angew.*

Physiol. 31. 173-85, 1972.
683. Molina, C. & E. Giorgi. Il metabolismo respiratorio dei soggetti anziani durante l'esercizio muscolare. *Med. Lavoro* 42: 315-25, 1951.
684. Monroe, R.T. *Diseases in old age,* pp. 253-62. Cambridge, Mass.: Harvard University Press, 1951.
685. Montoye, H.J. *Physical activity and health: an epidemiologic study of an entire community.* Englewood Cliffs, N.J.: Prentice-Hall, 1975.
686. Montoye, H.J., W.D. Van Huss, H. Olson, A. Hudec & E. Mahoney. Study of longevity and morbidity of college athletes. *J. Amer. Med. Ass.* 162: 1132-4, 1956.
687. Montoye, H.J., W.D. Van Huss, H. Olson, W.R. Pierson & A.J. Hudec. The longevity and morbidity of college athletes. *Phi. Epsilon Kappa Fraternity,* Michigan State University, 1957.
688. Montoye, H.J., W.D. Van Huss, W.D. Brewer, E.M. Jones, M.A. Ohlson, E. Mahoney & H. Olson. The effects of exercise on blood cholesterol in middle-aged men. *Amer. J. Clin. Nutr.* 7: 139-45, 1959.
689. Montoye, H.J., P.W. Willis & D.A. Cunningham. Heart rate response to sub-maximal exercise: relation to age and sex. *J. Gerontol.* 23: 127-33, 1968.
690. Montoye, H.J., P.W. Willis, G.E. Howard & J.B. Keller. Cardiac pre-ejection period: age and sex comparisons. *J. Gerontol.* 26: 208-16, 1971.
691. Morgan, J.E. (1873). Critical enquiry into the after-health of the men who rowed the Oxford and Cambridge boat race from the year 1829-1859. In *University Oars,* cited by Hartley & Llewellyn, 1939.
692. Morgan, P., M. Gildiner & G.R. Wright. Smoking reduction of adults who take up exercise: a survey of a running club for adults. *C.A.H.P.E.R. Journal* 42: 39-43, 1976.
693. Morgan, W.P. Psychological considerations. *J.H.P.E.R.* 39: 26, 1968.
694. Morgan, W.P. Psychological factors influencing perceived exertion. *Med. Sci. Sports* 5: 97-103, 1973.
695. Morgan, W.P., J.A. Roberts, F.R. Brand & A.D. Feinerman. Psychological effect of chronic physical activity. *Med. Sci. Sports* 2: 213-17, 1970.
696. Morris, J.N., S.P. Chave, C. Adam, C. Sirey & L. Epstein. Vigorous exercise in leisure-time and the incidence of coronary heart disease. *Lancet* i: 333-9, 1973.
697. Morris, J.N., J. Heady & P. Raffle. Physique of London busmen. *Lancet* ii: 569-70, 1956.
698. Morris, J.F., A. Koski & L.C. Johnson. Spirometric standards for healthy non-smoking adults. *Amer. Rev. Resp. Dis.* 103: 57-67, 1971.
699. Mortensen, J.D., L.B. Woolner & W.H. Bennett. Gross and microscopic findings in normal thyroid glands. *J. Clin. Endocrinol.* 15: 1270-80, 1955.
700. Most, A.S., T.R. Hornsten, V. Hofer & R.A. Bruce. Exercise ST changes in healthy men. *Arch. Int. Med.* 121: 225-9, 1968.
701. Muggleton, A. & J.F. Danielli. Inheritance of the 'life-spanning' phenomenon in Amoeba proteus. *Exp. Cell. Res.* 49: 116-20, 1968.
702. Müller, E.A. & R. Hettinger. Arbeitsphysiologische Untersuchungen verschiedener Oberschenel Kunstbeine. *Ztsch. Op.* 81: 525, 1952.
703. Munnichs, J.M.A. & A. Bigot. Psychology of aging, long-term illness and death. In *Textbook of geriatric medicine & gerontology,* ed. J.C. Brocklehurst, pp. 725-41. London: Churchill-Livingstone, 1973.
704. Murrell, K.F.H. & S. Griew. Age, experience and speed of response. In *Behaviour, aging and the nervous system,* ed. A.T. Welford & J.E. Birren, pp. 54-64. Springfield, Illinois.: C.C. Thomas, 1965.
705. Myhre, L.G. & W.V. Kessler. Body density and K^{40} measurements of body composition as related to age. *J. Appl. Physiol.* 21: 1251-5, 1966.

324   *References*

706.   Nagle, F.J. Physiological assessment of maximal performance. In *Exercise and sport science reviews*, vol. 1, ed. J.H. Wilmore, pp. 313-38. New York: Academic Press, 1973.
707.   Nakamura, M., H. Yamanota, Y. Kikuchi, Y. Isihara, T. Sata & S. Yoshimura. Cerebral atherosclerosis in Japanese: 1. Age related to atherosclerosis. *Stroke* 2: 400-8, 1971.
708.   Nakhjavan, F.K., W.H. Palmer & M. McGregor. Influence of respiration on venous return in pulmonary emphysema. *Circulation* 33: 8-16, 1966.
709.   Nandy, K. Further studies on the effects of centrophenoxine on the lipofuxin pigment in the neurons of senile guinea pigs. *J. Gerontol.* 23: 82-90, 1968.
710.   National Adult Physical Fitness Survey. *Newsletter.* President's Council on Physical Fitness and Sports, May 1973.
711.   National Adult Physical Fitness Survey. In *Physical Fitness Res. Digest,* ed. H.H. Clarke. 4 (2): April, 1974.
712.   Naughton, J.P., H.K. Hellerstein & I.C. Mohler. *Exercise testing and exercise training in coronary heart disease.* New York: Academic Press, 1973.
713.   Neary, G.J., R.J. Munson & R.N. Mole. *Chronic irradiation of mice by fast neutrons.* Oxford: Pergamon Press, 1957.
714.   Needham, C.D., M.C. Rogan & I. McDonald. Normal standards for lung volumes, intra-pulmonary gas mixing, and maximum breathing capacity. *Thorax* 9: 313-25, 1954.
715.   Neuberger, A., J.C. Perrone & H.G.B. Slack. Relative metabolic inertia of tendon collagen in the rat. *Biochem. J.* 49: 199-204, 1951.
716.   Neugarten, B.L. & R.J. Havighurst. Disengagement reconsidered in a cross-national context. In *Adjustment to retirement*, ed. R.J. Havighurst, M.A. Munnich, B. Neugarten & H. Thomae, pp. 138-46. Assen: Van Gorcum, 1969.
717.   Neugarten, B.L., R.J. Havighurst & S.S. Tobin. The measurement of life satisfaction. *J. Gerontol.* 16: 134-43, 1961.
718.   New, P.K., A.T. Ruscio & L.A. George. Toward an understanding of the rehabilitation system. *Rehab. Lit.* 30: 130-9, 1969.
719.   Newman, F., B.F. Smalley & M.L. Thompson. Effect of exercise, body and lung size on CO diffusion in athletes and nonatheletes. *J. Appl. Physiol.* 17: 649-55, 1962.
720.   Newman, G. & C.R. Nichols. Sexual activities and attitudes in older persons. *J. Amer. Med. Assoc.* 173: 33-5, 1960.
721.   Nicholas, J.J., R. Gilbert, R. Gabe & J.H. Auchincloss. Evaluation of an exercise therapy program for patients with chronic obstructive pulmonary disease. *Amer. Rev. Resp. Dis.* 102: 1-9, 1970.
722.   Nichols, A.B., C. Ravenscroft, D.E. Lamphiear, L.D. Ostrander, Jr. Independence of serum lipid levels and dietary habits. The Tecumseh Study. *J. Amer. Med. Assoc.* 236: 1948-53, 1976.
723.   Niinimaa, V & R.J. Shephard. Training and oxygen conductance in the elderly. I. The respiratory system. II. The cardiovascular system. *J. Gerontol.* In press, 1978.
724.   Nikkila, E.A., M.R. Taskinen, T. Miettinen, R. Pelkonen & H. Poppius. Effect of muscular work on insulin secretion. In *Physical activity and aging,* ed. D. Brunner & E. Jokl, pp. 121-25. Baltimore: University Park Press, 1970.
725.   Nikkila, E.A., M.R. Taskinen, T.A. Miettinen, R. Pelkonen & H. Poppius. Effects of muscular exercise on insulin secretion. *Diabetes* 17: 209-18, 1968.
726.   Nisbet, N.H. Who benefits? *Lancet* i: 133-4, 1970.
727.   Noble, B.J., K.F. Metz, K.B. Pandolf, C.W. Bell, E. Cafarelli & W.E. Sime. Perceived exertion during walking and running. *Med. Sci. Sports* 5:

116-20, 1973a.
728. Noble, B.J., K.F. Metz, K.B. Pandolf & E. Cafarelli. Perceptual responses to exercise: a multiple regression study. *Med. Sci. Sports* 5: 104-9, 1973b.
729. Nordgren, R.A., G.P. Hirsch, R.A. Menzies, D.D. Hendley, R. Kutsky & B.L. Strehler. Evidence for long-lived components in developing mouse tissues labelled with leucine.*Exp. Gerontol.* 4: 7-16, 1969.
730. Norris, A.H., T. Lundy & N.W. Shock. Trend in selected indices of body composition in men between the ages 30 & 80 years. *Ann. N.Y. Acad. Sci.* 110: 623-39, 1963.
731. Norris, A.H., C. Mittman & 'N.W. Shock. Changes in ventilation with age. In *Ageing of the lung*, ed. L. Cander & J.H. Moyer, pp. 136-42. New York: Grune & Stratton, 1964.
732. Norris, A.H. & N.W. Shock. Exercise in the adult years – with special reference to the advanced years. In *Science and medicine of exercise and sports*, ed. W.R. Johnson, pp. 466-90. New York: Harper & Row, 1960.
733. Norris, A.H., N.W. Shock, M. Landowne & J.A. Falzone. Pulmonary function studies: age differences in lung volumes and bellows function.*J. Gerontol.* 11: 379-87, 1956.
734. Norris, A.H., N.W. Shock & M.J. Yiengst. Age changes in heart rate and blood pressure responses to tilting and standardized exercise. *Circulation* 8: 521-6, 1953a.
735. Norris, A.H., N.W. Shock & G.H. Wagman. Age changes in the maximum conduction velocity of motor fibers of human ulnar nerves. *J. Appl. Physiol.* 5: 589-93, 1953b.
736. Norris, A.H., N.W. Shock & M.J. Yiengst. Age differences in ventilatory and gas exchange responses to graded exercise in males. *J. Gerontol.* 10: 145-55, 1955.
737. Novak, L.P. Aging, total body potassium, fat-free mass, and cell mass in males and females between ages 18 and 85 years. *J. Gerontol.* 27: 438-43, 1972.
738. Nutrition Canada. Nutrition a national priority; a report by Nutrition Canada to Dept. National Hlth. & Welfare, Ottawa, 1973.
739. Nutrition Canada. *Food consumption patterns report.* Ottawa: Health and Welfare, Canada, 1976.
740. Obrist, W.R. Electro-encephalographic approach to age changes in response speed. In *Behaviour, aging and the nervous system*, ed. A.T. Welford and J.E. Birren, pp. 259-72. Springfield, Illinois: C.C. Thomas, 1965.
741. Officer, J.E. Procaine – HCI growth enhancing effects on aged mouse, embryo fibroblasts cultured in vitro. In *Theoretical aspects of aging*, ed. M. Rockstein. New York: Academic Press, 1974.
742. Ogilvie, C.M., R.E. Forster, W.S. Blakemore & J.W. Morton. A standardized breath-holding technique for the clinical measurement of the diffusing capacity of the lung for carbon monoxide. *J. Clin. Invest.* 36: 1-17, 1957.
743. Olesun, K.H. Body composition in normal adults. In *Human body composition*, ed. J. Brozek, pp. 177-90. Oxford: Pergamon Press, 1963.
744. Oscai, L.B. The role of exercise in weight control. In *Exercise and sport science reviews*, vol. 1, ed. J.H. Wilmore, pp. 103-23. New York: Academic Press, 1973.
745. Oscai, L.B. & J.O. Holloszy. Effects of weight changes produced by exercise, food restriction or overeating on body composition. *J. Clin. Invest.* 48: 2124-8, 1969.
746. Ostrander, L.D., R.L. Brandt, M.O. Kjelsberg & F.H. Epstein. Electrocardiographic findings among the adult population of a total natural community.

Tecumseh, Michigan. *Circulation* 31: 888-98, 1965.
747.   Overstall, P.W., A.N. Exton-Smith, F.J. Imms & A.L. Johnson. Falls in the elderly related to postural imbalance. *Brit. Med. J.* i: 261-4, 1977.
748.   Paez, P.N., E.A. Phillipson, M. Maasengkay & B.J. Sproule. The physiological basis of training patients with emphysema. *Amer. Rev. Resp. Dis.* 95: 944-53, 1967.
749.   Paffenbarger, R.S. & W.E. Hale. Work activity and coronary heart mortality. *New Engl. J. Med.* 292: 545-50, 1975.
750.   Paffenbarger, R.S. & A.L. Wing. Characteristics in youth predisposing to fatal stroke in later years. *Lancet* i: 253-4, 1967.
751.   Paillat, P. The cost of the advancement of retirement age in industrialized countries. In *Work and aging. 2nd international course in social gerontology.* Paris: International Centre of Social Gerontology, 1971.
752.   Palmore, E. Health practices and illness among the aged. *Gerontologist* 10: 313-6, 1970.
753.   Pářizková, J. Impact of age, diet and exercise on man's body composition. *Ann. N.Y. Acad. Sci.* 110: 661-74, 1963.
754.   Pářizková, J. Impact of age, diet and exercise on man's body composition. In *International research in sport and physical education,* ed. E. Jokl and E. Simon, pp. 238-53. Springfield, Illinois: C.C. Thomas, 1964.
755.   Pářizková, J. & E. Eiselt. Body composition and anthropometric indicators in old age and the influence of exercise. *Human Biol.* 38: 351-63, 1966.
756.   Pářizková, J. & E. Eiselt. Longitudinal study of changes in anthropometric indicators and body composition in old men of various physical activity. *Human Biol.* 40: 331-44, 1968.
757.   Pářizková, J., E. Eiselt, S. Sprynarova & M. Wachtlova. Body composition, aerobic capacity and density of muscle capillaries in young and old men. *J. Appl. Physiol.* 31: 323-5, 1971.
758.   Parker, J.O., S. DiGiorgi & R.O. West. A haemodynamic study of coronary insufficiency precipitated by exercise. With observations on the effects of nitroglycerine. *Amer. J. Med.* 17: 470-83, 1966.
759.   Parker, S.R., C.G. Thomas, N.D. Ellis & W.E.T. McCarthy. *Effects of the redundancy payments act.* London: HMSO, 1971.
760.   Parkes, C.M. Psycho-physical transitions: a field for study. *Soc. Sci. and Med.* 5: 101-15, 1971.
761.   Patsch, J. Erfahrungen mit der Bestimmung der Diffusionkapazität der Lunge in Rühe und nach Belastung. *Wiener Med. Wschr.* 123: 435-8, 1973.
762.   Paul, P. Uptake and oxidation of substrates in the intact animal during exercise. In *Muscle metabolism during exercise,* ed. B. Pernow & B. Saltin, pp. 225-48. New York: Plenum Press, 1971.
763.   Pearl, R. *The rate of living: Being an account of some experimental studies on the biology of life duration.* New York: A.A. Knopf, 1928.
764.   Perley, M.M. & D.M. Kipnis. Differential plasma insulin responses to oral and infused glucose in normal weight and obese non-diabetic and diabetic subjects. *J. Lab. Clin. Med.* 66: 1009, 1965.
765.   Perley, M. & D.M. Kipnis. Plasma insulin responses to oral and intravenous glucose: studies in normal and diabetic subjects. *J. Clin. Invest.* 46: 1954-62, 1967.
766.   Perry, J. The mechanics of walking in hemiplegia. *Clin. Orthop. & Related Research* 63: 23-31, 1969.
767.   Pestalozza, G. & I. Shore. Clinical evaluation of presbyacusis on the basis of different test of auditory function. *Laryngol.* 65: 1136-63, 1955.
768.   Pett, L.B. & G.F. Ogilvie. The Canadian weight-height survey. *Human*

Biol. 28: 177-88, 1956.

769. Petty, T.L., G.A. Brink, M.W. Miller & P.R. Corsello. Objective functional improvement in chronic airway obstruction. *Chest* 57: 216-223, 1970.

770. Pickering, G.W. The peripheral resistance in persistent arterial hypertension *Clin. Sci.* 2: 209-35, 1936.

771. Pierce, A.K., P.N. Paez & W.F. Miller. Exercise training with the aid of a portable oxygen supply in patients with emphysema. *Amer. Rev. Resp. Dis.* 91: 653-9, 1965.

772. Pierce, A.K. & H.F. Taylor. Exercise training in the rehabilitation of patients with severe respiratory insufficiency due to pulmonary emphysema: The role of oxygen breathing. *Southern Med. J.* 55: 1216-21, 1962.

773. Pirie, A. Colour and solubility of the proteins of human cataracts. *Invest. Ophthalmol.* 7: 634-50, 1968.

774. Pitskelauri, G.Z. Some factors of longevity in Soviet Georgia. *Proc., 7th Int. Congress Gerontology*, Vienna, 26 June-July 2 1966.

775. Plutchik, R., H. Conte & M.B. Weiner. Studies on body image. II. Dollar values of body parts. *J. Gerontol.* 28: 89-91, 1973.

776. Plutchik, R., M.B. Weiner & H. Conte. Studies on body image. I. Body worries and body discomforts. *J. Gerontol.* 26: 334-50, 1971.

777. Polednak, A.P. Longevity and cause of death among Harvard College athletes and their class mates. *Geriatrics* 27: 53-64, 1972a.

778. Polednak, A.P. Longevity and cardiovascular mortality among former college athletes. *Circulation* 46: 649-54, 1972b.

779. Polednak, A.P. & A. Damon. College athletics, longevity and cause of death. *Human Biol.* 42: 28-46, 1970.

780. Pollock, M.L. The quantification of endurance training programs. In *Exercise and sport science reviews,* vol. 1, ed. J.H. Wilmore, pp. 155-88. New York: Academic Press, 1973.

781. Pollock, M.L. Physiological characteristics of older champion track athletes. *Res. Quart.* 45: 363-73, 1974.

782. Pollock, M.L., H.S. Miller, R. Janeway, A.C. Linnerud, B. Robertson & R. Valentino. Effects of walking on body composition & cardiovascular function of middle-aged men. *J. Appl. Physiol.* 30: 126-30, 1971.

783. Pollock, M.L., H.S. Miller, A.C. Linnerud & K.H. Cooper. Frequency of training as a determinant for improvement in cardiovascular function and body composition of middle-aged men. *Arch. Phys. Med. Rehab.* 56: 141-5, 1975.

784. Pomerance, A. Pathology of the heart with and without failure in the aged. *Brit. Heart. J.* 27: 697-710, 1965.

785. Pomeroy, W.C. & P.D. White. Coronary heart disease in former football players. *J. Amer. Med. Assoc.* 167: 711-16, 1958.

786. Popejoy, D.I. Unpublished doctoral dissertation. Univ. of Illinois, Urbana, 1967. Cited by R. Martens, 1972.

787. Post, F. Sex and its problems. IX. Disorders of sex in the elderly. *Practitioner* 199: 377-82, 1967.

788. Post, F. Learning from old age. *Proc. Roy. Soc. Med.* 63: 359-64, 1969.

789. Post, F. Psychiatric disorders. In *Textbook of geriatric medicine & gerontology*, ed. J.C. Brocklehurst, pp. 190-209. Edinburgh: Churchill-Livingstone, 1973.

790. Potter, W.A., S. Olafson & R.E. Hyatt. Ventilatory mechanics and expiratory flow limitation during exercise in patients with obstructive lung disease. *J. Clin. Invest.* 50: 910-19, 1971.

791. Powell, D.E.B., J.H. Thomas & P. Mills. Serum iron in elderly hospital patients. *Geront. Clin.* 10: 21-9, 1968.

792. Powell, R.R. Psychological effects of exercise therapy upon institu-

tionalized geriatric mental patients. *J. Gerontol.* 29: 157-61, 1974.

793.   President's Council on Fitness and Sports. National adult physical fitness survey. *Newsletter.* Special Ed. (May) pp. 1-27, 1973.

794.   Profant, G.R., R.G. Early, K.L. Nilson, F. Kusumi, V. Hofer & R.A. Bruce. Responses to maximal exercise in healthy middle-aged women. *J. Appl. Physiol.* 33: 595-9, 1972.

795.   Prout, C. Life expectancy of college oarsmen. *J. Amer. Med. Assoc.* 220: 1709-11, 1972.

796.   Pruett, E.D.R. Glucose and insulin during prolonged work stress in men living on different diets. *J. Appl. Physiol.* 28: 199-208, 1970.

797.   Pryor, W.A. Free radical reactions and their importance in biochemical systems. *Fed. Proc.* 32: 1862-9, 1973.

798.   Punsar, S., K. Pyolora & P. Siltanen. Classification of electrocardiographic S-T segment changes in epidemiological studies of coronary heart disease. *Ann. Med. Int. Fenn.* 57: 53-63, 1968.

799.   Pyorala, K., M.J. Karvonen, P. Taskinen, J. Takkunen & H. Kyronseppa. Cardiovascular studies on former endurance athletes. In *Physical activity and the heart,* ed. M.J. Karvonen & A.J. Barry, pp. 301-10. Springfield, Illinois: C.C. Thomas, 1967.

800.   Quetelet, A. *Sur l'homme et le developpement de ses facultés.* Paris: Bachelier Imprimeur-Libraire, 1835.

801.   Quigley, T.B. Life expectancy of Ivy-league rowing crews. *J. Amer. Med. Assoc.* 205: 652, 1968.

802.   Raab, W. Training, physical activity and the cardiac dynamic cycle. *J. Sports Med. Phys. Fitness* 6: 38-47, 1966.

803.   Rabbit, P.M.A. Age and time for choice between stimuli and between responses. *J. Gerontol.* 19: 307-12, 1964.

804.   Rabbit, P.M.A. Age and discrimination between complex stimuli. In *Behaviour, aging and the nervous system,* ed. A.T. Welford & J.E. Birren, pp. 35-53. Springfield, Illinois: C.C. Thomas, 1965.

805.   Raeder, S. Follow-up of the diabetic population in Bergen, Norway 1956-1966/68. *Nordic Council Arct. Med. Res. Rep.* 15: 19-21, 1976.

806.   Ralston, H.J. Some observations on energy expenditure and work tolerance of the geriatric subjects during locomotion. In *Conference on the geriatric amputee, Washington, 1961.* Washington NAS: NRC Publ. 919: 151-3, 1961.

807.   Ralston, H.J. Effects of immobilization of various body segments on the energy cost of human locomotion. *Ergonomics. Proc. 2nd Int. Ergonomics Assoc.* pp. 53-60. Dortmund: 1964.

808.   Reed, L.J. & A.G. Love. Biometric studies of U.S. army officers. I. Longevity in relation to physical fitness. *Proc. Amer. Life Convention,* May 1931.

809.   Reid, L. Chronic bronchitis and hypersecretion of mucus. *Lectures on the scientific basis of medicine.* 8: 235-55, 1960. London: Athlone Press (University of London).

810.   Reid, L. The aged lung. In *The pathology of emphysema.* London: Lloyd-Luke, 1967.

811.   Reindell, H., H. Klepzig, H. Steim, K. Musshof, H. Roskamm & E. Schildge. *Herz Kreislaufkrankheiten und Sport.* Munich: Johann Ambrosius Barth, 1960.

812.   Retzlaff, E. & J. Fontaine. Functional and structural changes in motor neurons with age. In *Behaviour, aging and the nervous system,* ed. A.T. Welford & J.E. Birren, pp. 340-52. Springfield, Illinois: C.C. Thomas, 1965.

813.   Réville, P. Sport for all. *Physical activity and the prevention of disease.* Strasbourg: Council of Europe, 1970.

814:    Richards, D.W. Pulmonary changes due to aging. In *Handbook of physiology*. Respiration, vol. II, ch. 66, pp. 1525-9. Washington DC: American Physiological Society, 1965.

815.   Richardson, I.M. *Age and need: a study of older people in North East Scotland*. London: Livingstone, 1964.

816.   Richardson, J.F. Heart rate in middle-aged men. *Amer. J. Clin. Nutr.* 24: 1476-81, 1971.

817.   Rice, D.P. Estimating the cost of illness. *Amer. J. Publ. Health* 57: 424-40, 1967.

818.   Ridge, M.D. & V. Wright. The aging of skin. *Gerontologia* 12: 174-92, 1966.

819.   Riley, C.P., A. Oberman, T.D. Lampton & D.C. Hurst. Submaximal exercise testing in a random sample of an elderly population. *Circulation* 42: 43-51, 1970.

820.   Rinzler, S.H. Primary prevention of coronary heart disease by diet. *Bull. N.Y. Acad. Med.* 44: 936-49, 1968.

821.   Rizzato G. & L. Marrazini. Thoracoabdominal mechanics in elderly men. *J. Appl. Physiol.* 28: 457-60, 1970.

822.   Robb, G.P. & H.H. Marks. Latent coronary artery disease. Determination of its presence and severity by the exercise electrocardiogram. *Amer. J. Cardiol.* 13: 603-18, 1964.

823.   Robb, G.P. & H.H. Marks. Post-exercise electrocardiogram in arteriosclerotic heart disease. *J. Amer. Med. Assoc.* 200: 918-26, 1967.

824.   Roberts, P.H., C.H. Kett & M.A. Ohlson. Nutritional status of older women; nitrogen, calcium, phosphorus retention of nine women. *J. Amer. Diet. Assoc.* 24: 292-9, 1948.

825.   Robertson, J.D. & D.D. Reid. Standards for the basal metabolism of normal people in Britain. *Lancet* i: 940, 1952.

826.   Robinson, S. Experimental studies of physical fitness in relation to age. *Arbeitsphysiol.* 4: 251, 1938.

827.   Robinson, S. Physical fitness in relation to age. In *Ageing of the lung*, ed. L. Cander & J.H. Moyer, pp. 287-301. New York: Grune & Stratton, 1964.

828.   Robinson, S., D.B. Dill, J.C. Ross, R.D. Robinson, J.A. Wagner & S.P. Tzankoff. Training and physiological aging in man. *Fed. Proc.* 32: 1628-34, 1972.

829.   Rochmis, P. & H. Blackburn. Exercise tests. A survey of procedures, safety, litigation experience in approximately 170,000 tests. *J. Amer. Med. Assoc.* 217: 1061-6, 1971.

830.   Rockstein, M. The role of molecular genetic mechanisms in the aging process. In *Molecular genetic mechanisms in development and aging*. New York: Academic Press, 1972.

831.   Rockstein, M. *The genetic basis for longevity. Theoretical aspects of aging*, pp. 1-10. New York: Academic Press, 1974.

832.   Rockstein, M. & K.F. Brandt. Changes in phosphorus metabolism of the gastrocnemius muscle in aging white rats. *Proc. Soc. Exp. Biol., N.Y.* 107: 377-80, 1961.

833.   Rodahl, K., N.C. Birkhead, J. Blizzard, B. Issekutz & E.D.R. Pruett. Physiological changes during prolonged bed rest. In *Nutrition and physical activity*, ed. G. Blix, p. 107. Stockholm: Almqvist & Wiksell, 1967.

834.   Rode, A. & R.J. Shephard. Cardiorespiratory fitness of an Arctic community. *J. Appl. Physiol.* 31: 519-26, 1971.

835.   Rode, A. & R.J. Shephard. Growth, development, and fitness of the Canadian Eskimo. In *Circumpolar Health*, ed. R.J. Shephard & S. Itoh, pp. 230-8. Toronto: University of Toronto Press, 1976.

836.   Rodstein, M. & F.D. Zeman. Postural blood pressure changes in the

330   References

eldery. *J. Chron. Dis.* 6: 581-8, 1957.
837.   Roessler, G.S. & B.G. Dunavant. Comparative evaluation of whole-body counter potassium[40] method for measuring lean body mass. *Amer. J. Clin. Nutr.* 20: 1171-8, 1967.
838.   Romo, M. Factors related to sudden death in acute ischaemic heart disease. A community study in Helsinki. *Acta. Med. Scand. Suppl.* 547: 7-92, 1972.
839.   Rook, A. An investigation into the longevity of Cambridge sportsmen. *Brit. Med. J.* i: 773-7, 1954.
840.   Root, A.W. & F.A. Oski. Effects of human growth hormone in elderly males. *J. Gerontol.* 24: 97-104, 1969.
841.   Rose, L.I., H.S. Friedman, S.C. Beering & K.H. Cooper. Plasma cortisol changes following a mile run in conditioned subjects. *J. Clin. Endocrinol.* 31: 339-41, 1970.
842.   Rosenberg, E. Effect of physical training on single breath diffusing capacity measured at rest. *Int. Z. angew. Physiol.* 24: 246-53, 1967.
843.   Rosin, A.J. & M.M. Glatt. Alcohol excess in the elderly. *Quart. J. Stud. Alcohol* 32: 53-9, 1971.
844.   Roskamm, H. Optimum patterns of exercise for healthy adults. In Proc. international symposium on physical activity & cardiovascular health, *Canad. Med. Assoc. J.* 96: 895-9, 1967.
845.   Rosow, I. Old people: their friends and neighbours. *Amer. Behav. Sci.* 14: (1) 56-69, 1970.
846.   Ross, M.H. Length of life and nutrition in the rat. *J. Nutrit.* 75: 197-210, 1961.
847.   Rothfels, K.H., E.B. Kupelwieser & R.C. Parker. Effects of X-irradiated feeder layers on mitotic activity and development of aneuploidy in mouse-embryo cells in vitro. *Canadian Cancer Conference* 5: 191-223, 1963.
848.   Rothman, R.H. & W.W.Parke. The vascular anatomy of the rotator cuff. *Clin. Orthop.* 14: 176-86, 1965.
849.   Rothman, R.H. & S. Slogoff. The effect of immobilization on the vascular bed of the tendon. *Surg. Gynecol. Obstet.* 122: 1064-6, 1967.
850.   Rousseau, M.F., L.A. Brasseur & J.M.R. Detry. Hemodynamic determinants of maximal oxygen intake in patients with healed myocardial infarction. *Circulation* 48: 943-9, 1973.
851.   Rowell, L.B. Visceral blood flow and metabolism during exercise. In *Frontiers of fitness*, ed. R.J. Shephard. Springfield, Illinois: C.C. Thomas, 1971.
852.   Rowlatt, C. & L.M. Franks. *Aging in tissues and cells.* Edinburgh: Churchill-Livingstone, 1973.
853.   Roy, C.S. The elastic properties of the arterial wall. *J. Physiol.* 3: 125-59, 1880.
854.   Roylance, P.J., I.R.A. Hanna & R.G. Tarbutt. Changes with age in the cell proliferation of rat bone marrow. *J. Anat.* 104: 191, 1969.
855.   Royce, J. Isometric fatigue curves in human muscle with normal and occluded circulation. *Res. Quart.* 29: 204-12, 1959.
856.   Rubin, I. *Sexual life after sixty.* London: George Allen & Unwin, 1966.
857.   Rübner, M. Das Wachsthumsproblem und die Lebensdauern des Menschen und einiger Säugethiere vom energetischen Standpunkte aus betrachtet. *Sber. Preuss. Akad. Wiss.* pp. 32-8, 1908.
858.   Rumball, A. & E.D. Acheson. Latent coronary heart disease detected by electro-cardiogram before and after exercise. *Brit. Med. J.* 5328: 423-8, 1963.
859.   Růžička, V. Beiträge zum Studium der Protoplasmahysteresis und der hysteretischen Vorgange (zur Kausalität des Alterns). I. Die Protoplasma-Hysteresis als Entropieerscheinung. *Arch. Mikr. Anat.* 101: 459-82, 1924.

860.   Ryan, A. Role of skills and rules in the prevention of sports injuries. In *Sports medicine*, ed. A.J. Ryan & F.L. Allman. New York: Academic Press, 1974.

861.   Ryhming, I. A modified Harvard step test for the evaluation of physical fitness. *Arbeitsphysiologie* 15: 235-50, 1953.

862.   Sacher, E.J., J. Finkelstein & L. Hellman. Growth hormone responses in depressive illnesses. *Arch. Gen. Psychiatr.* 25: 263-9, 1971.

863.   Sacher, G.A., D. Gralin, K. Hamilton, J. Gurian & S. Lesher. Survival of LAF mice exposed to Co^{60} γ rays for the duration of life at dosages of 6-20,000 r/day. *Radiat. Res.* 9: 175-6, 1958.

864.   Sachuk, N.N. The ageing worker's abilities and disabilities in relation to industrial production. In *Work and aging*, ed. J. Huet, pp. 147-62. Paris: Internat. Centre of Social Gerontology, 1971.

865.   Saltin, B. Energy metabolism in skeletal muscle fibres of man with exercise. In *Proceedings of XXth World congress of sports medicine*, ed. A.H. Toyne. Melbourne: Australian Sports Medicine Federation, 1974.

866.   Saltin, B. & G. Grimby. Physiological analysis of middle-aged and old former athletes. Comparison of still active athletes of the same ages. *Circulation* 38: 1104-15, 1968.

867.   Saltin, B., G. Blomqvist, J.H. Mitchell, R.L. Johnson, K. Wildenthal & C.B. Chapman. Response to exercise after bed rest and after training. *Amer. Heart Ass. Monograph No. 23*, pp. 1-68. Suppl. 7 to *Circulation*, vols. 37-8, 1968.

868.   Saltin, B., L.H. Hartley, Å. Kilböm & I. Åstrand. Physical training in sedentary middle-aged and older men. II. Oxygen uptake, heart rate, and blood lactate concentration at submaximal and maximal exercise. *Scand. J. Clin. Lab. Invest.* 24: 323-34, 1969.

869.   Salvosa, C.B., P.R. Payne & E.F. Wheeler. Energy expenditure of elderly people living alone or in local authority homes. *Amer. J. Clin. Nutr.* 24: 1467-70, 1971.

870.   Salzman, S.H., H.K. Hellerstein, J.D. Radke, H.W. Maistelman & R. Ricklin. Quantitative effects of physical conditioning on the exercise electrocardiogram of middle-aged subjects with arteriosclerotic heart disease. In *Measurement in exercise electrocardiography*, ed. H. Blackburn, chapter 23, pp. 388-410. Springfield, Illinois: C.C. Thomas, 1969.

871.   Sanne, H. & R. Sivertsson. The effect of exercise on the development of collateral circulation after experimental occlusion of the femoral artery in the cat. *Acta Physiol. Scand.* 73: 257-63, 1968.

872.   Sandhofer, F., F. Dienstl, K. Bolzano & H. Schwingschackl. Severe cardiovascular complication associated with prolonged starvation. *Brit. Med. J.* i: 462-3, 1973.

873.   Sauvy, A. The passage from activity to inactivity. In *First international course in gerontology*, ed. J.A. Huet, pp. 37-56. Paris: International Centre of Gerontology, 1970a.

874.   Sauvy, A. Demographic and economic aspects of the retirement problem. In *1st international course in social gerontology*, ed. J.A. Huet, pp. 15-36. Paris: Int. Centre of Social Gerontology, 1970b.

875.   Sawin, C.S., J.A. Rummel & E.L. Michel. Instrumental personal exercise during long duration space flights. *Aviat. Space Environ. Med.* 46: 394-400, 1975.

876.   Sayed, J., O. Schaefer, J.A. Hildes & M.A. Lobban. Biochemical indices of nutrient intake by Eskimos of Northern Foxe Basin, NWT. In *Circumpolar health*, ed. R.J. Shepard & S. Itoh. Toronto: University of Toronto Press, 1976.

877.   Schaer, H. Die periarthritis humeroscapularis. *Ergebnisse Chir. Orthop.* 21: 211-309, 1936.

878.   Schlesinger, Z., U. Goldbourt, J.H. Medalie, D. Oron, H.N. Neufeld & E. Riss. Pulmonary function ventilation values for healthy men aged 45 years and over. *Chest* 63: 520-4, 1973.

879.   Schmidt, C.D., M.L. Dickman, R.M. Gardner & F.K. Brough. Spirometric standards for healthy elderly men and women. 532 subjects, ages 55 through 94 years. *Amer. Rev. Resp. Dis.* 108: 933-9, 1973.

880.   Schmukler, M. & C.H. Barrows. Age differences in lactic and malic dehydrogenase in the rat. *J. Gerontol.* 21: 109-11, 1966.

881.   Schneider, H. *Die Abnutzungserkrankungen der Sehnen und ihre Therapie.* Stuttgart: Thieme, 1959.

882.   Schnohr, P. Longevity and causes of death in male athletic champions. *Lancet.* ii 1364-6, 1971.

883.   Schrijen, F. & V. Jezek. Constitution et maintien d'un état stable hémodynamique et ventilatoire au cours d'un exercise de 40 watts chez les pulmonaires chroniques. *Bull. Physiopath. Resp.* 6: 819-32, 1970.

884.   Schulze, W. *3rd international congress of gerontology,* London, p. 122, 1954. Cited by Durnin, 1973.

885.   Schwenger, C. *Future needs in retirement. National nutrition seminar, Toronto:* General Foods, Toronto, 1976.

886.   Scott, M.G. The contributions of physical activity to psychological development. *Res. Quart.* 31: 307, 1960.

887.   Seeman, P. The membrane actions of anesthetics and tranquilizers. *Pharm. Rev.* 24: 583-655, 1972.

888.   Selye, H. *Calciphylaxis.* Chicago, Illinois: University of Chicago Press, 1962.

889.   Semple, T. (ed.). *Myocardial infarction. How to prevent. How to rehabilitate.* Council of Rehabilitation, Int. Soc. of Cardiology, 1973.

890.   Shanas, E. Disengagement and work: myth and reality. In *Work and aging,* ed. J.A. Huet. Paris: International Centre of Social Gerontology, 1971a.

891.   Shanas, E. Measuring the home health needs of the aged in five countries. *J. Gerontol.* 26: 37-40, 1971b.

892.   Shanas, E., P. Townsend, D. Wedderburn, H. Friis, J. Stehouwer & P. Milhøj. *Old people in three industrial societies.* London: Routledge & Kegan Paul, 1968.

893.   Sheehan, G.A. Longevity of athletes. *Amer. Heart J.* 86: 425-6, 1973.

894.   Sheffield, L.T. & D. Roitman. Systolic blood pressure, heart rate & treadmill work at anginal threshold. *Chest* 63: 327-35, 1973.

895.   Sheldon, J.H. *The social medicine of old age.* London: Oxford University Press, 1948.

896.   Sheldon, J.H. On the natural history of falls in old age. *Brit. Med. J.* 5214: 1685-90, 1960.

897.   Shephard, R.J. World standards of cardiorespiratory performance. *Arch. Environ. Hlth.* 13: 664-72, 1966a.

898.   Shephard, R.J. Oxygen cost of breathing during vigorous exercise. *Quart. J. Exp. Physiol.* 51. 336-50, 1966b.

899.   Shephard, R.J. Intensity, duration and frequency of exercise as determinants of the response to a training regimen. *Int. Z. angew Physiol.* 26: 272-8, 1968a.

900.   Shephard, R.J. The heart and circulation under stress of Olympic conditions. *J. Amer. Med. Assoc.* 205: 150-5, 1968b.

901.   Shephard, R.J. Learning, habituation and training. *Int. Z. angew Physiol.* 28: 38-48, 1969a.

902.   Shephard, R.J. The working capacity of the older employee. *Arch. Environ. Hlth.* 18: 982-7, 1969b.

903. Shephard, R.J. Standard tests of aerobic power. In *Frontiers of fitness,* ed. R.J. Shephard, pp. 233-64. Springfield, Illinois: C.C. Thomas, 1971.
904. Shephard, R.J. *Alive man!* Springfield, Illinois: C.C. Thomas, 1972.
905. Shephard, R.J. Sudden death – a significant hazard of exercise? *Brit. J. Sports Med.* 8: 101-10, 1974.
906. Shephard, R.J. *Men at work. Applications of ergonomics to performance and design.* Springfield, Illinois: C.C. Thomas, 1974b.
907. Shephard, R.J. Future research on the quantifying of endurance training. *J. Hum. Ergol.* 3: 163-81, 1975.
908. Shephard, R.J. Exercise and chronic obstructive lung disease. *Exercise Sport Sci. Rev.* 4: 263-96, 1976.
909. Shephard, R.J. Do risks of exercise justify costly caution? *Physician & Sports Med.* 5: (2), 58-65, 1977a.
910. Shephard, R.J. Work physiology and activity patterns. In *IBP synthesis volume, Circumpolar peoples,* ed. F. Milan. Cambridge: Cambridge University Press, 1977b.
911. Shephard, R.J. *The fit athlete.* Oxford: Oxford University Press, 1977c.
912. Shephard, R.J. *Endurance fitness.* 2nd edition Toronto: University of Toronto Press, 1977d.
913. Shephard, R.J. *Human physiological work capacity. IBP human adaptability project,* Synthesis, vol. 4. Cambridge: Cambridge University Press, 1978.
914. Shephard, R.J. & J.R. Brown. Some observations on the fitness of a Canadian population. *Canad. Med. Assoc. J.* 98: 977-84, 1968.
915. Shephard, R.J., J. Hatcher & A. Rode. On the body composition of the Eskimo. *Europ. J. Appl. Physiol.* 32: 3-15, 1973.
916. Shephard, R.J., G. Jones, K. Ishii, M. Kaneko & A.J. Olbrecht. Factors affecting body density and thickness of subcutaneous fat. *Amer. J. Clin. Nutr.* 22: 1175-89, 1969.
917. Shephard, R.J. & T. Kavanagh. Predicting the exercise catastrophe in the post-coronary patient. *Canad. Fam. Phys.* In press, 1978.
918. Shephard, R.J. & T. Kavanagh. Characteristics of the master athlete. *Physician & Sports Med.* In press, 1978.
919. Shephard, R.J. & R. LaBarre. Attitudes of the public towards cigarette smoke in public places. *Can. J. Publ. Health.* In press, 1978.
920. Shephard, R.J. & K.H. Sidney. Effects of physical exercise on plasma growth hormone and cortisol levels in human subjects. *Ex. Sport Sci. Rev.* 3: 1-30, 1975.
921. Sheppard, H. The importance of the older worker in the economy of a nation (2). *Work and aging,* ed. J.A. Huet. Paris: Internat. Centre of Social Gerontology, 1971.
922. Shmavonian, B.M., A.J. Yarmat & S.I. Cohen. Relationships between the autonomic nervous system and central nervous system in age differences in behavior. In *Behaviour, aging and the nervous system,* ed. A.T. Welford & J.E. Birren, pp. 235-58. Springfield, Illinois: C.C. Thomas, 1965.
923. Shneidman, N.N. Soviet studies in the fitness of the aged. *Canad. Fam. Phys.* Oct. 1972.
924. Shock, N.W. Metabolism and age. *J. Chron. Dis.* 2: 687-703, 1955.
925. Shock, N.W. Physiological aspects of aging in man. *Ann. Rev. Physiol.* 23: 97-166, 1961.
926. Shock, N.W. An essay on aging. In *Ageing of the lung,* ed. L. Cander & J.H. Moyer, pp. 1-12. New York: Grune & Stratton, 1964.
927. Shock, N.W. Physical activity and the 'rate of ageing'. In: Proc. of international symposium on physical activity and cardiovascular health. *Canad. Med. Assoc. J.* 96: 836-42, 1967.

928.   Shock, N.W. & A.H. Norris. Neuromuscular coordination as a factor in age changes in muscular exercise. In *Physical activity and aging*, ed. D. Brunner & E. Jokl. Baltimore, Md.: University Park Press, 1970.

929.   Shreeve, W.W. Transfers of carbon -14 and tritium from substrates to CO_2, water, and lipids in obese and diabetic subjects in vivo. *Ann. N.Y. Acad. Sci.* 131: 464-75, 1965.

930.   Shuey, C.B., A.K. Pierce & R.L. Johnson. An evaluation of exercise tests in chronic obstructive pulmonary disease. *J. Appl. Physiol.* 25: 21-7, 1968.

931.   Sidney, K.H. Responses of elderly subjects to a program of progressive exercise training. Ph.D. Thesis – University of Toronto, 1976.

932.   Sidney, K.H. & R.J. Shephard. Maximum and submaximum exercise tests in men and women in the seventh, eighth and ninth decades of life. *J. Appl. Physiol.* 43: 280-7, 1977.

933.   Sidney, K.H. & R.J. Shephard. Attitudes towards health and physical activity in the elderly. Effects of a physical training programme. *Med. Sci. Sports* 8: 246-52, 1977a.

934.   Sidney, K.H. & R.J. Shephard. Perception of exertion in the elderly. Effects of aging, mode of exercise and physical training. *Percept. Motor Skills* 44: 999-1010, 1977b.

935.   Sidney, K.H. & R.J. Shephard. Frequency and intensity of exercise training for elderly subjects. *Med. Sci. Sports.* In press, 1978a.

936.   Sidney, K.H. & R.J. Shephard. Growth hormone and cortisol – age differences, effects of exercise and training. *Can. J. Appl. Sports Sci.* In press, 1978b.

937.   Sidney, K.H. & R.J. Shephard. Activity patterns of elderly men and women. *J. Gerontol.* 32: 25-32, 1977c.

938.   Sidney, K.H. & R.J. Shephard. Training and e.c.g. abnormalities in the elderly. *Brit. Heart J.* 39: 1114-20, 1977d.

939.   Sidney, K.H., R.J. Shephard & J. Harrison. Endurance training and body composition of the elderly. *Amer. J. Clin. Nutr.* 30: 326-33, 1977.

940.   Silver, H.M. & M. Landowne. The relation of age to certain electro-cardiographic responses of normal adults to a standardized exercise. *Circulation* 8: 510-20, 1953.

941.   Silverstone, F.A., M. Brandfonbrener, N.W. Shock & M.J. Yiengst. Age differences in the intravenous glucose tolerance tests and the response to insulin. *J. Clin. Invest.* 36: 504-14, 1957.

942.   Simms, H.S. The use of a measurable cause of death (heamorrhage) for the evaluation of aging. *J. Gen. Physiol.* 26: 169-78, 1942.

943.   Simons, P. & L. Reid. Muscularity of pulmonary artery branches in the upper and lower lobes of the normal young and aged lung. *Brit. J. Dis. Chest* 63: 38-44, 1969.

944.   Simonson, E. Changes in physical fitness and cardiovascular functions with age. *Geriatrics* 12: 28-39, 1957.

945.   Simonson, E. Functional capacities of older individuals. *J. Gerontol.* 13 (Suppl. 2): 18, 1958.

946.   Simonson, E. *Physiology of work capacity & fatigue*. Springfield, Illinois: C.C. Thomas, 1971.

947.   Simonson, E., W.M. Kearns & N. Enzer. Effects of methyl testosterone treatment on muscular performance and the central nervous system of older men. *J. Clin. Endocrin. Metab.* 4: 528-34, 1944.

948.   Simonson, E. & A. Keys. Working capacity in patients with orthopedic handicaps from poliomyelitis. *Amer. J. Physiol.* 151: 405-14, 1947.

949.   Simmons, R. & R.J. Shephard. Effects of physical conditioning upon the central and peripheral circulatory responses to arm work. *Int. Z. angew*

Physiol. 30: 73-84, 1971a.
950.   Simmons, R. & R.J. Shephard. Measurement of cardiac output in maximum exercise. *Int. Z. angew Physiol.* 29: 159-72, 1971b.
951.   Sinclair, H.M. Assessment and results of obesity. *Brit. Med. J.* (ii): 1404-7, 1953.
952.   Sinex, F.M. The mutation theory of aging. In *Theoretical aspects of aging,* ed. M. Rockstein. New York: Academic Press, 1974.
953.   Singer, A. & C. Rob. The fate of the claudicator. *Brit. Med. J.* ii: 633-6, 1960.
954.   Siperstein, M.D. In *Pathogenesis of diabetes mellitus,* ed. E. Cerasi & R. Luft, p. 81. New York: Wiley, 1970.
955.   Sjöstrand, T. The relationship between the heart frequency and the ST level of the electrocardiogram. *Acta Med. Scand.* 138: 200-10, 1950.
956.   Skerlj, B., J. Brozek & F.E. Hunt. Subcutaneous fat and age changes in body build and body form in women. *Amer. J. Phys. Anthropol.* 11: 577-600, 1953.
957.   Skinner, J.S. The cardiovascular system with aging and exercise. In *Medicine and sport,* vol. 4. *Physical activity and aging,* ed. D. Brunner & E. Jokl, pp. 100-8. Basel: Karger, 1970.
958.   Skrobak-Kaczynski, J. & T. Lewin. Secular changes in Lapps of Northern Finland. In *Circumpolar health,* ed. R.J. Shephard & S. Itoh, pp. 239-47. Toronto: University of Toronto Press, 1976.
959.   Smith, D.A., I. Harrison, B.E.C. Nordin, J. MacGregor & M. Jordan. Mineral metabolism in relation to ageing. *Proc. Nutr. Soc.* 27: 201-10, 1968.
960.   Smith, E.B. The influence of age and atherosclerosis on the chemistry of aortic intima. Part 1. The lipids. *J. Atheroscler. Res.* 5: 224-40, 1965.
961.   Smith, E.L. Bone, changes with age and physical activity. Unpublished Ph.D. dissertation, University of Madison, Wisconsin, 1971.
962.   Smith, E.L. & S.W. Babcock. Effects of physical activity on bone loss in the aged. Abstract 20th annual meeting of the Amer. College Sports Med., Seattle. *Med. Sci. Sports* 5: 68, 1973.
963.   Society of Actuaries. *Build and blood pressure study.* Chicago, Illinois: 1959.
964.   Soll, A.H., C.R. Kahn, D.M. Neville & J. Roth. Insulin receptor deficiency in genetic and acquired obesity. *J. Clin. Invest.* 56: 769-80, 1975.
965.   Sonka, J.I., I. Gregorova, Z. Tomosova, A. Pavlova, A. Zbirkova, R. Rath, J. Urbanek & M. Josifko. Plasma androsterone, dehydroepiandrosterone and 11-hydroxycorticoids in obesity. *Steroid Lipid Res.* 3: 65-74, 1972.
966.   Sorenson, J.A. & J.R. Cameron. A reliable in vivo measurement of bone-mineral content. *J. Bone Joint Surg.* 49: 481-97, 1967.
967.   Southgate, D.A.T. & J.V.G.A. Durnin. Calorie conversion factors. An experimental reassessment of the factors used in the calculation of the energy value of human diet. *Brit. J. Nutr.* 24: 517-35, 1970.
968.   Spain, D.M., D.F. Nathan & M. Gelles. Weight, body type and the prevalence of coronary atherosclerotic heart disease in males. *Amer. J. Med. Sci.* 245: 63-9, 1963.
969.   Speigel, P.M. Theories of aging. In *Developmental physiology and aging,* ed. P.S. Timiras. New York: Macmillan, 1972.
970.   Spencer, I.O.B. Death during therapeutic starvation for obesity. *Lancet* i: 1288-90, 1968.
971.   Spira, E. Orthopedic observations with physically active elderly subjects. In *Physical activity and aging.* Baltimore, Md.: University Park Press, 1970.
972.   Spiro, S.G., H.L. Hahn, R.L.T. Edwards & N.B. Pride. Cardio-

respiratory adaptations at the start of exercise in normal subjects and patients with chronic obstructive bronchitis. *Clin. Sci.* 47: 165-72, 1974.

973.   Spiro, S.G., H.L. Hahn, R.L.T. Edwards & N.B. Pride. An analysis of the physiological strain of submaximal exercise in patients with chronic obstructive bronchitis. *Thorax* 30: 415-25, 1975.

974.   Spitaels, G. The attitude of the working world with regard to the problems of age and retirement. In *Work and aging*, ed. J.A. Huet, pp. 55-72. Paris: International Centre of Social Gerontology, 1971.

975.   Stamford, B.A. Physiological effects of training upon institutionalized geriatric men. *J. Gerontol.* 27: 451-5, 1972.

976.   Stamford, B.A. Effects of chronic institutionalization on the physical working capacity and trainability of geriatric men. *J. Gerontol.* 28: 441-6, 1973.

977.   Stamford, B.A., W. Hambacker & A. Fallica. Effects of a daily physical exercise on the psychiatric state of institutionalized geriatric mental patients. *Res. Quart.* 45: 34-41, 1974.

978.   Stamler, J., D.M. Berksom & H.A. Lindberg. In *The pathogenesis of atherosclerosis*, chapter 3, ed. R.W. Wissler & J. Greer. Baltimore: Williams & Wilkins, 1972.

979.   Stamler, J., R. Stamler & T.N. Pullman. *The epidemiology of hypertension.* New York: Grune & Stratton, 1967.

980.   Starr, I. An essay on the strength of the heart and on the effect of aging upon it. *Amer. J. Cardiol.* 14: 771-83, 1964.

981.   Statistics Canada Survey (Unpublished 1972). Preliminary findings reported in Medical Post, 1972.

982.   Stauffacher, W., O.B. Crofford, B. Jeanrenaud & A.E. Renold. Comparative studies of muscle and adipose tissue metabolism in lean and obese mice. *Ann. N.Y. Acad. Sci.* 131: 528-40, 1965.

983.   Stehouwer, L.J. The role of the family and the community in the care of the elderly. In *Symposium on research and welfare policies for the elderly.* New York. United Nations, 1970.

984.   Stein, D. Arlidin. A clinical evaluation of a peripheral vasodilator with selective action on the muscle vessels. *Ann. Int. Med.* 45: 185, 1956.

985.   Steina, A. (1970). Cited by Beverfelt, 1971.

986.   Steinhardt, R.W., F.D. Zeman, J. Tuckman & I. Lorge. Appraisal of physical and mental health of the elderly: use of Cornell Medical Index and supplementary health questionnaire. *J. Amer. Med. Assoc.* 151: 378, 1953.

987.   Stelmach, G.E. & G.L. Diewert. Aging, information processing and fitness. In *Physical work and effort*, ed. G. Borg. Oxford: Pergamon Press, 1977.

988.   Stevenson, J.A.F. Exercise, food intake and health in experimental animals. *Canad. Med. Assoc. J.* 96: 862-6, 1967.

989.   Stevenson, J.A.F., B.M. Box, V. Feleki & J.R. Beaton. Bouts of exercise and food intake in the rat. *J. Appl. Physiol.* 21: 118-222, 1966.

990.   Stiles, M.H. Motivation for sports participation in the community. In Proc. of international symposium on physical activity and cardiovascular health. *Canad. Med. Assoc. J.* 96: 889-92, 1967.

991.   Stoboy, H., B.W. Rich & M. Lee. Workload and energy expenditure during wheelchair propelling. *Paraplegia* 8: 223-30, 1971.

992.   Stokes, W.R. Sexual functioning in the aging male. *Geriatrics* 6: 304-8, 1951.

993.   Strandell, T. Circulation during exercise in healthy old men. In *Physical fitness in relation to age & sex*, proceedings of a scientific seminar, Stockholm, 1962.

994.   Strandell, T. Circulatory studies in healthy old men. *Acta Med. Scand.*

Suppl. 141: 1-44, 1964a.

995. Strandell, T. Heart rate and work load at maximal working intensity in old men. *Acta Med. Scand.* 176: 301-18, 1964b.

996. Strandell, T. Total hemoglobin, blood volume and hemoglobin concentrations at rest and circulatory adaptation during exercise in relation to some anthropometric data in old men compared with young men. *Acta. Med. Scand.* 176: 219-32, 1964c.

997. Strandell, T. Heart rate, arterial lactate concentration and oxygen uptake during exercise in old men compared with young men. *Acta Physiol. Scand.* 60: 197-216, 1964d.

998. Strehler, B.L., D.D. Marks, A.S. Mildvan & M.V. Gee. Rate and magnitude of age pigment accumulation in the human myocardium. *J. Gerontol.* 14: 430-9, 1959.

999. Sundström, G. Influence of body position on pulmonary diffusing capacity in young and old men. *J. Appl. Physiol.* 38: 418-23, 1975.

1000. Suter, F. Ueber das Verhalten des Aortenumfanges unter physiologischen und pathologischen Bedingungen. *Arch. f. Exp. Path. u. Pharmakol.* 39: 289-332, 1897.

1001. Sutton, J.R., M.J. Coleman, J. Casey & L. Lazarus. Androgen responses during physical exercise. *Brit. Med. J.* (i): 520-22, 1973.

1002. Sutton, J.R., J.D. Young, L. Lazarus, J.B. Hickie & J. Maksvytis. The hormonal response to physical exercise. *Aust. Ann. Med.* 18: 84-90, 1969.

1003. Swendseid, M.E. & S.G. Tuttle. *Publicn. Nat. Res. Counc. Washington*, 843: 1969. Cited by Durnin, 1973.

1004. Sylven, B. & H. Malmgren. On alleged metachromasia of hyaluronic acid. *Lab. Invest.* 1: 413-31, 1952.

1005. Szafran, J. Decision processes and ageing. In *Behaviour, aging and the nervous system*, ed. A.T. Welford & J.E. Birren, pp. 21-34. Springfield, Illinois: C.C. Thomas, 1965.

1006. Szanto, S. Metabolic studies in physically outstanding elderly men. *Age & Ageing* 4: 37-42, 1975.

1007. Szilard, L. On the nature of the aging process. *Proc. Nat. Acad. Sci.* 45: 30-45, 1959.

1008. Tabakin, B.S., J.S. Hanson & A.M. Levy. Effects of physical training on the cardiovascular and respiratory response to graded upright exercise in distance runners. *Brit. Heart. J.* 27: 205-10, 1965.

1009. Talland, G.A. Effect of aging on the formation of sequential and spatial concepts. *Percept. Motor Skills* 13: 210, 1961.

1010. Tanner, J.M. *Growth at adolescence*, 2nd ed. Oxford: Blackwell Scientific Publications, 1962.

1011. Tanner, J.M. *The physique of the Olympic athlete*. London: Allen & Unwin, 1964.

1012. Taylor, G.F. A clinical survey of elderly people from a nutritional standpoint. In *Vitamins in the elderly*, ed. A.N. Exton-Smith & D.L. Scott, pp. 51-6. Bristol: J. Wright, 1968.

1013. Taylor, H.L., H.L. Blackburn, A. Keys, R.W. Parlin, C. Vasquez & T. Puchner. Coronary heart disease in seven countries. IV. Five-year follow-up of employees of selected U.S. railroad companies. *Circulation* 41, Suppl, I: 20-39, 1970.

1014. Taylor, H.L., A. Henschel, J. Brozek & A. Keys. The effect of bed rest on cardiovascular function and work performance. *J. Appl. Physiol.* 2: 223-39, 1949.

1015. Taylor, H.L., R.W. Parlin, H. Blackburn & A. Keys. Problems in the analysis of the relationship of coronary heart disease to physical activity or its lack, with special reference to sample size and occupational withdrawal. In *Physical activity in health and disease,* ed. K. Evang & K.L. Andersen. Baltimore: Williams & Wilkins, 1966.

1016. Taylor, J.A. A personality scale of manifest anxiety. *J. Abnormal Soc. Psych.* 48: 285-90, 1953.

1017. Taylor, R.R., J.W. Covell & J. Ross. Influence of the thyroid state on left ventricular tension-velocity relations in the intact, sedated dog. *J. Clin. Invest.* 48: 775-84, 1969.

1018. Tenney, S.M. & R.M. Miller. Dead space ventilation in old age. *J. Appl. Physiol.* 9: 321-7, 1956.

1019. Teraslinna, P., T. Partanen, P. Oja & A. Koskela. Some social characteristics and living habits associated with willingness to participate in a physical activity intervention study. *J. Sports Med.* 10: 138-44, 1970.

1020. Theorell, H., M. Béznak, R. Bonnichsen, K.G. Paul & A. Åkeson. On the distribution of injected radioactive iron in guinea pigs and its rate of appearance in some hemoproteins and ferritins. *Acta Chem. Scand.* 5: 445-75, 1951.

1021. Thomae, H. & U. Lehr. *Altern. Probleme und Tatsachen.* Frankfurt, 1968. Cited by Fulgraff, 1971.

1022. Thompson, W.E. & G.W. Streib. Situational determinants: Health and economic deprivation in retirement. *J. Soc. Issues* 14: (2): 18-34, 1958.

1023. Timiras, P.S. *Developmental physiology and aging.* ch. 28. New York: Macmillan, 1972.

1024. Timiras, P.S. & A. Vernadakis. Structural, biochemical and functional aging of the nervous system. In *Developmental physiology and aging.* New York: Macmillan, 1972.

1025. Tissue, T. Another look at self-rated health among the elderly. *J. Gerontol.* 27: 91-4, 1972.

1026. Tlusty, L. Physical fitness in old age. I. Aerobic capacity and other parameters of physical fitness followed by means of exercise in ergometric examination of elderly individuals. *Respiration* 26: 161-81, 1969a.

1027. Tlusty, L. Physical fitness in old age. II. Anaerobic capacity, anaerobic work in graded exercise, recovery after maximum work performance in elderly individuals. *Respiration* 26: 287-99, 1969b.

1028. Toscani, A. Physiology of muscular work in the aged. In *Work and aging. Second int. course in social gerontology*, ed. J.A. Huet, pp. 185-220. Paris: Int. Centre of Social Gerontology, 1971.

1029. Toth, S.E. The origin of lipofuscin age pigments. *Exptl. Gerontol.* 3: 19-30, 1968.

1030. Townsend, P. *The needs of the elderly and the planning of hospitals.* Cited by Wedderburn, 1973.

1031. Townsend, P. (1957). Cited by Munnicks, J.M.A. & A. Bigot. Psychology of aging, long-term illness and death. In *Textbook of geriatric medicine and gerontology*, ed. J.C. Brocklehurst. Edinburgh: Churchill-Livingstone, 1973b.

1032. Trotter, M. & R.R. Peterson. Ash weight of human skeletons in per cent of their dry, fat-free weight. *Anat. Rec.* 123: 341-58, 1955.

1033. Tunbridge, R.E. & J.H. Wetherill. Reliability and cost of diabetic diets. *Brit. Med. J.* ii: 78-80, 1970.

1034. Tunstall, J. *Old and alone*, pp. 64-72. London: Routledge & Kegan Paul, 1966.

1035. Turino, G.M., M. Brandfonbrener & A.P. Fishman. The effect of changes in ventilation and pulmonary blood flow on the diffusing capacity of the lung. *J. Clin. Invest.* 38: 1186-201, 1959.

1036. Turner, J.M., J. Mead & M.E. Wohl. Elasticity of human lungs in relation to age. *J. Appl. Physiol.* 25: 664-71, 1968.

1037. Turpeinen, O., M. Miettinen, M.J. Karvonen, P. Roine, M. Pekkarinen, E.J. Lehtosuo & P. Alivirta. Dietary prevention of coronary heart disease: long term experiment. I. Observations on male subjects. *Amer. J. Clin. Nutr.* 21: 255-76, 1968.

1038. Tuttle, S.G., S.H. Bassett, W.H. Griffith, D.B. Mulcare & M.E. Swendseid. Further observations on the aminoacid requirements of older men. II. Methionine and lysine. *Amer. J. Clin. Nutr.* 16: 229-31, 1965.

1039. Tzankoff, S.P., S. Robinson, F.S. Pyke & C.A. Brawn. Physiological adjustments to work in older men as affected by physical training. *J. Appl. Physiol.* 33: 346-50, 1972.

1040. Ufland, J.M. Einfluss des Lebensalters, Geschlechts, der Konstitution und des Berufs auf die Kraft verschiedenen Muskelgruppen. I. Mitteilung über den Einfluss des Lebensalters auf die Muskelkraft. *Arbeitsphysiol.* 6: 653-63, 1933.

1041. U.S. Department of Health, Education and Welfare Reports. Hearing levels of adults by age and sex. U.S.A. 1960-1962. *Nat. Cent. for Health Stat. Series* 11: (11), 1965.

1042. United States Senate. A Report of the Special Committee on Aging. *Developments in aging. Every tenth American*, p. 21. Report 92-784, 1972.

1043. Van Mervenne. Life span of athletes. *Ned. Tidj. Voor Geneslskunde* 85: 535-43, 1941.

1044. Vedin, J.A., C.D. Wilhelmsson, L. Wilhelmsen, J. Bjure & B. Ekström-Jodal. Relation of resting and exercise-induced ectopic beats to other ischaemic manifestations and to coronary risk factors. Men born in 1913. *Amer. J. Cardiol.* 30: 25-30, 1972.

1045. Verzár, F. Aging of the collagen fiber. *Int. Rev. Conn. Tiss. Res.* 2: 244-300, 1964.

1046. Viidik, A. Experimental evaluation of the tensile strength of isolated rabbit tendons. *Bio. Med. Engng.* 2: 64-7, 1967.

1047. Vitali, M. & R.G. Redhead. The modern concept of the general management of amputee rehabilitation. *Ann. Roy. Coll. Surg. Engl.* 40: (4), 251-60, 1967.

1048. Viru, A. & H. Akke. Effects of muscular work on cortisol and corticosterone content in the blood and adrenals of guinea pigs. *Acta Endocrinol. (Copenhagen)* 62: 385-90, 1969.

1049. Vogt, C. & O. Vogt. Aging of nerve cells. *Nature* 158: 304, 1946.

1050. Voigt, E-D. Discussion in: Rehabilitation von Patienten mit orthopädischen Erkrankungen und posttraumatischen Schäden. In *10 Jahre Rehabilitation als Schlüssel zum Dauerarbeitsplatz*, pp. 259-65. Stuttgart: Gentner Verlag, 1968.

1051. Von Euler, U.S. Sympatho-adrenal activity in physical exercise. *Med. Sci. Sports* 6: 165-73, 1974.

1052. Vranic, M., R. Kawamori & G.A. Wrenshall. The role of insulin and glucagon in regulating glucose turnover in dogs during exercise. *Med. Sci. Sports* 7: 27-33, 1975.

1053. Vyas, M.N., E.W. Banister, J.W. Morton & S. Grzybowski. Response to exercise in patients with chronic lung disease. *Amer. Rev. Resp. Dis.* 110: 395-402, 1974.

1054. Wade, G. & J.M. Bishop. *Cardiac output and regional blood flow.* Oxford: Blackwell, 1962.

1055. Wagenvoort, C.A. & N. Wagenvoort. Age changes in muscular pulmonary arteries. *Arch. Path.* 79: 524-8, 1965.

1056. Wagner, J.A., S. Robinson & R.P. Marino. Age and temperature regulation of humans in neutral and cold environments. *J. Appl. Physiol.* 37: 562-5, 1974.

1057. Wahren, J., P. Felig, J. Ahlborg & L. Jorfeldt. Glucose metabolism during leg exercise in man. *J. Clin. Invest.* 50: 2715-25, 1971.

1058. Wahren, J., P. Felig, R. Hendler & G. Ahlborg. Glucose and amino acid metabolism during recovery after exercise. *J. Appl. Physiol.* 34: 838-45, 1973.

1059. Wahren, J., B. Saltin, L. Jorfeldt & B. Pernow. Influence of age on the local circulatory adaptation to leg exercise. *J. Clin. Lab. Invest.* 33: 79-86, 1974.

1060. Wakefield, M.C. A study of mortality among the men who have played in the Indiana High School State Final basketball tournaments. *Res. Quart.* 15: 3-11, 1944.

1061. Walford, R.L. *The immunologic theory of aging.* Copenhagen: Munksgaard, 1964.

1062. Wallace, J.G. Some studies of perception in relation to age. *Brit. J. Psychol.* 47: 283-97, 1956.

1063. Warren, R. & R.B. Kihn. A survey of lower extremity amputations for ischaemia. *Surgery* 63: 107-20, 1968.

1064. Warren, S. Longevity and cause of death from irradiation in physicians. *J. Amer. Med. Assoc.* 162: 464-8, 1956.

1065. Wasserman, K., B.J. Whipp, S.N. Koyal & W.L. Beaver. Anaerobic threshold and respiratory gas exchange during exercise. *J. Appl. Physiol.* 35: 236-43, 1973.

1066. Watkin, D.M. In *Mammalian protein metabolism*, vol. 2, chapter 17, ed. H.N. Monro & J.B. Allison, pp. 247-63. New York: Academic Press, 1964.

1067. Watson, J.D. & F.H.C. Crick. Molecular structure of nucleic acids. A structure for deoxyribose nucleic acid. *Nature* 171: 737-8, 1953.

1068. Watts, J.H., A.N. Mann, L. Bradley, *et al.* Nitrogen balances of men over 65 fed the FAO and milk patterns of essential amino acids. *J. Gerontol.* 19: 370-4, 1964.

1069. Watts, J.H., A.N. Mann, L. Bradley, D.J. Thompson. Hypothermia in the aged: a study of the rôle of cold sensitivity. *Env. Research* 5: 119-26, 1972.

1070. Weale, R.A. Retinal illumination and age. *Trans. Illum. Eng. Soc.* 26: 95-100, 1961.

1071. Weale, R.A. On the eye. In *Behaviour, aging and the nervous system,* ed. A.T. Welford & J.E. Birren, pp. 307-25. Springfield, Illinois: C.C. Thomas, 1965.

1072. Wechsler, D. *The measurement and appraisal of adult intelligence.* Baltimore: Williams & Wilkins, 1958.

1073. Wedderburn, D. The aged and society. In *Textbook of geriatric medicine & gerontology,* ed. J.C. Brocklehurst, pp. 692-717. Edinburgh: Churchill-Livingstone, 1973.

1074. Weg, R.B. Sexual inadequacy in the elderly. In *The physiology and pathology of human aging,* ed. R. Goldman & M. Rockstein. New York: Academic Press, 1975.

1075. Weinblatt, E., S. Shapiro & C.W. Frank. Prognosis of women with newly diagnosed coronary heart disease – a comparison with course of disease among men. *Amer. J. Publ. Health* 63: 577-93, 1973.

1076. Weiner, J.S. & J.A. Lourie. *Human biology. A guide to field methods.* Oxford: Blackwell, 1969.

1077. Weiss, A.D. Sensory functions. In *Handbook of aging and the individual.* ed. J.E. Birren, pp. 503-42. Chicago: University of Chicago Press, 1959.

1078. Welford, A.T, Performance, biological mechanisms and age: a theoretical sketch. In *Behaviour, aging and the nervous system,* ed. A.T. Welford & J.E. Birren, pp. 3-20. Springfield, Illinois: C.C. Thomas, 1965.

1079. Welford, A.T. Age and skill: motor, intellectual and social. *Gerontologia* 4: 1-22, 1969.

1080. Welford, A.T. & J.E. Birren. *Behaviour, aging and the nervous system.* Springfield, Illinois: C.C. Thomas, 1973.

1081. Wessel, J.A., D.A. Small, W.D. Van Huss, D.J. Anderson & D.S. Cederquist. Age and physiological responses to exercise in women 20-69 years of age. *J. Gerontol.* 23: 269-78, 1968.

1082. Wessel, J.A., D.A. Small, W.D. Van Huss, W.W. Heusner & D.C. Cederquist. Functional responses to submaximal exercise in women 20-69 years. *J. Gerontol.* 21: 168-81, 1966.

1083. Wessel, J.A., A. Ufer, W.D. Van Huss & D. Cederquist. Age trends of various components of body composition and functional characteristics of women aged 20-69 years. *Ann. N.Y. Acad. Sci.* 110: 608-22, 1963.

1084. Wessel, J.A. & W.D. Van Huss. The influence of physical activity and age on exercise adaptation of women, 20-69 years. *J. Sports Med.* 9: 173-80, 1969.

1085. Westlund, K. *Mortality of diabetics.* Oslo: Universitetsforlaget, 1969.

1086. Westura, E.E. & J.A. Ronan. Comparison of heart rate, oxygen consumption and electrocardiographic responses to submaximal step exercise and near maximal exercise on a treadmill and bicycle ergometer. In *Measurement in exercise electrocardiography. The Ernst Simonson conference*, ed. H. Blackburn, pp. 342-62. Springfield, Illinois: C.C. Thomas, 1969.

1087. Whisnant, J.P., J.P. Fitzgibbons, L.T. Kurland & G.P. Sayre. Natural history of stroke in Rochester, Minnesota 1945 through 1954. *Stroke* 2: 11-22, 1971.

1088. Widdowson, E.M. & G.C. Kennedy. Rate of growth, mature weight and life span. *Proc. Roy. Soc. B.* 156: 96-108, 1962.

1089. Wikland, B. Medically unattended fatal cases of ischaemic heart disease in a defined population. *Acta Med. Scand.* 524: 3-78, 1971.

1090. Wilens, S.L. The post-mortem elasticity of the adult human aorta. Its relation to age and to the distribution of atheroma. *Amer. J. Path.* 13: 811-34, 1937.

1091. Wilkins, L.T. *The prevalence of deafness in the population of England, Scotland and Wales.* London: Central Office of Information, 1947.

1092. Will, G. & B.M. Groden. Benign hypochronic anaemia in the adult male. *Scot. Med. J.* 10: 21-3, 1965.

1093. Williams, W.E., D. Webster, M.P. Dixon & W. MacKenzie. Red cell longevity in old age. *Gerontol. Clin.* 4: 183-93, 1962.

1094. Williamson, J. Aging in modern society. *Proc. Roy. Soc. Health*, Edinburgh: 9 Nov. 1966.

1095. Wilmore, J., J. Royce, R. Girandola, F. Katch & V. Katch. Physiological alterations resulting from a 10-week program of jogging. *Med. Sci. Sports* 2: 7-14, 1970.

1096. Wilson, D.L. The programmed theory of aging. In *Theoretical aspects of aging*, ed. M. Rockstein, pp. 11-21. New York: Academic Press, 1974.

1097. Wilson, R.H., R.S. Meador, B.E. Jay & E. Higgins. The pulmonary pathologic physiology of persons who smoke cigarettes. *New Engl. J. Med.* 262: 956-61, 1960.

1098. Wilson, R.H.L. & N.L. Wilson. Obesity and cardiorespiratory stress. In *Obesity*, ed. N.L. Wilson, pp. 141-51. Philadelphia: F.A. Davis, 1969.

1099. Wirths, Von W. Die Relation von Arbeits und Grundumsatz zum Gesamtumsatz bei alteren Personen mit körperlicher Belastung. *Gerontologia* 8: 209-32, 1963.

1100. Wissler, R.W., D. Vesselinovitch, R. Hughes & T. Roth. Atherosclerosis and blood lipids in rhesus monkeys confined in a widely varying space. *Fed. Proc.* 28: 447, 1969.

1101. Wolf, E., D. Tzivoni & S. Stern. Comparison of exercise tests and 24 hour ambulatory electrocardiographic monitoring in detection of ST-T changes. *Brit. Heart J.* 36: 90-95, 1974.

1102. Wood, V., M.L. Wylie & B. Sheafor. An analysis of a short self-report measure of life satisfaction: correlation with rater judgements. *J. Gerontol.* 24: 465-9, 1969.

1103. Woolf, C.R. & J.T. Suero. Alteration in lung mechanics following training in chronic obstructive lung disease. *Dis. Chest.* 55: 37-44, 1969.

1104. Woolf, C.R. A rehabilitation programme for improving exercise tolerance of patients with chronic lung disease. *Canad. Med. Assoc. J.* 106: 1289-

1106. World Health Organisation. Cerebrovascular diseases: prevention, treatment and rehabilitation. *WHO Tech. Rept. Series* 469, 1971.

1107. World Health Organisation. Energy and protein requirements. Report of a joint FAO/WHO ad hoc expert committee. *Tech. Report* 522, 1973.

1108. Wright, G.R. & R.J. Shephard. Brake reaction time – effects of age, sex and carbon monoxide. *Arch. Env. Health.* In press, 1978.

1109. Wright, G.R., K.H. Sidney & R.J. Shephard. Variance of direct and indirect measurements of aerobic power. *J. Sports Med. Phys. Fitness.* In press, 1978.

1110. Wyndham. C.H., N.B. Strydom, J.S. Maritz, J.F. Morrison, J. Peter & Z.U. Potgieter. Maximum oxygen intake and maximum heart rate during strenuous work. *J. Appl. Physiol.* 14: 927-36, 1959.

1111. Wyndham, C.H., M. Watson & G.K. Sluis-Cremer. The relationship between weight and height of South African males of European descent between the ages of 20 and 60 years. *S. Afr. Med. J.* 44: 406-9, 1970.

1112. Yamaji, K. & R.J. Shephard. *Longevity and causes of death of athletes: A review of the literature. J. Hum. Ergol.* In press, 1978.

1113. Yiengst, M.J. & N.W. Shock. Blood & plasma volume in adult males. *J. Appl. Physiol.* 17: 195-8, 1962.

1114. York, C.M. Behavioral efficiency in a visual monitoring task as a function of signal rate and observer age. *Percept. Mot. Skills* 15: 404, 1962.

1115. Young, C.M. Body composition and body weight: criteria of over-nutrition. *Canad. Med. Assoc. J.* 93: 900-10, 1965.

1116. Young, C.M., J. Blondin, R. Tensuan & J.H. Fryer. Body composition studies of 'older' women, thirty to seventy years of age. *Ann. N.Y. Acad. Sci.* 110: 589-607, 1963.

1117. Zaborowski, M. Aging and recreation. *J. Gerontol.* 17: 302-9, 1962.

1118. Zohman, L.R. & R.E. Phillips. *Medical aspects of exercise testing and training.* New York: Intercontinental Medical Book Corporation, 1973.

1119. Zohman, L.R. & J.S. Tobis. *Cardiac rehabilitation.* New York: Grune & Stratton, 1970.

1120. Zuti, W.B. & L.A. Golding. Comparing diet and exercise as weight reduction tools. *Physician & Sports Medicine* 4: 49-53, 1976.

INDEX